Immunotherapy in Myeloma: A Theme Issue in Honor of Prof. Dr. Gösta Gahrton

Immunotherapy in Myeloma: A Theme Issue in Honor of Prof. Dr. Gösta Gahrton

Editors

Nicolaus Kröger
Laurent Garderet

MDPI • Basel • Beijing • Wuhan • Barcelona • Belgrade • Manchester • Tokyo • Cluj • Tianjin

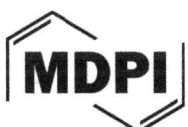

Editors
Nicolaus Kröger
Department of Stem Cell
Transplantation,
University Medical Center
Hamburg-Eppendorf
Germany

Laurent Garderet
Service d'Hématologie,
Hôpital Pitié Salpêtrière
France

Editorial Office
MDPI
St. Alban-Anlage 66
4052 Basel, Switzerland

This is a reprint of articles from the Special Issue published online in the open access journal *Hemato* (ISSN 2673-6357) (available at: http://www.mdpi.com).

For citation purposes, cite each article independently as indicated on the article page online and as indicated below:

LastName, A.A.; LastName, B.B.; LastName, C.C. Article Title. *Journal Name* **Year**, *Volume Number*, Page Range.

ISBN 978-3-0365-2906-6 (Hbk)
ISBN 978-3-0365-2907-3 (PDF)

© 2021 by the authors. Articles in this book are Open Access and distributed under the Creative Commons Attribution (CC BY) license, which allows users to download, copy and build upon published articles, as long as the author and publisher are properly credited, which ensures maximum dissemination and a wider impact of our publications.

The book as a whole is distributed by MDPI under the terms and conditions of the Creative Commons license CC BY-NC-ND.

Contents

About the Editors vii

Preface to "Immunotherapy in Myeloma: A Theme Issue in Honor of
Prof. Dr. Gösta Gahrton" by Per Ljungman ix

Nicolaus Kröger and Laurent Garderet
Immunotherapy in Myeloma: A Theme Issue in Honor of Prof. Dr. Gösta Gahrton
Reprinted from: *Hemato* **2022**, 3, 1, doi:10.3390/ hemato3010001 1

Luis Gerardo Rodríguez-Lobato, Aina Oliver-Caldés, David F. Moreno,
Carlos Fernández de Larrea and Joan Bladé
Why Immunotherapy Fails in Multiple Myeloma
Reprinted from: *Hemato* **2021**, 2, 1, doi:10.3390/hemato2010001 3

Juan Luis Reguera-Ortega, Estefanía García-Guerrero and Jose Antonio Pérez-Simón
Current Status of CAR-T Cell Therapy in Multiple Myeloma
Reprinted from: *Hemato* **2021**, 2, 43, doi:10.3390/hemato2040043 45

Nico Gagelmann and Nicolaus Kröger
Donor Lymphocyte Infusion to Enhance the Graft-versus-Myeloma Effect
Reprinted from: *Hemato* **2021**, 2, 12, doi:10.3390/hemato2020012 57

Marie Thérèse Rubio, Adèle Dhuyser and Stéphanie Nguyen
Role and Modulation of NK Cells in Multiple Myeloma
Reprinted from: *Hemato* **2021**, 2, 10, doi:10.3390/hemato2020010 67

Christie P. M. Verkleij, Wassilis S. C. Bruins, Sonja Zweegman and
Niels W. C. J. van de Donk
Immunotherapy with Antibodies in Multiple Myeloma: Monoclonals, Bispecifics,
and Immunoconjugates
Reprinted from: *Hemato* **2021**, 2, 7, doi:10.3390/hemato2010007 83

Benedetto Bruno, Giuseppe Lia, Francesca Bonifazi and Luisa Giaccone
Decades of Progress in Allogeneic Stem Cell Transplantation for Multiple Myeloma
Reprinted from: *Hemato* **2021**, 2, 5, doi:10.3390/hemato2010005 99

About the Editors

Nicolaus Kröger is Professor of Medicine and Medical Director of the Department of Stem Cell Transplantation at the University Medical Center Hamburg-Eppendorf, Germany. Prof. Kröger is board certified in hematology, oncology and internal medicine. Since 2018, he has been the President of the European Society of Blood and Marrow Transplantation (EBMT). He also served as the Chairman of the German Stem Cell Working Group (DAG-KBT) from 2014 until 2020, and is a member of several editorial boards such as Blood, Haematologica, Bone Marrow Transplantation, and Transplantation and Cellular Therapy (former Biology of Blood and Marrow Transplantation). He is also a member of numerous Scientific Committees such as ASH, EHA, and ESH. He has received several awards for his work to dat,e including the prestigious EBMT van Bekkum Award in 2015. In 2020, he was awarded a doctor honoris causa from the University Belgrade. Prof. Kröger has published extensively in his area of expertise and has contributed to more than 750 publications in peer-reviewed journals such as NEJM, Lancet, JCO, JNCI, PNAS, Blood, and Leukemia.

Laurent Garderet is a French hematologist working in the hematology department at Pitié Salpêtrière Hospital in Paris, France. He did his medical studies as well as his training in Paris. He also did a post-doctoral internship in the transplant department of the M.D Anderson Cancer Center in Houston under the supervision of Dr Richard Champlin. His main interests focus on myeloma treatment and biology. He is a board member of the Intergroupe Francophone du Myélome and a previous chairman of the Plasma Cell Disorder subcommittee of the EBMT Chronic Malignancies Working Party. He is also a member of the International Myeloma Society (IMS) as well as the International Kidney Monoclonal Gammopathy (IKMG) research group.

Preface to "Immunotherapy in Myeloma: A Theme Issue in Honor of Prof. Dr. Gösta Gahrton"

It is a great honor for me to write this introduction to celebrate the achievements of my mentor, colleague, and friend Prof. Gösta Gahrton. It is very fitting that he is celebrated with this issue on the topic "immunotherapy of multiple myeloma".

Gösta Gahrton was born in 1932 in the provincial town of Kristianstad in the southern part of Sweden, where his father was a physician as well. He studied medicine in Lund, where he also started his research before moving to Stockholm in 1961 to continue his research in the laboratory of Torbjörn Caspersson, a very well-known Swedish researcher who, among other achievements, developed the Q-binding technique to visualize human chromosomes. During the subsequent decade, he spent two years in Boston at the Children's Cancer Research Foundation and worked as a hematologist at Karolinska Hospital. In 1974, Gösta Gahrton moved to Huddinge Hospital, later Karolinska University Hospital Huddinge, where he, together with a group of colleagues, especially Prof. Carl-Gustav Growth, performed the first bone marrow transplantation in Sweden in 1975. Gösta Gahrton became Professor of Medicine at Huddinge Hospital in 1985, a position he held until his retirement in 1997. During his time there, the Section of Hematology, later the Department of Hematology, flourished and became an important center for hematological research in Sweden.

Gösta Gahrton has also held other important scientific positions, both in Sweden and internationally. He was a member of the Nobel committee for several years and was also its chairman for one year. He has been president of the EBMT, and president of the WMDA, to name a few international positions. In these organizations, he has shown his diplomatic talents in developing and enabling collaboration.

Gösta Gahrton's most prominent characteristic as a scientist is his inquisitiveness and willingness to investigate and develop new fields. Looking back over more than 60 years as a scientist, he has addressed and studied several different fields. His first studies were in cellular biology, later developing into the field of cytogenetics, and he ran a cytogenetic laboratory for many years. In 1990, he was the senior author on a paper describing the prognostic subgroups in B-cell CLL defined by specific cytogenetic abnormalities published in New England Journal of Medicine. He was also one of the founders of the first study group for the treatment of AML in Sweden, a group in which he was involved for many years, including as its chairman.

Bone Marrow Transplantation became another major interest after the start of the program at Huddinge Hospital and Gösta was one of the key drivers for the development of the largest transplant program in Sweden. His interest in bone marrow transplantation, today stem cell transplantation, has continued for several decades and he has been able to combine this with one of his other main interests, namely, multiple myeloma, the topic of this celebratory issue. At Huddinge Hospital, in 1985, we performed one of the first allogeneic transplants for multiple myeloma in the world and we published the experience of three patients in 1986. He has, since then, been very active in the field, including as the chairman of the myeloma subcommittee of the EBMT for many years, resulting in many important papers, including the seminal paper "Allogeneic bone marrow transplantation in multiple myeloma" published in New England Journal of Medicine in 1991. In the late 1980s, he became interested in gene therapy when the field was in the very early phase of its development, an interest that he has held ever since.

One of Gösta Gahrton's strongest qualities is his role as a mentor and tutor for students, collaborators, junior researchers, and colleagues. The first time I spoke to him was in approximately 1980 in the staff lunchroom at the Hematology ward at, what was then, Huddinge Hospital in Stockholm, Sweden. I was then a Junior Resident in internal medicine with the goal of becoming an Infectious Disease Specialist. He had never met me before and sat down with a cup of coffee and asked me who I was, what my goals were, and if I wanted to conduct research. After 10 minutes, he said: "Why don't you study CMV infection after allogeneic bone marrow transplantation. I will call my friend, who is a virologist" and after this moment, my career plans were changed and instead of an Infectious Disease Specialist, I became a Hematologist. This is very typical of Gösta Gahrton, who, among his many achievements, has inspired many young physicians to combine clinical hematology with research. He is always interested and willing to help but also critical in a constructive way. Another very important quality is his willingness to let more junior people grow. As mentioned above, he has had many interests during his scientific career and when a junior colleague has developed into an independent researcher, Gösta Gahrton has repeatedly stepped back and allowed others to take over responsibility in that area of research and allow for their growth as scientists and clinicians. However, we have always known that we can count on his help and support when we needed it. Many of his former students, therefore, hold or have held important positions in Swedish hematology.

Thanks Gösta!

Per Ljungman
Professor (em) in Hematology

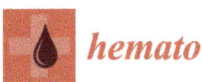

Editorial

Immunotherapy in Myeloma: A Theme Issue in Honor of Prof. Dr. Gösta Gahrton

Nicolaus Kröger [1,*] and Laurent Garderet [2]

1 Department of Stem Cell Transplantation, University Medical Center Hamburg-Eppendorf, 20246 Hamburg, Germany
2 Service d'Hématologie, Hôpital Pitié Salpêtrière, 47–83 Boulevard de L'hôpital, F-75013 Paris, France; laurent.garderet@aphp.fr
* Correspondence: nkroeger@uke.uni-hamburg.de

Immunotherapy has become a major pillar in the treatment of multiple myeloma. This Special Issue of *Hemato* addresses the increasing role of immunotherapy-based treatment options in multiple myeloma and is dedicated to Prof. Gösta Gahrton, former president of the European Society for Blood and Marrow Transplantation (EBMT), who, in 1987, published results of allogeneic stem cell transplantation as one of the most effective immunotherapies in patients with multiple myeloma [1]. Even if allogeneic stem cell transplantation has not found its definitive role in the treatment of multiple myeloma, our understanding of the immunological interaction of myeloma cells and the microenvironment and the improving techniques of monoclonal or bispecific antibodies and CAR-T technology as well as translational research on myeloma has rapidly developed in the last 30 years and immunotherapy has become a major backbone in the treatment of multiple myeloma.

After a personal introduction to Prof. Gahrton by Per Ljungman, Juan Luis Reguera-Ortega from José A. Pérez-Simón's group in Sevilla presents an overview of the rapidly growing field of chimeric antigen receptor T-cells (CAR-T) in myeloma [2], before Nico Gagelmann, from the Hamburg group, summarizes the effect of donor T-cells (DLI) after allogeneic stem cell transplantation to enhance the graft-versus-myeloma effect [3]. The increasing role of natural killer cells is highlighted and reviewed by Marie Therese Rubio, Adèle Dhuyser, and Stéphanie Nguyen from Nancy [4].

The development of monoclonal, bispecific, and immune conjugated antibodies is described by Christie Verkleij, Wassilis Bruins, Sonja Zweegman, and Niels van de Donk from Amsterdam [5], while Benedetto Bruno together with Giuseppe Lia, Francesca Bonifazi, and Luisa Giaccone describe the development and progress in allogeneic stem cell transplantation for myeloma in the last decades [6]. This Special Issue closes with an article by Luis Gerardo Rodríguez-Lobato from Joan Bladé's group in Barcelona summarizing the current knowledge about the failure of immunotherapy in multiple myeloma [7].

All the contributions are excellent state-of-the-art studies and the editors express their deep gratitude to the authors and hope that readers will enjoy this Special Issue on this exciting field in the treatment of multiple myeloma.

Funding: This research received no external funding.

Conflicts of Interest: The authors declare no conflict of interest.

Citation: Kröger, N.; Garderet, L. Immunotherapy in Myeloma: A Theme Issue in Honor of Prof. Dr. Gösta Gahrton. *Hemato* **2022**, *3*, 1–2. https://doi.org/10.3390/hemato3010001

Received: 13 December 2021
Accepted: 13 December 2021
Published: 22 December 2021

Publisher's Note: MDPI stays neutral with regard to jurisdictional claims in published maps and institutional affiliations.

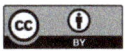

Copyright: © 2021 by the authors. Licensee MDPI, Basel, Switzerland. This article is an open access article distributed under the terms and conditions of the Creative Commons Attribution (CC BY) license (https://creativecommons.org/licenses/by/4.0/).

References

1. Gahrton, G.; Tura, S.; Flesch, M.; Gratwohl, A.; Gravett, P.; Lucarelli, G.; Michallet, M.; Reiffers, J.; Ringdén, O.; van Lint, M.T.; et al. Transplantation in Multiple Myeloma: Report from the European Cooperative Group for Bone Marrow Transplantation. *Blood* **1987**, *4*, 1262–1264. [CrossRef]
2. Reguera-Ortega, J.L.; García-Guerrero, E.; Pérez-Simón, J.A. Current Status of CAR-T Cell Therapy in Multiple Myeloma. *Hemato* **2021**, *2*, 660–671. [CrossRef]
3. Gagelmann, N.; Kröger, N. Donor Lymphocyte Infusion to Enhance the Graft-versus-Myeloma Effect. *Hemato* **2021**, *2*, 207–216. [CrossRef]
4. Rubio, M.T.; Dhuyser, A.; Nguyen, S. Role and Modulation of NK Cells in Multiple Myeloma. *Hemato* **2021**, *2*, 167–181. [CrossRef]
5. Verkleij, C.P.M.; Bruins, W.S.C.; Zweegman, S.; van de Donk, N.W.C.J. Immunotherapy with Antibodies in Multiple Myeloma: Monoclonals, Bispecifics, and Immunoconjugates. *Hemato* **2021**, *2*, 116–130. [CrossRef]
6. Bruno, B.; Lia, G.; Bonifazi, F.; Giaccone, L. Decades of Progress in Allogeneic Stem Cell Transplantation for Multiple Myeloma. *Hemato* **2021**, *2*, 89–102. [CrossRef]
7. Rodríguez-Lobato, L.G.; Oliver-Caldés, A.; Moreno, D.F.; Fernández de Larrea, C.; Bladé, J. Why Immunotherapy Fails in Multiple Myeloma. *Hemato* **2021**, *2*, 1–42. [CrossRef]

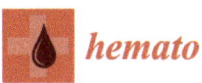 *hemato*

Review

Why Immunotherapy Fails in Multiple Myeloma

Luis Gerardo Rodríguez-Lobato [1,2,†], **Aina Oliver-Caldés** [1,2,†], **David F. Moreno** [1,2], **Carlos Fernández de Larrea** [1,2,‡] and **Joan Bladé** [1,2,*,‡]

1. Amyloidosis and Multiple Myeloma Unit, Department of Hematology, Hospital Clínic of Barcelona, 08036 Barcelona, Spain; lgrodriguez@clinic.cat (L.G.R.-L.); oliver@clinic.cat (A.O.-C.); dfmoreno@clinic.cat (D.F.M.); cfernan1@clinic.cat (C.F.d.L.)
2. Institut d'Investigacions Biomèdiques August Pi i Sunyer (IDIBAPS), 08036 Barcelona, Spain
* Correspondence: jblade@clinic.cat; Tel.: +34-93-227-54-28; Fax: +34-93-227-54-84
† These authors contributed equally to this manuscript.
‡ These authors share senior authorship.

Abstract: Multiple myeloma remains an incurable disease despite great advances in its therapeutic landscape. Increasing evidence supports the belief that immune dysfunction plays an important role in the disease pathogenesis, progression, and drug resistance. Recent efforts have focused on harnessing the immune system to exert anti-myeloma effects with encouraging outcomes. First-in-class anti-CD38 monoclonal antibody, daratumumab, now forms part of standard treatment regimens in relapsed and refractory settings and is shifting to front-line treatments. However, a non-negligible number of patients will progress and be triple refractory from the first line of treatment. Antibody-drug conjugates, bispecific antibodies, and chimeric antigen receptors (CAR) are being developed in a heavily pretreated setting with outstanding results. Belantamab mafodotin-blmf has already received approval and other anti-B-cell maturation antigen (BCMA) therapies (CARs and bispecific antibodies are expected to be integrated in therapeutic options against myeloma soon. Nonetheless, immunotherapy faces different challenges in terms of efficacy and safety, and manufacturing and economic drawbacks associated with such a line of therapy pose additional obstacles to broadening its use. In this review, we described the most important clinical data on immunotherapeutic agents, delineated the limitations that lie in immunotherapy, and provided potential insights to overcome such issues.

Keywords: multiple myeloma; immunotherapy; daratumumab; BCMA; bi-specific T cell engagers; chimeric antigen receptor; relapse; cytokine-release syndrome

Citation: Rodríguez-Lobato, L.G.; Oliver-Caldés, A.; Moreno, D.F.; Fernández de Larrea, C.; Bladé, J. Why Immunotherapy Fails in Multiple Myeloma. *Hemato* 2021, 2, 1–42. https://dx.doi.org/10.3390/hemato2010001

Received: 15 November 2020
Accepted: 18 December 2020
Published: 22 December 2020

Publisher's Note: MDPI stays neutral with regard to jurisdictional claims in published maps and institutional affiliations.

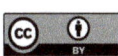

Copyright: © 2020 by the authors. Licensee MDPI, Basel, Switzerland. This article is an open access article distributed under the terms and conditions of the Creative Commons Attribution (CC BY) license (https://creativecommons.org/licenses/by/4.0/).

1. Introduction

Multiple myeloma (MM) is a neoplastic plasma cell disease that accounts for 1.8% of all cancers diagnosed annually in the United States (US) and a similar proportion of all cancers diagnosed annually in Western Europe. MM is considered the second most common hematological malignancy after lymphoma or chronic lymphocytic leukemia [1–3].

Clonal plasma cells arise on the basis of an initial event—like cytogenetic (CG) abnormalities—that occur in early development of the B-cell maturation process [4]. Once a non-malignant plasma cell acquires a primary CG abnormality, namely trisomies or IgH translocations, the potential clone is able to remain for many years. From a clinical perspective, monoclonal gammopathy of undetermined significance (MGUS) is a well-defined pre-MM stage for detection of CG abnormalities [5–7]. However, multiple ways can trigger clonal plasma cells, like the well-recognized "second hits" that include monosomies, 1q aberrations, or del17p. Additionally, with the bone marrow (BM) microenvironment playing a key role, disease progression is characterized by a parallel, altered immune response. Among the most relevant cytokines in MM are interleukin 6 (IL-6) [8,9], B cell activating factor belonging to the TNF family (BAFF), transmembrane activator and calcium-modulator and cytophilin ligand interactor (TACI) [10], and insulin-like growth factor I (IGF-1) [11]. In advanced stages involving extramedullary disease, there appears to be an independent IL-6 pathway that facilitates migration outside the BM [12,13]. Other cytokines involved in MM include interleukin 8 (IL-8), interleukin (IL-10), vascular endothelial growth factor (VEGF), and transforming growth factor-beta (TGF-β), all of which induce tumor growth and inhibit T cell activity [14]. T cell exhaustion relies on the basis of T cell activity loss and sustained expression of inhibitory receptors. Moreover, IL-10 can increase expression of immune checkpoints on T cells such as programmed cell-death-protein-1 (PD-1), T cell immunoglobulin and ITIM domain (TIGIT), and cytotoxic T-lymphocyte antigen 4 (CTLA-4) and thereby reduce their effector activity [15–17]. Other immune interactions include stimulation of T-helper 17 (Th-17) by TGF-β or IL-6 to produce bone disease [18]. In summary, multiple interactions from the BM microenvironment and MM cells lead to immune escape and suppression of T cell effector capacity. Cyclical recruitment of exhausted T cells helps maintain the pathological immune microenvironment.

Treatment strategies are based on the combination of proteasome inhibitors (PI) and immunomodulatory drugs (IMiDs) [19,20]; however, in relapse and refractory (R/R) MM scenarios, immunotherapy may play an even stronger role in inhibiting immune checkpoints, targeting plasma cell surface antigens, and even developing cancer vaccines [21,22]. Given post-procedure immune restoration with better immune surveillance, another option for patients with high-risk disease and good performance status is allogeneic transplantation [23]. However, toxicity related to this procedure may not be well tolerated in many patients.

For this reason, designing chimeric antigen receptor (CAR) T cells is an innovative therapeutic option, especially in individuals with R/R MM [24]. While improvements have been made in treatment strategies, MM continues to be an almost incurable disease and novel therapeutic strategies are necessary. In this review, we described the most important clinical data on immunotherapeutic agents (Table 1 and Figure 1), delineated the limitations that lie in immunotherapy, and provided potential insights to overcome such issues.

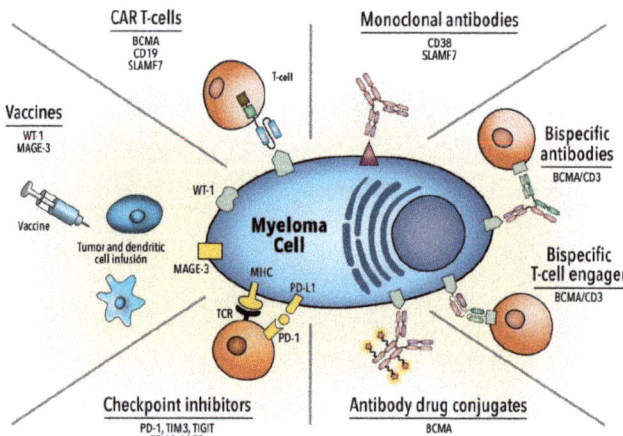

Figure 1. Different immunotherapeutic strategies to treat multiple myeloma. BCMA, B-cell maturation antigen; CAR, chimeric antigen receptor; LAG3, lymphocyte activation gene-3; PD-1, programmed cell death protein 1; PD-L1, programmed death-ligand 1; SLAMF7, signaling lymphocyte activation molecule family 7; TCR, T cell receptor; TIGIT, T cell immunoglobulin and ITIM domain; TIM3, T cell immunoglobulin and mucin domain-containing protein 3; WT-1, Wilms' tumor 1 protein; MAGE-3, melanoma-associated antigen 3.

Table 1. Outcomes of the most important clinical trials using immunotherapy against multiple myeloma.

Agent	Target	Specification	Prior Lines	Response	Prognosis	Toxicity
Monoclonal antibodies	CD38	First-in-human, phase I/II. Monotherapy 16 mg/kg [25,26]	≥3	ORR 31.1% sCR 4.7%	PFS 4 mo OS 20.1 mo	IRR 48% (2.7% ≥ grade 3)
		GEN 503. Part 2: dose expansion with DRd [27,28]	2	ORR 81% sCR 25%	PFS 72% OS 90%	IRR 56% (6.3% ≥ grade 3)
		POLLUX phase III DRd vs. Rd. R refractory were excluded [29]	1	CR 43.1 vs. 19.2% ($p < 0.001$) sCR 22.4 vs. 4.6% ($p < 0.001$) (DRd vs. Rd)	12 m PFS 83.2 vs. 60.1% OS 91.2 vs. 76.4% ($p < 0.001$)	IRR 47.7% (6.3% ≥ grade 3); 92% occurring during the first infusion
		CASTOR phase III DVd [30,31]	2	ORR 83.8 vs. 63.2% ($p < 0.0001$) CR or better 28.8 vs. 9.8% ($p < 0.0001$) sCR 8.8 vs. 2.6% (DVd vs. Vd)	18 m PFS 48 vs. 7.9% In high-risk cytogenetics PFS 11.2 vs. 7.2%	IRR 45.3% (8.3% ≥ grade 3)
	SLAMF7/CS-1	E monotherapy. Phase I, dose escalation 0.5–20 mg/kg [32]	≥2	No maximum tolerated dose ORR 0% SD 26.5%	NA	IRR 52% before the initiation of prophylaxis
		Vd +/− E, randomized phase II [33]	≥1	ORR 65 vs. 63% CR 4 vs. 4% (EVd vs. Vd)	PFS 9.7 vs. 6.9 mo OS 85 vs. 74%	IRR 7% (0% ≥ grade 3)
		ELOQUENT-2 Rd +/− E, randomized phase III [34]	1–3	ORR 79 vs. 66% ($p = 0.0002$) (ERd vs. Rd)	3 y PFS (3y) 26 vs. 18% 3 y-OS 60 vs. 53% ($p = 0.026$)	Comparable between groups
		Pd +/− E, randomized phase II [35]	≥2	ORR 53 vs. 26% (EPd vs. Pd)	PFS 10.3 vs. 4.7 mo	IRR 5% (0% ≥ grade 3)
ADC	BCMA	GSK-2857916 conjugated to MMAF; phase I [36,37]	≥3	ORR 60% CR 9% sCR 6%	PFS 12 mo	Thrombocytopenia 35% Eye-related events: Blurry vision 52%, dry eyes 37%, photophobia 29%
	CD138	Indatuximab ravtansine linked to maytansinoid; phases I/II [38,39]	≥2	ORR 5.9% CR 0% SD 42.9%	PFS 3 mo	Fatigue 47% Diarrhea 43%
	CD56	Lorvotuzumab-mertansine; phase I [40]	≥1	ORR 5.7% CR 0% SD 42.9%	PFS 26.1 weeks in evaluable	Peripheral neuropathy 5.3%
	CD74	Milatuzumab doxorubicin; phase I [41]	≥2	No objective responses. SD 5/19 (26%) for 3 mo	NA	$n = 1$ grade 3 IRR

Table 1. Cont.

Agent	Target	Specification	Prior Lines	Response	Prognosis	Toxicity
Bispecific antibodies	BCMA/CD3	AMG 420: First-in-human, phase I, dose escalation: maximum tolerated 400 µg/day. No extramedullary disease [42,43]	≥2	Dose 400 µg/day ORR 70% sCR 50%	Dose 400 µg/day PFS 9 mo	CRS 38.1% (grade ≥ 3 7.1%) Dose-limiting peripheral neuropathy n = 2
		Teclistamab; phase I; dose range: 0.3–270 µg/kg [44]	6	ORR 78% in patients receiving highest dose	-	CRS 56% (all grade 1/2) Neurotoxicity 8% (3% grade ≥ 3) IRR 9%
Immune checkpoint inhibitors	PD-1	Nivolumab monotherapy; phase I including several neoplasms [45]	≥1	ORR 4% SD 63%	-	Drug-related AEs 52% any grade, 19% ≥ grade 3
		KEYNOTE-183; phase III, randomized Pd +/− Pembrolizumab [46]	≥2	ORR 34 vs. 40% (Pembrolizumab + Pd vs. Pd)	PFS 5.6 vs. 8.4 (median time to progression 8.1 vs. 8.7 mo) (Pembrolizumab + Pd vs. Pd)	Serious AE 63 vs. 46% (Pembrolizumab + Pd vs. Pd) TRM n = 4: unknown cause, neutropenic sepsis, myocarditis, Stevens–Johnson syndrome
		KEYNOTE-185; phase III, randomized Rd +/− Pembrolizumab [46]	Newly-diagnosed ASCT in-eligible	ORR 64 vs. 62% (Pembrolizumab + Rd vs. Rd)	PFS not reached	Serious AE 54 vs. 39% (Pembrolizumab + Rd vs. Rd) Terminated because of the uneven number of deaths between groups
CAR T cell	BCMA	NCI scFv murine/CD28 [47]	9.5	ORR 81% (≥CR 13%)	mEFS 7.2 mo	CRS 94% (grade ≥ 3 38%) ICANS NA (grade ≥ 3 19%)
		UPenn/CART-BCMA scFv human/4-1BB [48]	7	ORR 64% (≥CR 11%)	mPFS 4.2 mo	CRS 88% (grade ≥ 3 32%) ICANS 32 (grade ≥ 3 12%)
		LCAR-B38M VHH llama/4-1BB [49,50]	3	ORR 88% (≥CR 74%)	mPFS 20 mo 18 m OS 68%	CRS 89% (grade ≥ 3 7%) ICANS 2 (grade ≥ 3 0%)
		LCAR-B38M VHH llama/4-1BB [51]	4	ORR 88% (≥CR 77%)	1 y PFS 53% 1 y OS 82%	CRS 100% (grade ≥ 3 41%) ICANS NA (grade ≥ 3 NA)

Table 1. Cont.

Agent	Target	Specification	Prior Lines	Response	Prognosis	Toxicity
		Ciltacabtagene Autolecuel (LCAR-B38M/JNJ68284528) CARTITUDE-1 [52]	6	ORR 97% (sCR 67%)	1 y PFS 76.6% 1 y OS 88.5%	CRS 95% (grade ≥ 3 4%) ICANS 21% (grade ≥ 3 10%)
		Idecabtagene Vicleucel (bb2121)/scFv murine/4-1BB [24]	7–8	ORR 85% (≥CR 45%)	mPFS 11.8 mo	CRS 76% (grade ≥ 3 6%) ICANS 42% (grade ≥ 3 3%)
		Idecabtagene Vicleucel (bb2121)/scFv murine/4-1BB KarMMA [53]	6	ORR 73% (≥CR 33%)	mPFS 8.8 mo mOS 19.4 mo	CRS 84% (grade ≥ 3 6%) ICANS 18% (grade ≥ 3 3%)
		Orvacabtagene Autoleucel (JCARH125)/scFv human 4-1BB EVOLVE [54]	6	ORR 92% (≥CR 36%)	mPFS 9.3 mo	CRS 89% (grade ≥ 3 3%) ICANS 13% (grade ≥ 3 3%)
Vaccines	Dendritic cells/tumor fusions	Vaccine composed of autologous dendritic cells and patient-derived myeloma cells; 16 patients included [55]	4	SD: 11	-	Site reaction (grade 1)
	hTERT/Survivin	NCT00499577 [56]	1	IR 36%	mEFS 20 mo	Chills 57% Rash > 85% (grades 1–2)
	Dendritic cells/tumor fusions	Two cohorts: 24 patients vaccinated post-ASCT 12 patients vaccinated pre- and post- ASCT [57]	-	ORR 78% (CR 47%)	2 y PFS 57%	Site reaction (grade 1) Myalgia (grade 1)
	MAGE-A3	NCT01245673 [58]	1–5	IR 88%	2 y OS 74% 2 y EFS 56%	Site reaction >90%
	XBP1 CD138 CS1	NCT01718899: SMM patients; two cohorts: Monotherapy Combination with IMiDs [59]	1	IR 95%	mTTP: 36 w mTTP: not reached	Site reaction 58–100% (grades 1–2)
	MAGE-A3	NCT01380145: vaccinated post ASCT [60]	1–2	IR 100%	mPFS 27 mo mOS not reached	Site reaction 54% (grade 1)Myalgia 33% (grades 1–2)

ADC, anti-drug conjugate; AE, adverse events; ASCT, autologous stem cell transplantation; BCMA, B-cell maturation antigen; BiTEs: bi-specific T cell engagers; CAR, chimeric antigen receptor; CR, complete response; CRS, cytokine-release syndrome; D, daratumumab; d, dexamethasone; E, elotuzumab; EFS, event-free survival; ICANS, immune effector cell-associated neurotoxicity syndrome; IMiD, immunomodulatory drug; IR, immune response; IRR, infusion-related reactions; m, median; MMAF, monomethyl auristatin F; mo, months; NA, not available; NCI, National Cancer Institute; ORR, overall response rate; OS, overall survival; P, pomalidomide; PFS, progression-free survival; R, lenalidomide, R/R, relapsed-refractory; SD, stable disease; scFv, single-chain variable fragment; sCR, stringent complete response; TTP, time to progression; UPenn, University of Pennsylvania; V, bortezomib; w, weeks.

2. Monoclonal Antibodies

2.1. Anti-CD38

CD38 was first discovered in 1980 when Reinherz and Schlossman were studying the human lymphocyte surface using monoclonal antibodies (MoA) in search of the T cell receptor. A glycoprotein highly expressed in MM cells, CD38 is also found at lower levels in normal lymphoid and myeloid cells, including NK cells, B cells, and activated T cells, and in non-hematological tissues in some cases [61]. The role of CD38 can be observed in several functions. It acts as an adhesion molecule, interacting with the endothelial ligand CD31. It also plays a role in extracellular NAD^+ and cytoplasmic NADP metabolism, mobilizing cyclic adenosine diphosphate (ADP) ribose, ADP ribose (ADPR), and nicotinic acid adenine dinucleotide phosphate [62,63].

The high expression of CD38 on MM cells led to the development of several anti-CD38 MoA in the 1990s, with daratumumab (fully human) and isatuximab (chimeric) being the most studied ones. The antitumoral effect of these antibodies correlates with their capacity to induce antibody-dependent cellular toxicity (ADCC), complement-dependent toxicity (CDC), and antibody-dependent cellular phagocytosis (ADCP) of $CD38^+$-opsonized cells. Further, the inhibition of the ectoenzymatic function of CD38 and the induction of direct apoptosis may contribute to the efficacy of these antibodies against MM [64]. Daratumumab interacts with CD38 present in monocytes and can inhibit in vitro osteoclastogenesis and bone resorption, which may improve bone-related alterations in these patients.

Developed in 2008 and approved as a single agent in 2015 and 2016 by the US Food and Drug Administration (FDA) and European Medicines Agency (EMA), respectively, daratumumab administered as monotherapy to heavily pretreated patients with MM showed an overall response rate (ORR) of 31.1%, with 4.7% having a complete response (CR). The median duration of the response was 4 months and median overall survival (mOS) was 20.1 months. This study reported responses in all subgroups, including patients with extramedullary disease and high-risk cytogenetics [25,26].

An ex vivo assay and in vivo xenograft mouse model demonstrated the efficacy of daratumumab when combined with IMiDs such as lenalidomide, proving its capacity to increase daratumumab-mediated lysis and thereby activate the effector function of autologous immune cells. Such improvement in efficacy was also observed when daratumumab was administered in combination with bortezomib and lenalidomide even in bortezomib- and lenalidomide-resistant MM cells. Similarly, the use of lenalidomide in this study proved capable of increasing daratumumab-mediated lysis through activation of NK cells [65].

The number of regimens incorporating daratumumab together with other backbone combinations is increasing. Daratumumab was further tested in a randomized phase II study with lenalidomide and dexamethasone (n = 152)(GEN503) [27,28], in which 88% of patients achieved at least a partial response (PR) and the CR rate was 25%. In the POLLUX [29] phase III study, investigators compared lenalidomide plus dexamethasone (Rd) against daratumumab plus both drugs (DRd). In both groups, patients with lenalidomide-refractory MM were excluded. In the DRd group, 12-month progression-free survival (PFS) and 12-month OS were 83.2% and 91.2%, respectively, whereas 12-month PFS and 12-month OS were 60.1% and 76.4%, respectively, in the Rd group ($p < 0.001$). Patients treated with the DRd scheme achieved a CR of 43.1%, of which 22.4% were negative minimal residual disease (MRD); patients treated with the Rd scheme achieved a CR of 19.2%, with the stringent complete response (sCR) being 4.2% ($p < 0.001$). In the CASTOR study, patients with R/R MM receiving bortezomib and dexamethasone (Vd) with or without daratumumab (DVd) were compared. Findings revealed 18-month PFS of 48% and 7.9% in the DVd and Vd groups, respectively, [30] and a benefit conferred in high-risk cytogenetic patients, with a median PFS of 11.2 and 7.2 months in the DVd and Vd groups, respectively [31]. More recently, daratumumab is approved for first-line treatment for patients with MM, including candidates for autologous stem cell transplantation (ASCT) (with bortezomib, thalidomide, and dexamethasone [66]) and non-candidates (with melphalan, bortezomib, and prednisone [67] or lenalidomide and dexamethasone [68]). More combinations in the relapse setting are now in clinical trials, such as daratumumab plus pomalidomide [69] or carfilzomib [70], and results are encouraging.

Isatuximab (chimeric) has shown strong pro-apoptotic activity, independent of cross-linking agents and antitumor activity related to CDC, ADCC, and ADCP. Activity of this antibody is enhanced by pomalidomide; a phase III trial comparing pomalidomide and dexamethasone with or without isatuximab obtained a PFS of 11.5 vs. 6.5 months (isatuximab vs. control, respectively) [71].

The main mechanisms of action of daratumumab include (Table 2):

- Complement-dependent cytotoxicity (CDC): Binding between the Fc tail of the antibody and C1q activates the complement cascade to end with the formation of the membrane attack complex (MAC) [72];
- Antibody-dependent cell-mediated cytotoxicity (ADCC): Binding between FC-gamma receptors on effector cells (T and NK cells) and the Fc tail of daratumumab releases cytotoxic molecules, leading to MM cell death [65];
- Antibody-dependent cellular phagocytosis (ADCP): Opsonization of the tumor cell occurs when the Fc tail of the CD38 antibody binds to the Fc-gamma receptor of phagocytic cells such as monocytes or macrophages [73];
- Direct effects such as programmed cell death, induction of nanotube formation and mitochondrial transfer, inhibition of ectoenzyme functions, or inhibition of adhesion molecules occur after antibody-mediated cross-linking [74,75];
- Immunomodulatory effects related to the fact that CD38 is expressed in several immune cells other than MM cells: Regulatory T cells, B cells, and myeloid-derived suppressor cells (MDSC), along with their immunosuppressive functions, are eliminated after treatment with daratumumab [76,77].

Thus, several mechanisms of resistance of daratumumab have been described:

- CD38 expression: Tests performed on modified MM cell lines that express different levels of CD38 have shown greater CDC and ADCC in cells expressing high levels of CD38 compared to cells with low expression. In MM plasma cells, expression is heterogenic and daratumumab activity is correlated with such expression levels [78]. Analysis performed on samples of patients who had been enrolled in daratumumab clinical trials showed a quick and marked decrease in CD38 levels after treatment in all patients; a decrease in CDC and ADCC was also observed in ex vivo tests. Downregulation of CD38 of this type also occurs in cell subsets other than MM cells and mechanisms are not fully understood. Some strategies to overcome such resistance have been proposed and are based on combinations with other drugs capable of increasing CD38 levels such as IMiDs, panobinostat, all-trans retinoic acid (ATRA), and ricolinostat [79–81]. The ability of ATRA to resynthesize CD38 is being analyzed in a clinical trial (NCT02751255);
- Complement inhibitory proteins: Tumor cells are known to be capable of increasing soluble and membrane-bound complement regulatory proteins such as C4-binding protein, CD55, or CD59 to protect themselves from complement attacks, similar to the way in which immune checkpoint inhibitor receptors function [82]. Ex vivo analysis using MM cell lines with low expression of CD55 and CD59, and MM cell lines treated with phospholipase-C to remove GPI-anchored proteins (CD55 and CD59) showed increased daratumumab CDC. These observations were not confirmed with MM cells obtained from daratumumab-naïve patients. In addition, an increase in CD55 and CD59 expression was detected in MM cells obtained from patients who were progressing under monotherapy treatment. In this case, ATRA combination may also decrease upregulation of complement inhibitors [78]. Panobinostat, which has shown to increase CD38 levels, also increases CD55 and CD59 levels, possibly explaining the lack of benefit in terms of CDC, although ADCC improved [83];
- CD47-SIRPα interaction: CD47 expressed in tumor cells of solid tumors and hematological malignancies interacts with regulatory transmembrane protein SIRPα that

is expressed on dendritic cells and macrophages, decreasing their phagocytic function [84]. Upregulation of CD47 has been observed in drug-resistant MM cells and blocking the interaction between SIRPα and CD47 restores phagocytosis [85]. Anti-CD47 therapies are under evaluation in other lymphoid malignancies and low-dose cyclophosphamide may decrease CD47 expression to improve ADCP [86–88];
- Polymorphisms on Fc-gamma receptors: Mechanism of action of daratumumab ADCC and ADCP depend on the activation of Fc-gamma receptors on effector cells [89]. Affinity may differ based on allelic variants of these receptors. Fc-gamma receptors were genotyped in samples of patients with MM included in daratumumab clinical trials, demonstrating a positive correlation between polymorphisms 3A and 2B and outcome in terms of PFS, albeit not OS [90];
- The way in which the microenvironment plays a crucial role in MM has been well studied. Bone marrow stromal cells (BMSC) protect MM cells from drugs and effector cells such as cytotoxic T cells [91]. Interaction between BMSC and MM cells may upregulate anti-apoptotic molecules like survivin, which could contribute to resistance against daratumumab;
- Soluble CD38 (sCD38) may have a draining effect on daratumumab function and diminish efficacy; however, the presence of sCD38 has been observed in only a few patients and in such cases, did not correlate with response. There are no published data about other CD38 antibodies and the impact of sCD38 [82];
- NK cells play a crucial role in ADCC. Some studies have shown a correlation between daratumumab-induced ADCC and NK cell-to-MM cell ratio [78]. Due to their capacity to activate NK cells, IMiDs could improve NK function and ADCC, even in patients with IMiD-refractory MM [65,92]. An increase in ADCC was observed in ex vivo experiments when interaction between NK inhibitory receptors KIR (KIR2DL-1, -2, -3) and their respective ligands was blocked. Similarly, ADCC was reported to improve synergistically with the addition of lenalidomide to the experiment. As NK cells express CD38 on their surface, fratricide and a diminished effector function can arise. When studied in patients, the reduction in NK levels was similar in responders and non-responders to daratumumab and no correlation with outcome was observed. Some measures have nonetheless been proposed to diminish this eventual effect, including the administration of ex vivo-expanded autologous NK cells to increase the count, and pretreatment of such cells with F(ab')2 fragments of daratumumab to avoid fratricide [93,94].

Table 2. Mechanisms of action and resistance to daratumumab.

Mechanisms of Action	Mechanisms of Resistance
- Complement-dependent cytotoxicity (CDC) - Antibody-dependent cell-mediated cytotoxicity (ADCC) - Antibody-dependent cellular phagocytosis (ADCP) - Direct effects - Immunomodulatory effects	- CD38 expression - Complement inhibitory proteins - CD47-SIRPα interaction - Polymorphisms on Fc-gamma receptors - Bone marrow microenvironment - Soluble CD38 (sCD38) - NK cells

2.2. Anti-SLAMF7

Signaling lymphocytic molecule F7 (SLAMF7) or cell-surface glycoprotein CD2 subset 1 (CS1) is a glycoprotein expressed on healthy plasma cells, MM cells, and NK-cells, and absent in other tissue. Expression of such is found in more than 95% of MM plasma cells independent of cytogenetics. This molecule belongs to the immunoglobulin superfamily within the SLAM family subgroup [95]. For this reason, generating a MoA directed at this target has been of great interest, with elotuzumab being the most relevant one. Elotuzumab is a humanized immunoglobulin G1 immunostimulatory MoA that works by activating signals in NK cells via interaction with protein EAT-2, and is capable of directly activating NK cells by ADCC via CD16 [96]. In MM plasma cells, this mechanism is compromised by the lack of EAT-2 expression found in tumor cells. For this reason, elotuzumab does not induce proliferation in MM cells.

In a phase I study (n = 35), the maximum tolerated dose of elotuzumab was not reached and the drug was administered at 20 mg/kg iv once every 2 weeks for 8 weeks total. None of the patients achieved a PR or better; 26.5% achieved stable disease; and the rate of infusion-related reactions before prophylaxis initiation was 52% [32].

Elotuzumab is therefore not active in monotherapy. Yet, its potential activity in combination with PI and IMiDs, such as lenalidomide and pomalidomide, was explored. In a randomized phase II study with Vd with or without elotuzumab (n = 152) [33], 63% of patients achieved at least a PR with median PFS (mPFS) of 6.9 months and 1-year OS of 74%, while 65% of patients in the elotuzumab group achieved a PR or better with a PFS of 9.7% and 1-year OS of 85%. No mechanisms of resistance to elotuzumab were described. Furthermore, in a randomized phase III ELOQUENT-2 study testing the combination of Rd +/− elotuzumab in patients with R/R MM, ORR were 79% vs. 66% in the elotuzumab vs. control groups (p = 0.0002), with 1-year OS of 91% vs. 83%, 2-year OS of 73% vs. 69%, and 3-year OS of 60% vs. 53% (p = 0.026). Adverse events (AE) were comparable between groups [34]. Additionally, 117 subjects were enrolled in a multicenter, randomized, open-label phase II trial comparing pomalidomide and dexamethasone with or without elotuzumab in lenalidomide- and bortezomib-refractory patients with R/R MM. With a minimum follow-up of 9.1 months, mPFS were 10.3 and 4.7 months in the elotuzumab and control groups, respectively, and ORR were 53% and 26% in the elotuzumab and control groups, respectively. Infusion reactions were observed in 5% of patients (n = 3) and classified as grades 1 or 2 [35]. A phase III study performed by the German-speaking Myeloma Multicenter Group randomized patients to receive induction therapy based on bortezomib, lenalidomide, and dexamethasone with or without elotuzumab (Elo-VRD vs. VRD) obtaining an ORR of 82.4% vs. 85.6% (p = 0.35), respectively. AEs of grade 3 or higher occurred in 65.4% patients (Elo-VRD) and 66.5% (VRD) mainly related to nervous system disorders, infections, and blood disorders. There were 9 and 4 treatment-related deaths in the Elo-VRD and VRD groups, respectively [97]. At the last American Society of Clinical Oncology (ASCO) meeting, primary analysis of the phase II trial (SWOG-1211) comparing Elo-VRD vs. VRD for ND, high-risk MM patients were presented. One hundred and three patients were included, and after a median follow-up of 53 months, no difference in mPFS (31 vs. 34 months, 68 vs. not reached, respectively; p = 0.45) nor in OS (68 months vs. not reached; p = 0.48) was observed [98]. Recently, data from a phase III clinical trial evaluating Elo-Rd in transplant-ineligible newly diagnosed multiple myeloma (NDMM) patients (ELOQUENT-1) have not shown a benefit with the addition of elotuzumab as front-line therapy [99]. Thus, elotuzumab has shown limited activity in the treatment of MM in terms of response and survival in both first and further lines of therapy. In the future, it will be necessary to determine the best combination for elotuzumab and the best scenario for its use.

A main limitation of both anti-CD38 and anti-SLAMF7 MoAs are infusion-related reactions (IRR), which happen primarily during initial administration and consists of pyrexia, chills, nausea, vomiting, flushing, cough, and dyspnea. Specifically, with elotuzumab, such IRR were mainly observed prior to the administration of premedication based on corticosteroids, acetaminophen, and antihistamines [32]. The rate of IRR due to elotuzumab was 7–10% with proper prophylaxis. In the case of daratumumab, however, IRR were reported in more than 50% of patients during the first infusion, even with prophylaxis, decreasing to 7% in further infusions [27].

In conclusion, monoclonal antibodies, specially CD38 directed agents, have proved to improve outcomes in MM and have reached a starring role in first line treatments.

3. Antibody-Drug Conjugate

Antibody-drug conjugates (ADCs) are MoAs joined to a cytotoxic compound via a chemical linker. These antibodies selectively target specific antigens located on the cell surface of interest. By internalizing the compound, the cytotoxic part can induce cell death. Several targets in MM and their respective antibodies are under study. The most relevant ones are mentioned below:

BCMA (CD269)-targeted ADCs: B-cell maturation antigen is a transmembrane receptor expressed on malignant plasma cells. Belantamab mafodotin (GSK-2857916) is a humanized anti-BCMA IgG1 MoA conjugated to monomethyl auristatin F (MMAF), capable of inducing ADCC activity against myeloma cells. A multicenter, phase I trial with patients with R/R MM (n = 35) showed an ORR of 60%, with 14% CR and mPFS of 12 months. The most frequent AE was thrombocytopenia (35%); similarly, several eye-related events were observed, including blurry vision (52%), dry eyes (37%), and photophobia (29%) [36,37]. Phase II clinical trial for RR MM patients (DREAMM-2) showed 30% and 34% of ORR in the 2.5 and 3.4 mg/kg cohorts, respectively. The most common grade ≥3 AE were keratopathy, thrombocytopenia, and anemia [100]. The keratopathy was further studied in DREAMM-2 patients and microcyst-like epithelial changes were found in 72% of cases. The management of eye-related AEs included dose delays (47%), dose reductions (25%), and discontinuation in 1% of patients [101]. Further studies are being performed to elucidate efficacy of this compound in combination with other MM therapies.

CD138 ADCs: CD138 or syndecan-1 is an extracellular protein receptor involved in cell-to-cell adhesion [102]. It is present in malignant plasma cells and some epithelial neoplasms. Indatuximab ravtansine is a MoA targeting CD138, linked with a disulfide bond to maytansinoid cytotoxic compound. In a phase I/II trial, ORR was 5.9% with no CR; however, 61.8% of patients maintained stable disease, with a mPFS of 3 months [38]. The most frequent toxicities reported were fatigue (47%) and diarrhea (43%) [39].

CD56 ADCs: Neural cell adhesion molecule 1 (NCAM1), otherwise known as CD56, is expressed in 75% of malignant plasma cells, yet in less than 15% of normal plasma cells [103]. Lorvotuzumab-mertansine is a MoA targeting CD56, conjugated to a microtubule inhibitor (MD1) by a disulfide bond linker. In a phase I trial for patients with R/R MM, ORR was reported at 5.7%, with no CR; however, 42.9% of patients maintained stable disease for 15.5 months. Peripheral neuropathy was an AE reported in 5.3% of patients [40].

CD74 ADCs: CD74 is a type II transmembrane glycoprotein of the major histocompatibility complex (MHC) class II, with antigen presentation functions [104]. Milatuzumab doxorubicin is an ADC with a MoA, targeting the CD74 linked via a hydrazine linker to doxorubicin. In a phase I study, this drug showed no objective response; it did, however, maintain 5 of 19 patients in stable disease for at least 3 months [41].

To sum up, ADCs have shown limited clinical results in monotherapy, so further combination studies are required to elucidate their efficacy in MM. Keratopathy could be a limiting factor for its widespread use. It will be necessary to establish adequate preventive measures, make timely diagnoses, and administer effective treatments against this complication.

4. Bispecific Monoclonal Antibodies

Bispecific monoclonal antibodies (Bs MoA) are antibodies that have two different targets and an activating or neutralizing function. Diverse bispecific antibody platforms (BiTE®, DuoBody®, and Dual-Affinity Re-Targeting®) are available, all distinguishable by structural differences among constructs. However, the majority of clinical trial data related to MM treatment are limited to the BiTE® platform [105]. BiTEs (bi-specific T cell engagers) are constructs composed of two different single-chain variable fragments (scFv) obtained from MoA and joined by a flexible peptide linker. One of the scFv acts as a binding domain for tumor cells via recognition of surface antigens and can be modified to specifically bind the malignant cell of interest and the other MoA bound to CD3, the invariable site of the TCR [106]. The junction between tumor cell and T cell leads to proliferation and growth of effector cells. These cells release cytotoxic molecules such as perforin, which creates transmembrane pores in tumor cells, and granzyme B, which acts as an initiator of apoptosis with the consequent tumor cell lysis [107]. This therapy is cytotoxic even without requiring the function of antigen-presenting cells, costimulatory molecules, or MHC-1/peptide complex. In contrast to CAR T cell therapy, Bs MoA have come to be considered as an "off-the-shelf" treatment: Processing and manufacturing time are not necessary and patients can benefit immediately from therapeutic approach [108]. Blinatumomab—targeting CD19 and CD3 in acute lymphoblastic leukemia (ALL)—was the first worldwide-approved Bs MoA (initial approval was conferred in 2014 by the FDA and full approval in 2017) [109,110].

Currently, several target antigens have been studied to treat MM with Bs MoA, with BCMA and CD38 being the most promising ones [107]. AMG-420, a BCMA/CD3 Bs MoA, was tested in a first-in-human, phase I dose-escalation trial. Patients with R/R MM who had received two or more lines of treatment were recruited to obtain a maximum tolerated dose of 400 µg/daily. Of the 10 patients who received that dose, ORR was 70% and 5 (50%) patients achieved MRD-negative CR. Grade 2–3 cytokine release syndrome (CRS) was observed in three patients and non-treatment-related mortality was reported in two patients (pulmonary aspergillosis and fulminant adenovirus hepatitis). One patient developed a dose-limiting, grade 3 peripheral polyneuropathy at 400 µg/dose [42,43]. Due to the miniscule size of Bs MoA (5kDa), its serum half-life is short and results in the continuous need for intravenous administration. With a more extended half-life, BCMA/CD3 Bs MoA (AMG-701) can be administered once per week, having demonstrated in vitro proliferation of central memory and effector memory cells and in vivo MM cytotoxicity [111,112]. A phase I/II study for patients with MM who relapsed after three or more lines of therapy is in progress to estimate the maximum tolerated dose (MTD) and establish safety and tolerability (NCT03287908).

Similarly, teclistamab (JNJ-64007957) is an investigational bispecific antibody targeting both the BCMA and CD3 receptors on T cells. In preclinical studies, the drug proved capable of recruiting and activating T cells to direct their cytotoxicity against BCMA$^+$ MM cells from an MM cell line (H929) and in BM samples obtained from patients with MM as well [113]. Results obtained from these studies led to the development of a phase I clinical trial in patients with R/R MM, enrolling those adult patients who had received a median of 6 lines of treatment. Patients were treated with teclistamab at doses ranging from 0.3–270 µg/kg. Of the 78 patients who were administered teclistamab, 21 responded to treatment. Responses were found to be deep and persistent. Additionally, the treatment achieved an ORR of 67% among the 12 patients who received the highest dosage; three of the patients achieved a CR [44]. CRS was observed in 56% of patients (CRS events were all grades 1–2 and during initial doses). Neurotoxicity was seen in 8% of cases and 3% were grade 3 or higher. In addition, IRR were reported in 9% of patients. There were 2 dose-limiting toxicities: A case of grade 4 thrombocytopenia which resolved after one day and a grade 4 delirium, which resolved after 16 days. A grade 5 AE was reported, consisting of a respiratory failure in the context of pneumonia [44]. Recent results from the last European Hematology Association (EHA) meeting highlight the efficacy of CC-93269, an asymmetric 2 + 1 bispecific with bivalent BCMA binding and monovalent CD3 binding, with a half-life extended domain. This phase I trial (NCT03486067) included 30 patients (median of 5 prior lines of therapy). ORR was 43%, including 17% with a CR or sCR. Among 9 patients receiving 10 mg, the ORR was 89% (≥CR: 44%). The main AEs included cytopenias and infections. CRS was observed in 77% of patients, but most were grade 1 [114]. This study continues including patients in the dose-escalation phase.

GBR-1342 is a CD38/CD3 Bs MoA in current evaluation in a first-in-human, phase I/II study in PI-, IMiD-, and daratumumab-refractory patients with MM; the question of interest is whether subjects previously treated with daratumumab will respond to CD38-targeted Bs MoA. This study is currently recruiting patients (NCT03309111) [115]. Then, there is also the CD38/CD3 Bs MoA AMG-424, which has also shown potent activity against MM cell lines in spite of lower or higher CD38 expression in these cells. As inhibition of tumor growth in a murine model and acceptable toxicities in monkeys have been demonstrated (depletion of peripheral B-lymphocytes), a first-in-human, multi-center, phase I study for patients with R/R MM was approved (NCT03445663) and has, in recent times, finished (June 2020).

Recently, results on Cevostamab-BFCR4350A, a FcRH5-CD3 bispecific antibody have been presented at the last American Society of Hematology (ASH) meeting. The phase I, dose escalation study (NCT03275103), included 51 R/R MM patients (55% with high-risk cytogenetics). The median number of prior lines of therapy was 6. The ORR was 51.7%, including 3 sCRs and 3 CRs. Responses were observed in patients with high-risk cytogenetics, prior exposure to anti-CD38 MoA, ADC, and CAR T cell therapy. Regarding toxicity, CRS was observed in 75% of patients (grade $\geq$ 3: one patient). Other grade 3 or 4 AEs observed were lymphopenia (11.8%), anemia (5.9%), and thrombocytopenia (5.9%). No fatal (grade 5) AEs have been reported [116].

In addition, the last updated data of talquetamab-JNJ-64407564, a GPRC5D-CD3 Bs MoA, were presented at the last ASH meeting. One-hundred and thirty-seven patients have been included in the phase I trial (NCT03399799). The median number of prior lines was 6, and 15% of the patients had received prior BCMA-directed therapy. Respecting efficacy, this product showed ORRs of 78% and 67% with the IV and the SC route, respectively. CRS was observed in 47% of patients (mostly grades 1 or 2; grade 3 was seen only with the IV route) and neurotoxicity in 5% of patients. IRR have been reported in 14–15% of patients, all of them grades 1 or 2, and usually in the first cycle [117].

Impressive preclinical results are arousing interest in trispecific antibodies such as the trispecific T cell engager targeting CD38, CD3, and CD28, which has shown high killing capacity of MM tumor cell lines in *in vitro* tests and also suppressed MM growth in mice, with proliferation of memory and effector T cells and downregulation of regulatory T cells in primates [118]. Trispecific NK cell engagers are also under development, targeting the NK antigen CD16A, and BCMA and CD200 in MM cells [119].

The primary results obtained with Bs MoA show that this strategy is a promising approach in the treatment of patients with MMs, although drug-related toxicities, especially CRS and neurotoxicity, days of hospitalization, and patient surveillance should be taken into account.

5. Immune Checkpoint Inhibitors

The immune system plays a crucial role in cancer development and progression. However, cytolytic activity of immune cells during the initial phase of carcinogenesis is the predominant mechanism used to fight against malignant cells. A balance between cancer progression and cancer eradication is then reached during the intermediate phase, mediated by modulatory proteins denominated as checkpoint molecules. When the immune system grows tolerant to the presence of cancer after this phase, tumor cells escape and can progress and induce metastasis [120,121].

Immune checkpoint molecules are a family of proteins composed of receptors—mostly located in T cells and other immune effector cells—and ligands located in antigen-presenting cells (APCs), monocytes, and tumor cells as well. The function of checkpoint receptors is to promote a balance between activating and inhibitory signals [122]. Several examples of checkpoint receptors have been widely studied, such as PD-1, CTLA-4, LAG-3 [123], TIM-3, and TIGIT. Interaction with their respective ligands triggers an inhibitory signal capable of counteracting T cell-mediated immunity. In a physiological setting, checkpoints have a modulatory function that maintains balance between immune response and immune tolerance. This aspect is crucial, as it protects the organism from autoimmunity. Despite that, tumor cells can take advantage of this mechanism, expressing checkpoint ligands on their surface and inducing inhibitory signals, to promote tumor immune tolerance [124,125]. Blocking checkpoint inhibitors has shown impressive tumor response in heavily treated patients with melanoma, lung cancer, or Hodgkin lymphoma [126].

Several immune dysregulations have been described in MM. BM niche cells contribute to tumor growth and immune escape by creating a permissive microenvironment promoted by factors with immunosuppressive properties such as TGF-β, prostaglandin E2, IL-10, and IL-6 [127]. Additionally, an impaired maturation and differentiation pattern has been described in dendritic cells (DCs) of patients with MM [128,129]. Increased levels of PD-L1 have been found in MM plasma cells as well as an increased expression of PD-1 in circulating effector cells like T and NK cells [130,131]. The immunosuppressive role of other checkpoint receptors such as CD85j or TIGIT has also been shown in MM. A study demonstrated lower expression of CD85j, an inhibitory immune checkpoint for B-cell function, in patients with active MM and MGUS (a premalignant condition), suggesting that such a lower expression in malignant PCs may eliminate the inhibitory signal—causing an increase in PC resistance to NK cytotoxicity—and lead to immune escape [132]. TIGIT, an inhibitory checkpoint receptor expressed on lymphocytes, and its ligands poliovirus receptor (PVR) and Nectin-2, could also play a role in immune escape. In vitro functional assays demonstrated inhibition of $CD8^+$ T cell signaling and proliferation, which could be restored by TIGIT blockade. TIGIT blockade also showed an increased proliferation of IFN-γ-secreting $CD4^+$ [17,133]. Although preclinical data suggest that blockade of the PD-1/PD-L1 axis could be effective in the treatment of MM, clinical data published to date do not support such statement. A phase I study with pembrolizumab monotherapy, a PD-L1 blocker, from patients with R/R MM achieved stable disease as the best response [134]. A separate phase I study exploring the use of nivolumab (PD-1 blocker), which comprised patients with different hematological neoplasms, included 27 patients with R/R MM. Of these patients, 63% achieved stable disease, while only one patient achieved an objective response (4%) [45]. Despite the limited outcomes obtained with PD-1/PD-L1 blockers in monotherapy, some studies reported better efficacy when in combination with IMiDs like lenalidomide or pomalidomide, even in patients treated previously with IMiDs. The reason for such efficacy was the enhancing effect conferred by these agents on the PD-1/PD-L1 axis. In the KEYNOTE-183 study, a phase III randomized trial comparing pomalidomide and dexamethasone with or without pembrolizumab, ORR was 34% vs. 40% in the pembrolizumab-PD group and PD group, respectively. Immune-mediated AE occurred in 18% of patients in the pembrolizumab group, with the most frequent being pneumonitis, hyperthyroidism, and rash. Serious AE were reported in 63% vs. 46% of patients in the pembrolizumab group and control group, respectively, with treatment-related mortality occurring in four patients with the following etiologies: Unknown cause, neutropenic sepsis, myocarditis, and Stevens–Johnson syndrome. The FDA indicated that based on the data presented to the monitoring committee, risks associated with the pembrolizumab combination outweighed the benefits and the study was to be discontinued [46]. The phase III study KEYNOTE-185, which compared Rd administration with or without pembrolizumab (200 mg every 3 weeks) in patients with NDMM who were not eligible for ASCT, showed a high rate of immune-mediated AE and mortality, with an interim unplanned analysis suggesting an unfavorable benefit-risk profile [135].

The efficacy of PD-1/PD-L1 blockers seems to be related to a higher immune cell infiltration of the tumor [121]. Mutational burden and neo-antigen expression have also proven to play a crucial role in PD-L1 expression on solid tumors. Results obtained with checkpoint inhibitor blockers may be explained by the fact that MM is known to have a low burden of mutations when compared to other solid, hematological diseases, as well as low immune cell infiltrate [136]. Toxicities observed in KEYNOTE trials raised concerns in other trials that combined an immune checkpoint inhibitor with IMiDs; most were therefore suspended or terminated [137].

6. Chimeric Antigen Receptor T Cell Therapy

CARs are synthetic fusion proteins designed in a modular fashion that redirect lymphocytes to recognize and eliminate cells that express a target antigen on their surfaces. CARs are endowed with four fundamental components: Either the extracellular antigen-binding domain or scFv derived typically from the light and heavy chains of MoAs to provide antigen-specificity in a non-HLA-restricted manner; either the spacer or hinge based on CD8-, CD28-, IgG1-, or IgG4-derived domains; the transmembrane domain from CD8α or CD28 moieties; and intracellular or activation domains derived from the CD3ζ moiety of the TCR (first generation) and the addition of one (second generation) or two (third generation) costimulatory domains derived from CD28, 4-1BB moieties and others that are necessary for optimal T cell function, proliferation, and persistence. Armored or fourth-generation CARs include immune modulating capacities, suicide genes, controllable on–off protein switches, and molecules to reduce or overcome T cell dysfunction or exhaustion (Figure 2) [138–140]. Synthetically engineered T cells expressing CARs against the CD19 antigen have shown outstanding results in B-cell malignancies in clinical trials, and the FDA and EMA have approved the use of tisagenlecleucel, axicabtagene ciloleucel and brexucabtagene autoleucel [141–148]. Indeed, the results led to many more additional clinical trials in diverse hematological and solid cancers, and several encouraging results have been reported with the use of CAR T cell therapy-targeting BCMA in patients with MM. Due to the therapy's potential as a treatment strategy in patients with R/R MM, the first anti-BCMA CAR is expected to be approved within the coming months. However, an in-depth review of all the clinical trials that are being carried out using CAR T cell therapy in patients with myeloma goes beyond the scope of this manuscript. Exhaustive reviews have been published elsewhere [149–153]. The two most important BCMA CAR T cell products that are currently being evaluated in registration phase clinical trials include idecabtagene vicleucel and ciltacabtagene autoleucel (Table 1). Idecabtagene vicleucel is a second-generation CAR that includes a 4-1BB costimulatory domain and a murine scFv. The latest results from the phase II trial (KarMMa; NCT03361748) were presented at the last ASCO meeting. The trial enrolled 149 patients and the doses of 150 to 450 × 10^6 CAR T cells were analyzed. The ORR was 73% (CR rate 33%), with a mPFS and OS of 8.8 and 19.4 months, respectively. Patients treated at the highest dose level had an ORR of 82% and a mPFS of 12.1 months. Regarding safety profile, CRS and immune effector cell-associated neurotoxicity syndrome (ICANS) were observed in 84% and 18% of all patients, respectively [53]. Ciltacabtagene autoleucel is also a second-generation CAR that includes a 4-1BB costimulatory domain and two llama-derived variable-heavy chain only fragments against two different BCMA epitopes. The latest results from the phase Ib/II trial (CARTITUDE-1; NCT03548207) were presented at the last ASH meeting. The trial included 97 patients and a single infusion of the product at a target dose of 0.75 × 10^6 CAR T cell/kg was administered. The ORR was 96.9% (sCR rate 67%), with a one-year PFS and OS of 76.6% and 88.5%, respectively. In terms of toxicity, CRS was observed in 94.8% of all patients (grade ≥ 3 in 4.1%) and ICANS occurred in 20.6% of patients (grade ≥ 3 in 10.3%). Ten deaths occurred during the study due to adverse events (eight patients) and progressive disease (two patients) [52].

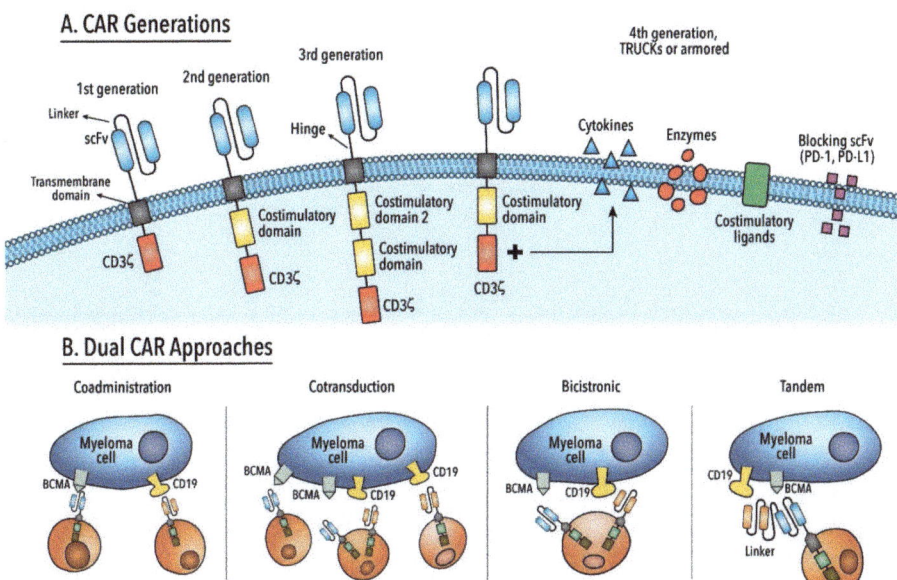

Figure 2. (**A**) Structure of a CAR and different generations of chimeric antigen receptors. (**B**) Schematic representations of different strategies targeting two target antigens simultaneously. TRUCKs, T cells redirected for antigen-unrestricted cytokine-initiated killing; scFv, single-chain variable fragment.

BCMA is by far the most predominant antigen used for targeted CAR T cell therapy in MM. Reasons for targeting BCMA include the antigen's high surface expression in malignant plasma cells, its exclusive expression in some mature B-cell subsets, and its non-expression in normal tissue and hematopoietic stem cells [154–156]. BCMA regulates B cell differentiation, survival, and maturation. However, in the malignant plasma cell, BCMA is associated with the cell's survival and proliferation, and contributes to the immunosuppressive BM microenvironment [157,158]. BCMA expression is higher in patients with MM when compared with non-malignant plasma cells; nevertheless, the levels vary [159,160]. In general, CAR T cells targeting BCMA have shown impressive results in heavily pretreated patients with MM, including achieving deep responses (ORR 60–97% ($\geq$CR in 10–86%)), manageable toxicity (CRS 60–100% (grade $\geq$ 3 in 0–41%), and ICANS 2–42% (grade $\geq$ 3 in 0–19%)), and a mPFS of 2–20 months [24,47–49,51–54,161–166]. These results are non-homogenous but can be explained by differences in patient inclusion protocols, CAR constructs, conditioning regimens, CAR T cell doses, and toxicity grading scales. Furthermore, despite these impressive remission rates, it should be noted that many patients are resistant and will relapse after CAR T cell therapy. No plateau is observed in PFS curves after CAR T cell infusion, as has been reported in other diseases such as diffuse large B-cell lymphoma or B-cell ALL. The following sections therefore provide a comprehensive analysis of the possible mechanisms of relapse as well as present potential strategies to overcome failure in this type of immunotherapy (Table 3). Table 4 details a summary of differences between BiTEs and CAR T cells. Finally, these sections briefly describe other difficulties, such as toxicity, manufacturing challenges, and economic burden, which could limit the widespread use of CAR T cell therapy.

Table 3. Obstacles of CAR T cell therapy and possible strategies to overcome them.

Limitation	Rationale	Approach
Antigen-positive escape	Impaired T cell persistence	Optimize CAR design (human scFv, hinge, costimulatory domains) to avoid antigen-independent tonic signaling and reduce antigenicity Younger T cell donors, transduction to stem cell memory T cell and central memory T cells, block T cell differentiation signaling, or use of non-viral transduction systems Genomic knock-in of the CAR sequence to the *TRAC* locus
	Impaired T cell potency	Fine-tuning CAR design (human scFv, hinge, costimulatory domains) Avoid antigen-independent tonic signaling Genomic knock-in of the CAR sequence to the *TRAC* locus Avoid T cell exhaustion (combine with immune check-point inhibitors or disrupt the checkpoint pathway) Reduce the amount of soluble target antigen Optimize lymphodepletion protocol
	Tumor microenvironment-induced immunosuppression	Boost T cell trafficking and migration Overcome inhibitory signals by blocking immune check-point pathways or switching inhibitory signals present in the TME into pro-inflammatory signals Targeting immunosuppressive immune cells (regulatory T cells, tumor-associated macrophages, myeloid-derived suppressor cells) Armored CAR T cells or TRUCKs
Antigen-negative escape	Immune selection pressure Gene mutations Lineage switching Trogocytosis Antigen masking	Identification and selection of the most suitable tumor antigen Fine-tuning antigen binding affinity Targeting multiple tumor antigens (sequential or co-administration of single-target CAR products, dual CARs, or tandem CARs) Upregulate surface density of the target antigen Targeting myeloma stem cells
Toxicities	CRS and ICANS	Optimizing reduction in the number of CAR T cells infused or dividing doses on different days Prompt recognition with the use of predictive biomarkers Use of tocilizumab or corticosteroids in early stages of the disease Tailored modifications of the construct, optimizing the costimulatory domain CAR T cells with suicide genes or "OFF-switches"
	On-target, off-tumor	Affinity tuning of the scFv Advanced CAR engineering: "AND" logic-gate, "ON-switch", "SPLIT", or inhibitory CARs
Manufacturing	Amount and quality of T cells Vein-to-vein time Production failure	Allogeneic CAR T cells (major concerns: GvHD and CAR T cell rejection)
Access and economic	Infrastructure, workflows, processes, regulatory requirements, and economic burden	Cooperation among multiple stakeholders Use of non-viral gene delivery with transposon/transposase systems Creation of community CAR T cell therapy centers Promote the outpatient setting Shift from centralized to decentralized manufacturing, namely "bedside manufacturing" Cost-effectiveness, cost-benefit, and quality-adjusted life-year analyses Outcome-based reimbursement or staged payment models Legitimate value of immunotherapy as shown by real-world evidence and longer follow-ups

CRS, cytokine-release syndrome; GvHD, graft-versus-host disease; ICANS, immune effector cell-associated neurotoxicity syndrome; scFv, single-chain variable fragment; TME, tumor microenvironment; TRAC, T cell receptor alpha constant; TRUCK, T cells redirected for antigen-unrestricted cytokine-initiated killing.

Table 4. Some differences between bispecific antibodies and CAR T cell.

	Bispecific Antibodies	CAR T Cell
Production	"Off-the-shelf": No need for manufacturing time, allowing for immediate treatment of the patient	Individual manufacturing for each patient, starting with autologous lymphapheresis. Approach: Allogeneic CAR T cells under development
Administration	Continuous intravenous infusion Approach: extended half-life bispecific antibodies	Punctual infusion of the product (dose is sometimes split up into several days to reduce AEs)
T cell phenotype and effector function	Binding of endogenous $CD8^+$ and $CD4^+$ T cells, which have a superior cytotoxic function than naïve T cells	The product is mostly composed of naïve $CD8^+$ and $CD4^+$ T cells; these cells have higher self-renewal, survival, and penetration in lymphoid tissues

AE: Adverse events; CAR: Chimeric antigen receptor.

6.1. Mechanisms or Relapse

Understanding the underlying mechanisms that determine or predict relapses is crucial in order to improve therapeutic approaches. Despite the high CR rates achieved with CD19-targeted CAR T cells (81–90% in B-cell ALL and 50% in B-cell non-Hodgkin lymphoma (NHL)), 10–20% of patients with B-cell ALL and 20–50% of patients with B-cell NHL will be refractory, while 30–60% of those with B-cell ALL who achieve CR and 20–30% of those with B-cell NHL who achieve CR will relapse [141,143,144,167,168]. With respect to BCMA-targeted CAR T cells in patients with MM, 3–40% of such patients will be refractory, while 15–50% of those patients who achieve CR will relapse during the first year of follow-up. Although the data are still very immature, there is evidence that a greater proportion of patients will relapse with longer follow-ups [24,47,48,50–54].

To date, two relapse patterns—antigen-positive and antigen-negative escapes—have been elucidated due to the high number and extensive follow-up period of patients who received CD19-targeted CAR T cells. Knowledge of such patterns may contribute to enhancing BCMA-targeted CAR T cell therapy in patients with MM.

6.1.1. Antigen-Positive Escape

Relapse of this nature most frequently occurs in CAR T cell immunotherapy. It is characterized by the maintenance of antigen expression on the tumor cell surface. Mechanisms found in such relapse underlie poor persistence and the low potency of CAR T cells, as well as mutations in survival or apoptosis pathways in tumor cells and the immunosuppressive tumor microenvironment (TME).

The use of non-human-derived scFv might contribute to CAR T cell inactivation due to the HLA-restricted T cell-mediated immune response and the presence of anti-CAR T cell antibodies [169]. Investigators Xu et al. found anti-CAR T cell antibodies in 6 patients with MM before or after relapse using a llama-derived bi-epitope-targeting BCMA CAR (LCAR-B38M). The presence of these antibodies was also associated with a notable reduction in the number of residual CAR T cells [51]. Different groups are therefore using fully human scFv to reduce antigenicity that would then increase persistence and improve efficacy [48,54,163–165,170–172]. This strategy may hold potential to re-challenge the targeted antigen and reinfuse the same or different CAR [171].

Intracellular signaling domains also play an important role in the persistence and efficacy of the product. Costimulatory CD28-based CARs enhance activation, proliferation, and cytotoxicity of T cells by promoting effector memory T cell differentiation and increasing aerobic glycolysis, albeit with reduced persistence. Meanwhile, 4-1BB-based CARs promote oxidative metabolism, bolster central memory T cell differentiation and improve T cell persistence [173–176]. Although the optimal costimulatory molecule to use in myeloma has yet to be elucidated, most products targeting BCMA are based on the 4-1BB moiety. Efforts are currently being undertaken to improve stimulatory signaling. Some examples include incorporating both CD28 and 4-1BB moieties into the CAR to maintain rapid activation kinetics and improved persistence, respectively [177,178]; mutating the activation motif in CD28 or encoding a single CD3ζ ITAM so as to hinder exhaustion and improve the persistence of T cells [179–181]; and, either incorporating new costimulatory domains (CD27 or ICOS) to enhance survival or differentiating CD4$^+$ T cells towards a Th1/Th17 phenotype [173,182,183].

T cell fitness and subset composition have been recognized as markers of expansion and response [48,139,184,185]. CAR T cells manufactured from older donor T cells had worst transduction efficiency and impaired effector functions when compared with younger donor T cells, reflected by gene expression, secretory pattern, and transcription factor balance [186]. Quality of harvested T cells might also be compromised due to the disease itself and the type, number, and intensity of prior treatments [187–190]. Therefore, harvesting T cells during the first line of treatment and not in subsequent relapses may have clinical potential [191], as well as administering CAR T cell therapy as an earlier intervention in patients with MM. There are, in fact, clinical trials underway, evaluating BCMA-targeted CAR T cells in first-line treatment in high-risk patients with MM (KarMMa-4, NCT04196491) and in second-line treatment with high-risk factors (KarMMa-2, NCT03601078). With respect to T cell subpopulations, random compositions of T cell subsets were used in initial BCMA clinical trials; however, growing evidence supports the belief that tailored composition of T cell subsets could increase efficiency and persistency [192]. A higher CD4$^+$/CD8$^+$ T cell ratio in the leukapheresis product was associated with better expansion and response, and less differentiated or more naïve stem cell memory and central memory T cells were predictive biomarkers of expansion and clinical response [48,184]. That stated, orvacabtagene autoleucel (JCARH125, NCT03430011) [154,155] and FCARH143 product (NCT03338972) [164] are manufactured using a 1:1 ratio (CD4$^+$/CD8$^+$) before and after gene transfer, respectively, to homogenize the amount of T cells infused among patients and enhance crosstalk between CD4$^+$ and CD8$^+$ T cells [192]. Another strategy to enrich memory-like T cells includes blocking T cell differentiation signaling derived from constitutive CD3ζ and the phosphoinositide 3-kinase (PI3K), AKT and mTOR activation pathway [193]. bb21217 (NCT03274219) is a next-generation product of idecabtagene vicleucel that adds PI3K inhibitor bb007 during ex vivo culture with the expectation to enhance persistence and potency [161]. The addition of IL-7 and IL-15 to CAR T cell cultures enhances cytolytic and proliferative capacities and enriches naïve central memory T cells [194]. Novel CAR T cell product P-BCMA-101 (NCT03288493), conceived using the non-viral piggyBac® DNA modification system, favors enrichment of T memory stem cells, providing a higher therapeutic index [163].

Ligand-independent chronic activation or tonic signaling leads to detrimental effects on CAR functionality. It is characterized by different growth and phenotype patterns of CAR T cells, and is associated with accelerated differentiation, exhaustion, and impaired anti-tumor effects [195,196]. Adjustments can be made in the configuration of the CAR to avoid it, though. For example, centyrin™ are small monomeric, thermostable, and less immunogenic proteins based on a tenascin fibronectin type III sequence that have binding affinities similar to scFv and no signs of tonic signaling thus far [197]. A clinical trial with such technology is currently underway (P-BCMA-101, NCT03288493) [163]. Additionally, the hinge/spacer is crucial in preventing tonic signaling. Appropriate length of IgG-derived spacers and the replacement of the N-glycosylation site by FcγR-binding might recover CAR T cell functionality [198,199]. However, most CAR myeloma trials use CD8α-derived spacers to reduce the presence of tonic signaling [47,48,200]. Another useful option in third-generation CARs is to place the 4-1BB costimulatory domain distal to the cell membrane [173]. Advancements in genome editing tools using CRISPR/Cas9 have allowed for the targeted genomic knock-in of the CAR sequence to the T cell receptor α constant (*TRAC*) locus, resulting in a homogeneous expression of the CAR, the prevention of tonic signaling, a delay in effector T cell differentiation and exhaustion, and the enhancement of T cell potency [201].

T cell dysfunction is associated with tumor progression and relapse. T cell exhaustion refers to effector T cells with a reduced capacity to secrete cytokines and is characterized by an increased expression of inhibitory receptors (PD1, TIM3, LAG3, CTLA4, and TIGIT), reduced proliferative capacity, an altered transcriptional factor program (NFAT, IRF4, NR4A, and TOX), and a unique epigenetic landscape. T cell senescence is defined as the terminal differentiation state due to excessive cell replication, and is associated with cell cycle arrest and telomere shortening [202–204]. Brudno et al. observed a higher fraction of CAR T cells expressing senescence (KLRG1 and CD57) and exhaustion (PD-1) markers after CAR T cell infusion with CD28-based BCMA CAR in patients with MM [47]. CAR T cell anti-tumor activity may be boosted by the disruption of the immune checkpoint signaling pathway [205], by either combining the cell product with an immune checkpoint inhibitor antibody [205–207] or genetic modulations. Several examples of such include deleting PD-1 in CAR T cells with gene silencing techniques such as CRISPR/Cas9 or short hairpins RNAs [208,209]; engineering CARs that secrete PD-L1-targeted IgG antibodies or PD-1-targeted scFv [210,211]; transducing a CAR with a truncated PD-1 receptor that lacks intracellular domains [208]; and transducing a PD-1 switch receptor fused with an intracellular CD28 domain and thus modifying a dominant-negative inhibitory signal via an activating costimulatory signal [212,213]. However, data are conflicting with respect to impairment of anti-tumor function and proliferation activity of CAR T cells due to PD-1 silencing [214,215]. Further investigation is therefore warranted to elucidate the specific role that each immune checkpoint receptor plays and the optimal time for its inhibition in MM [216].

The presence of a soluble target antigen in the bloodstream could be an obstacle in CAR T cell therapy. A reduction in the density of the selected antigen on the tumor cell surface would not make it possible to reach the threshold that triggers the effector functions of CAR T cells and would hamper the scFv domain of the CAR [217]. For example, the soluble fragment of BCMA protein (sBCMA) can be shed into the bloodstream due to cleavage performed by the gamma-secretase (GS) [218]. With respect to MM, sBCMA may have a role in the disease pathophysiology, with increased levels of sBCMA being associated with a worse prognosis [219–221]. Preclinical data suggest that high concentrations of sBCMA may interfere with cytokine production and cytolytic capacity of BCMA-targeted CAR T cells [222]. Conversely, though, preclinical [154,160] and clinical [24,47,48,54] evidence highlight that BCMA-targeted CAR T cell activity is not compromised and sBCMA could be an adjunctive biomarker to assess response and progression [47,48]. These differences could be explained by the different epitopes to which the CARs are redirected, as some epitopes could be cryptic or not accessible in the soluble conformation of BCMA [217]. A possible, recently elucidated strategy to reduce the amount of sBCMA is the addition of a GS inhibitor (GSI), which efficiently blocks BCMA shedding [222]. The next section will provide further details about the possible utility of inhibiting the GS in anti-BCMA immunotherapy.

Malignant plasma cells and dysregulated BM TME interactions contribute to the pathogenesis, progression, and therapy resistance in myeloma [223]. However, knowledge concerning the role of immunosuppressive TME in relapse after the use of CAR T cells in patients with myeloma is minimal. Evidence obtained from patients with solid tumors indicates that objective response to CAR T cell therapy is infrequent and ephemeral due to cell stroma and immunosuppressive modulators, aberrant vascularization, hypoxia, and lack of nutrients [224]. In response, a wide set of approaches are being conceived to overcome these challenges. Some examples are as follows: (1) Increasing expression of chemokine receptors (CCR4, CSF-1R, and CCR2b) in CAR T cells to improve migration and anti-tumor activity to boosting T cell trafficking to tumors [225–227]; (2) targeting protease activation protein (FAP)-expressing stromal cells or secreting extracellular matrix-modifying enzymes (anti-GD2 CAR) to degrade heparan sulfate proteoglycans to infiltrate physical barriers. However, targeting fibroblast could develop considerable on-target, off-tumor toxicities [228–230]; (3) either blocking immune checkpoint pathways as aforementioned;

(4) switching inhibitory signals (IL-4) present in the TME to pro-inflammatory signals (IL-2, IL-7 or IL-15) [231–233] to overcome T cell inhibitory signals, or disrupting the proapoptotic FAS signal pathway to impair the function as dominant-negative receptors [234]; (5) targeting immunosuppressive immune cells (regulatory T cells, tumor-associated macrophages, MDSC) with CAR T cells [224,235,236]; and (6) engineering bionic CAR T cells (armored CAR T cells or TRUCKs) to secrete stimulatory cytokines (IL-12, IL-15, IL-18) [237–240] that foster the effector activity of CAR T cells (third stimulatory signal) and propagate the anti-tumor immune response via recruitment of endogenous immune cells [241–243]. While the preclinical potential of such advanced engineering is great, clinical utility remains to be defined.

Conditioning regimens or lymphodepletion protocols based on chemotherapy prior to CAR T cell therapy aim to reduce tumor burden, eliminate immunosuppressive cells (Tregs and MDSC), remove homeostatic cytokine sinks (IL-2, IL-7, and IL-15), activate APC, downregulate indoleamine 2,3-dioxygenase in tumor cells, and enhance function, expansion, and persistence of CAR T cells [244–247]. Beneficial effects such as better clinical response and prognosis have been observed in B-cell malignancies and MM [48,248–251]. Although no current standard regimen has been established in MM clinical trials, the mainstream combination used is fludarabine plus cyclophosphamide. Further knowledge is needed to determine the most suitable regimen, dosing, and timing of drug administration.

6.1.2. Antigen-Negative Escape

This type of escape is characterized by the loss of or downregulation in the targeted antigen expression. It has been described with different targeted immunotherapies including CAR T cells [252]. Complete antigen loss may not be absolutely necessary to escape CAR T cells; however, decrease in the target antigen expression may suffice. Some evidence suggests that a minimum and individual threshold of antigen expression is needed for CAR T cell activation [252,253]. Apparently, within the MM setting, the antigen-negative or downregulation of the antigen is not the primary mechanism of escape, although some clinical trials using BCMA-targeted CAR T cells have reported it [47,48,164,254]. Investigators Brudno et al. described the case of one patient who lost BCMA expression at the time of progression. BM analysis showed the presence of a mixed cell population, with some maintaining BCMA expression and others losing it [47]. Likewise, Green et al. reported the case of one patient whose tumor biopsy at relapse revealed both a BCMA^{neg} myeloma cell population and 70% reduction in intensity of BCMA expression in remaining myeloma cells [164]. A separate study by Cohen et al. also showed similar findings, reporting a decrease in intensity of BCMA expression in 4 of 9 patients who did not achieve an objective response to the BCMA-targeted CAR [48]. Notably, after CAR T cell infusion, intensity of BCMA expression was minimal in residual myeloma cells; however, in most patients at progression, expression returned to baseline levels [48]. Martin et al. presented three cases of BCMA antigen loss after idecabtagene vicleucel; a biallelic deletion of chromosome 16p encompassing the BCMA locus was confirmed in one case [254,255].

Evidence obtained on CAR T cells targeting the CD19 antigen has elucidated some of the plausible mechanisms related to this subtype of relapse. These mechanisms include: (1) Immune selection pressure: Pre-existing target antigen-negative subclones prior to CAR T cell therapy may transform to dominant clones after selective stress generated by immune-targeted therapy [256,257]. This type of escape is highly probable in myeloma due to intratumor heterogeneity and clonal evolution [258]; (2) gene mutations: Frameshift and missense mutations have been described with the subsequent loss of expression of the targeted antigen. Furthermore, alterations have been identified in the splicing factor that could cause protein isoforms contributing to CAR T cell escape [259–261]; (3) lineage switching: Immunotherapy could induce conversion or reprogramming to a different leukemic cell lineage [262,263]; (4) trogocytosis and cooperative killing: Described only in in vitro and xenograft models, this mechanism of escape is characterized by the transfer of the target antigen to CAR T cells during the immune synapse. Such transfer subsequently decreases density of the antigen expressed on the tumor cell surface and triggers fratricide among CAR T cells, resulting in ensuing exhaustion [264,265]; and (5) antigen masking: This mechanism occurs when the CAR gene is unintentionally transduced into a leukemic B-cell during product manufacturing. CAR-transduced blasts will bind to the target antigen expressed on their own cell surface and result in the masking of and resistance to CAR T cells [266]. Overall, though, there may be some strategies to overcome this subtype of escape mechanism.

One of the most relevant and complex factors in determining CAR T cell therapy success is the identification and selection of the most suitable tumor antigens. Although no mainstream definition exists, the ideal tumor antigen should fulfill the following requirements: Have high, homogeneous expression on tumor cell surface; be involved in disease pathophysiology and maintain expression at different stages of the disease; be resistant to therapeutic pressure exerted by immunotherapy to avoid the downregulation or complete loss of the antigen; have no expression in normal tissue to avoid on-target, off-tumor toxicities; and if released into the bloodstream, should be minimal [267–270]. Potential molecules are currently being evaluated in clinical (e.g., BCMA, SLAMF7, CD19, CD38, CD44v6, GPRC5D) and preclinical (e.g., CD229, integrin β7) settings, and some have shown encouraging outcomes. Providing further details of these evaluations goes beyond the scope of this manuscript; however, comprehensive reviews that address this topic are available [152,153,271]. In all, finding the ideal antigen in myeloma is challenging and grand endeavors are being undertaken to find the balance between safety and effectiveness.

Targeting multiple tumor antigens may counteract antigen escape. Thus far, different approaches have been implemented including sequential treatment or co-administration of different single-target CAR T cell products; co-expression of two different CAR molecules on T cell surfaces using a single bicistronic vector (dual CARs); and expression of two scFvs in extracellular domains in "single-stalk" intracellular module (tandem CARs) (Figure 2) [272,273]. In the preclinical setting, different combinations have been shown to be useful (CD19/BCMA, BCMA/SLAMF7, and BCMA/GPRC5D [215,274–276]), while in the clinical setting, preliminary and encouraging results targeting BCMA/CD38, CD19/BCMA, and BCMA/TACI have been presented [277–280]. However, due to the selection of two antigens, special attention should be given to a potential increase in toxicity. Similarly, at the manufacturing level, bicistronic CARs require codon optimization if DNA recombination is not to occur, and engineering design of tandem CARs must be optimal if adequate antigen recognition and T cell activation are to be achieved [272].

Another plausible method to maintain or upregulate surface density of the target antigen is via in combination with different drugs. CD38 expression can be modulated with ATRA [78] and histone deacetylase inhibitors panobinostat and ricolinostat [80,81] to improve immunotherapy efficacy. BCMA expression could be enhanced with ATRA as an epigenetic modulator and improve CAR T cell efficacy [281]. As mentioned prior, the use of GSI in the preclinical setting reduces the shedding of sBCMA, leading to an increase in BCMA surface expression and improvement in BCMA-targeted CAR T cell therapy [222]. Currently, these findings are being verified in a clinical setting with crenigacestat as the inhibitor of GS. Outcomes of this clinical trial may prove promising, as initial results have been encouraging, especially in patients who relapsed after BCMA-targeted therapies [282].

Myeloma stem cells contribute to the high rates of refractoriness and relapse of this disease. These cells are able to remain in a quiescent state, undergo self-renewal and hold differentiation potential, be resistant to cell death mechanisms, and escape from immunosurveillance. Indeed, due to these characteristics, myeloma stem cells could be a target for CAR T cell therapy [283]. It has been suggested that these less differentiated, myeloma subclones do not express CD138, but they do express other antigens like CD19 and CD229 [284–287]. Designing CARs targeting these molecules may confer benefits [288,289], even though positive cell fraction is extremely scarce [290]. Nonetheless, while this type of treatment is interesting in theory, further, more comprehensive studies are warranted.

6.2. CAR T Cell-Related Toxicities

This novel therapy revealed new and potentially life-threatening toxicities that could limit its widespread use. The most prominent toxicities are CRS, ICANS and on-target, off-tumor toxicity [291,292]. CRS is characterized by the release of inflammatory cytokines associated with a wide range of symptoms such as fever, hypoxia, hypotension, and organ dysfunction. Treatment may include symptom support, corticosteroids, and IL-6 receptor antagonist tocilizumab [292–295]. ICANS is associated with the impairment of the blood–brain barrier and a subsequent elevation of cytokines in cerebrospinal fluid. Symptomatology varies from aphasia and confusion to seizures and cerebral edema. Clinical management may include appropriate supportive treatment and corticosteroids; the use of tocilizumab is justified only when CRS is co-existing [292,294–297]. Great efforts have been made to establish appropriate grading methods and treatment guidelines to improve the diagnosis and management of these complications [298–300]. With respect to on-target, off-tumor toxicity, this occurs due to recognition by CAR T cells of a targeted antigen expressed in non-tumor cells. A classic example of such toxicity is the development of B-cell aplasia and hypogammaglobulinemia during the use of CD19-targeted CAR T cells. However, other examples with potentially devastating outcomes have been reported [294–303].

In an MM setting using BCMA-targeted CAR T cells, CRS and ICANS rates are 60–100% and 2–42%, respectively, with the majority being grade ≤ 2 (59–100% and 81–100%, respectively). Tocilizumab and corticosteroids were required in 28–79% and 15–52% of patients, respectively [24,47,48,53,54,304]. Such data could translate into less severity when compared to CD-19 CARs.

As an in-depth review of different strategies mitigating toxicities has been published elsewhere [272,273,295], only some of the most prominent alternatives will be mentioned. The risk of CRS and ICANS is related to CAR T cell activation kinetics, the dose of CAR T cells infused, and baseline factors or comorbidities. Activation of CAR T cells are modulated by tumor burden, antigen expression, and the construct itself (affinity of scFv and costimulatory domains) [273]. The risk of toxicity may be attenuated by either reducing the number of CAR T cells infused or dividing the doses on different days. Prompt recognition of severe CRS and ICANS with the use of predictive biomarkers may also help. With respect to the construct, tailored modifications can be designed, including (1) optimizing the costimulatory domain (CD28 or 4-1BB), which depends on surface density of target antigen and the degree of expansion or persistence of CAR T cells [294,305]; and (2) engineering CARs with "suicide genes" using an apoptosis-triggering fusion protein comprising caspase 9 (iCasp9) [306] or "OFF-switches" like truncated epidermal growth factor receptor (EGFRt), which can be targeted with cetuximab [307] to dismiss CAR T cells. Dasatinib may also work as an on/off switch for CAR T cells by ablating the lymphocyte-specific protein tyrosine kinase (LCK)-signaling pathway [308]. Strategies designed to limit on-target, off-tumor toxicities include the following: Affinity tuning of the scFv to discern between normal and tumor cells per antigen density level [309–311]; "AND" logic-gate CARs that require simultaneous presence of two-cell surface antigens to activate the T cell [312]; "ON-switch" CARs, which need a small, heterodimerizing molecule to bind the dissociated antigen binding domain with the signaling domain for activation [313]; "SPLIT-CARs", the co-expression of two different CARs that recognize different antigens, in which one encloses the activation domain (CD3ζ) and the other the co-stimulation domain. Both antigens must be present for full T cell activation [314–316]; and inhibitory CARs (iCARs) bear an inhibitory signaling domain of immune-checkpoint proteins (CTLA-4 or PD-1) to inhibit T cell activation after recognition of the target antigen expressed in non-tumoral cells [317]. It remains to be determined which of all of these pre-clinical strategies may be useful in the clinical setting. Furthermore, the therapeutic/toxic window of each CAR construct is different; appropriate interventions may therefore differ and should be established for every CAR T cell [252,273].

6.3. Product Manufacturing, Access and Economic Challenges

Manufacturing CAR T cells from autologous T cells has certain limitations, as administration of CAR T cells may not be feasible in some patients. Some primary reasons for these limitations include difficulty in harvesting enough T cells from lymphopenic patients due to the disease itself and previous treatments; disease progression during manufacturing time; and failure in CAR T cell production due to T cell dysfunction [273,318]. To circumvent these hurdles, engineering CAR T cells from healthy allogeneic or "third-party" T cell donors has been proposed. This "off-the-shelf" strategy has many potential advantages, including cryopreserved batches to avoid treatment delays, less T cell quality issues, the possibility to redose and combine different target CAR T cells, possible decrease in manufacturing costs, and a greater number of patients possibly benefiting from such therapy [273,318]. Nevertheless, this approach is associated with two major concerns: (1) Graft versus host disease (GvHD) development and (2) rejection and removal of allogeneic T cells by the host immune system. To reduce the risk of GvHD, different therapeutical approaches are being used such as allogeneic donor-derived T cells in stem cell transplant recipients [319,320], non-$\alpha\beta$ T cells (NK cells or umbilical cord blood NK cells) [321,322], and gene-editing tools (zinc-finger, TALEN, and CRISPR/Cas9 technologies) to disrupt the endogenous TCR of CAR T cells [201,323,324]. To avoid allogeneic T cell rejection, it has been suggested to do the following: (1) Creating a T cell bank that matches the majority of HLA-subtypes [325]; (2) elongating the duration of lymphopenia by disrupting *TRAC* and *CD52* locus of CAR T cells to result in alemtuzumab-resistant CAR T cells [324]; (3) and disrupting *HLA-A* or *β2-microglobulin* genes on allogeneic CAR T cells [326]. Different promising BCMA (ALLO-715, ALLO-647, and P-BCMA-ALLO1) and SLAMF7 (UCARTCS1)-directed products are being evaluated in clinical trials [327–329]. Early data presented in the last ASH meeting showed that ALLO-715 and ALLO-647 have a manageable safety profile and clinical activity [330]. However, more robust data and longer follow-up are needed to determine the true potential and the target population of this strategy.

These "living drugs" are different from other oncological drugs, as various infrastructures, workflows, processes, and regulatory requirements are required to guarantee product quality and manufacturing time ("vein-to-vein time") [331]. The management of these patients require cooperation among multiple stakeholders and specialized teams with appropriate skill sets, standard operating procedures, and laborious site setup processes (extensive preparation and certifications) [332]. Another critical point in large-scale application is therapy costs. The Institute for Clinical and Economic Research (ICER) performed a cost-effectiveness analysis of previously authorized CAR T cells which are below the threshold to be considered cost effective ($150,000 per quality-adjusted life-year (QALY) gained) [333]. However, this analysis is not yet available for patients with myeloma. Long-term effectiveness will be a key outcome to possibly improve the cost-effectiveness ratio [334]. Other strategies that could reduce costs include non-viral gene delivery with "Sleeping Beauty" or "PiggyBac" transposon/transposase systems—which are more affordable than the use of viral vectors [335,336]—and the creation of community CAR T cell therapy centers and promotion of the outpatient setting to increase the number of patients who benefit from these treatments and improve hospital finances. A shift from centralized to decentralized manufacturing, namely "bedside manufacturing" could increase capacity, reduce costs, and lessen vein-to-vein time [332].

CAR T cell therapy has demonstrated excellent efficacy in clinical trials and some products are expected to be approved during this year. However, this strategy still has only a modest PFS. Therefore, in the near future, new strategies will be necessary to optimize these products.

7. Vaccines

Given the contribution of the immunological profile of MM pathogenesis, a vaccine may be able to stimulate a clinical response achieved with standard therapy. There are many mechanisms involved and clinical trials ongoing. However, this review will only present vaccines with published results. For example, patients treated with vaccines based on dendritic/patient-derived myeloma cells exhibited expansion of CD4$^+$ and CD8$^+$ lymphocytes; 11 of 16 patients achieved stable disease [55]. Furthermore, the same group reported that vaccination after ASCT resulted in expansion of myeloma-specific T cells and deeper minimal residual disease [57]. Other vaccines based on antigens overexpressed in myeloma, such as survivin and human telomerase reverse transcriptase (hTERT), which were transferred after ASCT, have led to higher cellular and humoral reconstitution as well as increased antitumor immunity and improved event-free survival [56]. MAGE-A3 (melanoma-associated antigen 3) is a protein detected in 50% of myeloma cells, becoming more frequent in the advanced stage of the disease. Two studies have therefore used MAGE-A3 as a peptide to conceive a vaccine. Both studies reported high specific T cell immunity after ASCT [58,60]. For smoldering MM, a vaccine targeting three myeloma peptides (XBP1, CD138, and CS1) was safe and well tolerated, achieving acceptable immune response alone and in combination with lenalidomide [59]. In summary, vaccines appear as a safe alternative to stimulate T cell response, possibly increasing or deepening such response after a transplant. A combination of vaccines with other strategies such as anti-PD1 antibodies may improve immune response [337]. The lack of longer follow-up trials to evaluate its real clinical impact and a high number of patients involved makes vaccines an ongoing field of interest, with still so many questions to answer within the coming years.

8. Personal Perspective

Immunotherapy is revolutionizing cancer treatment, uncovering new pathways to harness anti-tumor immune functions. Although novel immunotherapy approaches have proven effective in patients with myeloma, there are still concerns and hurdles that preclude their use. A major challenge is its unpredictable efficacy, namely whether such therapy will prove useful in only a minority of patients [338,339]. Such unpredictability could be due to interpersonal variability, tumor heterogeneity, and clonal evolution [216,258,340]. The reductionist approach that targets single molecular pathways or mutations might be upgraded with the use of combinatorial strategies targeting different pathways and possible synergistic effects [341]. Another way to improve the response would be to implement immunotherapy during the early stages of the disease, as restoration of robust anti-tumor activity would be easier than in advanced or heavily pretreated stages [339]. Additionally, the identification of potential biomarkers remains an unmet need in immunotherapy. Prognostic biomarkers are useful in predicting the likelihood of relapse and survival, irrespective of therapy, while predictive biomarkers foretell outcomes with a specific drug [342]. Molecular profiling technologies have allowed such identification. However, none of these biomarkers have been robustly validated in MM immunotherapy. It may be that, in the future, receptors and ligands of immune checkpoints, sBCMA levels, or the preinfused T cell subset will foresee accurate outcomes. Current medicine is evolving towards precision medicine, mainly in oncology, to personalize and refine health care in all its aspects. This includes medical decisions, diagnostic testing, and treatment selection, as well as elucidating prognosis in a subgroup of patients based on the molecular and cellular features of a tumor, overall environment, and individual lifestyle [343,344]. Several studies have already demonstrated the feasibility of adopting innovative approaches in precision oncology [345–347]. However, the percentage of patients who are eligible and will benefit for targeted-driven therapy remains a minority [348]. Different challenges will therefore have to be addressed. For example, as delayed responses could be observed with immunotherapy, traditional endpoints will need to be optimized for chemotherapy-based treatments [349]. Additionally, as progress is being made with biomarkers in precision oncology, next-generation clinical trials or master protocols (basket and umbrella trials) will be needed in order to evaluate specific molecular lesions in small cohorts of patients [350]. Finally, economic sustainability in immunotherapy has become a prominent concern. Immunotherapy agents are expensive, placing a great financial strain on the health system and, in some countries, the patient. Proper cost-effectiveness, cost-benefit, and QALY analyses will be required to resolve this matter of importance [339]. To make it more affordable, outcome-based reimbursement or staged payment models have been developed for gene therapies; however, if immunotherapy is to prove its legitimate value in terms of benefits and grow in accessibility, further real-world evidence and longer follow-ups with more patients will be necessary to leverage the therapeutic approach powerfully [351]. In the following years, close cooperation and coordination among different stakeholders will be necessary to preserve patient access and health care system sustainability.

Immunotherapy has generated a paradigm shift in the treatment of MM. MoA have shown minimal toxicity and outstanding efficacy, so it is expected that anti-CD38 MoA will be used in all standard front-line therapy for younger patients with NDMM and in non-transplant eligible patients. This will generate the need to seek specific therapeutic strategies in R/R patients, since the outcomes of patients with MM R/R to CD38-targeted MoA therapy are poor [352]. There is eagerness that novel immunotherapeutic strategies will provide clinical benefit in this challenging population. However, many BCMA-specific products and approaches are currently being explored in the R/R setting. ADC, Bs MoA, and CAR T cells will be a turning point in the therapeutic arsenal against MM. It will be necessary to analyze the advantages and disadvantages of each product and determine the best scenario to use them. Furthermore, there are currently no direct comparisons to determine which one is superior. Both ADC and Bs MoA are easy to use and available immediately; they do not require specialized centers for their administration, nor apheresis. ADC does not need a predefined number of T cells for their production. CAR T cell requires a few weeks to manufacture and specialized medical centers for administration, narrowing the number of patients who can receive it. Elderly and heavily pre-treated patients with lymphopenia could be a challenge in the manufacture of CAR T cells. T cell fitness could be of great importance for both Bs MoA and CAR T cell function. Regarding toxicities, both Bs MoA and CAR T cell products can develop CRS and ICANS, while ADC can develop keratopathy in the majority of patients. Respecting affordability, ADC and Bs MoA are less expensive when compared to CAR T cell products. So far, it remains unproven which BCMA-targeted strategy provides a better therapeutic index. Real-world data and longer follow-ups will provide new insights to clarify the proper way to integrate these therapies into current treatment algorithms.

9. Conclusions

In recent years, immunotherapy has positioned itself as a cutting-edge therapeutic strategy. It has become a game changer for patients with cancer. In patients with multiple myeloma, immunotherapy remains in a nascent stage; however, its therapeutic potential has already begun to be elucidated. Different products are expected to be approved in the short term. Nonetheless, this type of therapy faces different challenges, from efficacy and safety to manufacturing and economic affordability. To surmount these hurdles, more comprehensive knowledge is necessary to fully understand the mechanisms involved in relapse, boost "bench-to-bedside" research, enhance cooperation among various stakeholders, optimize manufacturing and scalability, and foster sustainability. It is our hope that this novel treatment approach could be used in early stages of the disease and become widely available. Restoring immune balance may just lead to long-lasting remissions long awaited.

Author Contributions: L.G.R.-L., A.O.-C., and D.F.M. wrote and reviewed the manuscript. C.F.d.L. and J.B. reviewed the manuscript. All authors have read and agreed to the published version of the manuscript.

Funding: L.G.R.-L. as a BITRECS fellow has received funding from the European Union's Horizon 2020 research and Innovation Programme under the Marie Sklodowska-Curie grant agreement No 754550 and from "La Caixa" Foundation. This work has been supported in part by grants from the Instituto de Salud Carlos III, Spanish Ministry of Health (FIS PI19/00669 and ICI19/00025), Fondo Europeo de Desarrollo Regional (FEDER), 2017SGR00792 (AGAUR; Generalitat de Catalunya).

Acknowledgments: The authors would like to thank Josep Solanes for his support in the graphic edition. We would like to thank Anthony Armenta for providing medical editing assistance.

Conflicts of Interest: The authors declare no conflict of interest.

References

1. Siegel, R.L.; Miller, K.D.; Jemal, A. Cancer statistics. *CA Cancer J. Clin.* **2020**, *70*, 7–30. [CrossRef]
2. Cowan, A.J.; Allen, C.; Barac, A.; Basaleem, H.; Bensenor, I.; Curado, M.P.; Foreman, K.; Gupta, R.; Harvey, J.; Hosgood, H.D.; et al. Global Burden of Multiple Myeloma: A Systematic Analysis for the Global Burden of Disease Study 2016. *JAMA Oncol.* **2018**, *4*, 1221–1227. [CrossRef]
3. Sant, M.; Allemani, C.; Tereanu, C.; De Angelis, R.; Capocaccia, R.; Visser, O.; Marcos-Gragera, R.; Maynadié, M.; Simonetti, A.; Lutz, J.M.; et al. Incidence of hematologic malignancies in Europe by morphologic subtype: Results of the HAEMACARE project. *Blood* **2010**, *116*, 3724–3734. [CrossRef]
4. Kumar, S.K.; Rajkumar, S.V. The multiple myelomas - current concepts in cytogenetic classification and therapy. *Nat. Rev. Clin. Oncol.* **2018**, *15*, 409–421. [CrossRef] [PubMed]
5. Lakshman, A.; Paul, S.; Rajkumar, S.V.; Ketterling, R.P.; Greipp, P.T.; Dispenzieri, A.; Gertz, M.A.; Buadi, F.K.; Lacy, M.Q.; Dingli, D.; et al. Prognostic significance of interphase FISH in monoclonal gammopathy of undetermined significance. *Leukemia* **2018**, *32*, 1811–1815. [CrossRef] [PubMed]
6. Merz, M.; Hielscher, T.; Hoffmann, K.; Seckinger, A.; Hose, D.; Raab, M.S.; Hillengass, J.; Jauch, A.; Goldschmidt, H. Cytogenetic abnormalities in monoclonal gammopathy of undetermined significance. *Leukemia* **2018**, *32*, 2717–2719. [CrossRef]
7. Mikulasova, A.; Wardell, C.P.; Murison, A.; Boyle, E.M.; Jackson, G.H.; Smetana, J.; Kufova, Z.; Pour, L.; Sandecka, V.; Almasi, M.; et al. The spectrum of somatic mutations in monoclonal gammopathy of undetermined significance indicates a less complex genomic landscape than that in multiple myeloma. *Haematologica* **2017**, *102*, 1617–1625. [CrossRef] [PubMed]
8. Klein, B.; Zhang, X.G.; Lu, Z.Y.; Bataille, R. Interleukin-6 in human multiple myeloma. *Blood* **1995**, *85*, 863–872. [CrossRef] [PubMed]
9. Gunn, W.G.; Conley, A.; Deininger, L.; Olson, S.D.; Prockop, D.J.; Gregory, C.A. A crosstalk between myeloma cells and marrow stromal cells stimulates production of DKK1 and interleukin-6: A potential role in the development of lytic bone disease and tumor progression in multiple myeloma. *Stem Cells* **2006**, *24*, 986–991. [CrossRef] [PubMed]
10. Hengeveld, P.J.; Kersten, M.J. B-cell activating factor in the pathophysiology of multiple myeloma: A target for therapy? *Blood Cancer J.* **2015**, *5*, e282. [CrossRef] [PubMed]
11. Sprynski, A.C.; Hose, D.; Caillot, L.; Réme, T.; Shaughnessy, J.D.; Barlogie, B.; Seckinger, A.; Moreaux, J.; Hundemer, M.; Jourdan, M.; et al. The role of IGF-1 as a major growth factor for myeloma cell lines and the prognostic relevance of the expression of its receptor. *Blood* **2009**, *113*, 4614–4626. [CrossRef]
12. Mitsiades, C.S.; McMillin, D.W.; Klippel, S.; Hideshima, T.; Chauhan, D.; Richardson, P.G.; Munshi, N.C.; Anderson, K.C. The role of the bone marrow microenvironment in the pathophysiology of myeloma and its significance in the development of more effective therapies. *Hematol. Oncol. Clin. N. Am.* **2007**, *21*, 1007–1034. [CrossRef] [PubMed]
13. Asaoku, H.; Kawano, M.; Iwato, K.; Tanabe, O.; Tanaka, H.; Hirano, T.; Kishimoto, T.; Kuramoto, A. Decrease in BSF-2/IL-6 response in advanced cases of multiple myeloma. *Blood* **1988**, *72*, 429–432. [CrossRef] [PubMed]
14. Görgün, G.T.; Whitehill, G.; Anderson, J.L.; Hideshima, T.; Maguire, C.; Laubach, J.; Raje, N.; Munshi, N.C.; Richardson, P.G.; Anderson, K.C. Tumor-promoting immune-suppressive myeloid-derived suppressor cells in the multiple myeloma microenvironment in humans. *Blood* **2013**, *121*, 2975–2987. [CrossRef] [PubMed]
15. Benson, D.M.; Bakan, C.E.; Mishra, A.; Hofmeister, C.C.; Efebera, Y.; Becknell, B.; Baiocchi, R.A.; Zhang, J.; Yu, J.; Smith, M.K.; et al. The PD-1/PD-L1 axis modulates the natural killer cell versus multiple myeloma effect: A therapeutic target for CT-011, a novel monoclonal anti-PD-1 antibody. *Blood* **2010**, *116*, 2286–2294. [CrossRef]
16. Minnie, S.A.; Kuns, R.D.; Gartlan, K.H.; Zhang, P.; Wilkinson, A.N.; Samson, L.; Guillerey, C.; Engwerda, C.; MacDonald, K.; Smyth, M.J.; et al. Myeloma escape after stem cell transplantation is a consequence of T-cell exhaustion and is prevented by TIGIT blockade. *Blood* **2018**, *132*, 1675–1688. [CrossRef]
17. Lozano, E.; Mena, M.P.; Díaz, T.; Martin-Antonio, B.; Leon, S.; Rodríguez-Lobato, L.G.; Oliver-Caldés, A.; Cibeira, M.T.; Bladé, J.; Prat, A.; et al. Nectin-2 Expression on Malignant Plasma Cells Is Associated with Better Response to TIGIT Blockade in Multiple Myeloma. *Clin. Cancer Res. Off. J. Am. Assoc. Cancer Res.* **2020**, *26*, 4688–4698. [CrossRef]
18. Prabhala, R.H.; Pelluru, D.; Fulciniti, M.; Prabhala, H.K.; Nanjappa, P.; Song, W.; Pai, C.; Amin, S.; Tai, Y.T.; Richardson, P.G.; et al. Elevated IL-17 produced by TH17 cells promotes myeloma cell growth and inhibits immune function in multiple myeloma. *Blood* **2010**, *115*, 5385–5392. [CrossRef]
19. Richardson, P.G.; Weller, E.; Lonial, S.; Jakubowiak, A.J.; Jagannath, S.; Raje, N.S.; Avigan, D.E.; Xie, W.; Ghobrial, I.M.; Schlossman, R.L.; et al. Lenalidomide, bortezomib, and dexamethasone combination therapy in patients with newly diagnosed multiple myeloma. *Blood* **2010**, *116*, 679–686. [CrossRef]
20. Rosiñol, L.; Oriol, A.; Rios, R.; Sureda, A.; Blanchard, M.J.; Hernández, M.T.; Martínez-Martínez, R.; Moraleda, J.M.; Jarque, I.; Bargay, J.; et al. Bortezomib, lenalidomide, and dexamethasone as induction therapy prior to autologous transplant in multiple myeloma. *Blood* **2019**, *134*, 1337–1345. [CrossRef]

21. Leblay, N.; Maity, R.; Hasan, F.; Neri, P. Deregulation of Adaptive T Cell Immunity in Multiple Myeloma: Insights Into Mechanisms and Therapeutic Opportunities. *Front. Oncol.* **2020**, *10*, 636. [CrossRef] [PubMed]
22. Garfall, A.L.; Stadtmauer, E.A. Cellular and vaccine immunotherapy for multiple myeloma. *Hematol. Am. Soc. Hematol. Educ. Program.* **2016**, *2016*, 521–527. [CrossRef] [PubMed]
23. Greil, C.; Engelhardt, M.; Ihorst, G.; Schoeller, K.; Bertz, H.; Marks, R.; Zeiser, R.; Duyster, J.; Einsele, H.; Finke, J.; et al. Allogeneic transplantation of multiple myeloma patients may allow long-term survival in carefully selected patients with acceptable toxicity and preserved quality of life. *Haematologica* **2019**, *104*, 370–379. [CrossRef] [PubMed]
24. Raje, N.; Berdeja, J.; Lin, Y.; Siegel, D.; Jagannath, S.; Madduri, D.; Liedtke, M.; Rosenblatt, J.; Maus, M.V.; Turka, A.; et al. Anti-BCMA CAR T-Cell Therapy bb2121 in Relapsed or Refractory Multiple Myeloma. *N. Engl. J. Med.* **2019**, *380*, 1726–1737. [CrossRef]
25. Lonial, S.; Weiss, B.M.; Usmani, S.Z.; Singhal, S.; Chari, A.; Bahlis, N.J.; Belch, A.; Krishnan, A.; Vescio, R.A.; Mateos, M.V.; et al. Daratumumab monotherapy in patients with treatment-refractory multiple myeloma (SIRIUS): An open-label, randomised, phase 2 trial. *Lancet* **2016**, *387*, 1551–1560. [CrossRef]
26. Usmani, S.Z.; Weiss, B.M.; Plesner, T.; Bahlis, N.J.; Belch, A.; Lonial, S.; Lokhorst, H.M.; Voorhees, P.M.; Richardson, P.G.; Chari, A.; et al. Clinical efficacy of daratumumab monotherapy in patients with heavily pretreated relapsed or refractory multiple myeloma. *Blood* **2016**, *128*, 37–44. [CrossRef]
27. Plesner, T.; Arkenau, H.T.; Lokhorst, H.M.; Gimsing, P.; Krejcik, J.; Lemech, C.; Minnema, M.; Lassen, U.N.; Laubach, J.P.; Ahmadi, T.; et al. Safety and Efficacy of Daratumumab with Lenalidomide and Dexamethasone in Relapsed or Relapsed, Refractory Multiple Myeloma. *Blood* **2014**, *124*, 84. [CrossRef]
28. Plesner, T.; Arkenau, H.T.; Gimsing, P.; Krejcik, J.; Lemech, C.; Minnema, M.C.; Lassen, U.; Laubach, J.P.; Palumbo, A.; Lisby, S.; et al. Daratumumab in Combination with Lenalidomide and Dexamethasone in Patients with Relapsed or Relapsed and Refractory Multiple Myeloma: Updated Results of a Phase 1/2 Study (GEN503). *Blood* **2015**, *126*, 507. [CrossRef]
29. Dimopoulos, M.A.; Oriol, A.; Nahi, H.; San-Miguel, J.; Bahlis, N.J.; Usmani, S.Z.; Rabin, N.; Orlowski, R.Z.; Komarnicki, M.; Suzuki, K.; et al. Daratumumab, Lenalidomide, and Dexamethasone for Multiple Myeloma. *N. Engl. J. Med.* **2016**, *375*, 1319–1331. [CrossRef]
30. Palumbo, A.; Chanan-Khan, A.; Weisel, K.; Nooka, A.K.; Masszi, T.; Beksac, M.; Spicka, I.; Hungria, V.; Munder, M.; Mateos, M.V.; et al. Daratumumab, Bortezomib, and Dexamethasone for Multiple Myeloma. *N. Engl. J. Med.* **2016**, *375*, 754–766. [CrossRef]
31. Weisel, K.C.; San Miguel, J.; Cook, G.; Leiba, M.; Suzuki, K.; Kumar, S.; Cavo, M.; Avet-Loiseau, H.; Quach, H.; Hungria, V.; et al. Efficacy of daratumumab in combination with lenalidomide plus dexamethasone (DRd) or bortezomib plus dexamethasone (DVd) in relapsed or refractory multiple myeloma (RRMM) based on cytogenetic risk status. *J. Clin. Oncol.* **2017**, *35* (Suppl. 15), 8006. [CrossRef]
32. Zonder, J.A.; Mohrbacher, A.F.; Singhal, S.; Van Rhee, F.; Bensinger, W.I.; Ding, H.; Fry, J.; Afar, D.E.; Singhal, A.K. A phase 1, multicenter, open-label, dose escalation study of elotuzumab in patients with advanced multiple myeloma. *Blood* **2012**, *120*, 552–559. [CrossRef] [PubMed]
33. Jakubowiak, A.; Offidani, M.; Pégourie, B.; De La Rubia, J.; Garderet, L.; Laribi, K.; Bosi, A.; Marasca, R.; Laubach, J.; Mohrbacher, A.; et al. Randomized phase 2 study: Elotuzumab plus bortezomib/dexamethasone vs bortezomib/dexamethasone for relapsed/refractory MM. *Blood* **2016**, *127*, 2833–2840. [CrossRef] [PubMed]
34. Dimopoulos, M.A.; Lonial, S.; White, D.; Moreau, P.; Palumbo, A.; San-Miguel, J.; Shpilberg, O.; Anderson, K.; Grosicki, S.; Spicka, I.; et al. Elotuzumab plus lenalidomide/dexamethasone for relapsed or refractory multiple myeloma: ELOQUENT-2 follow-up and post-hoc analyses on progression-free survival and tumour growth. *Br. J. Haematol.* **2017**, *178*, 896–905. [CrossRef] [PubMed]
35. Dimopoulos, M.A.; Dytfeld, D.; Grosicki, S.; Moreau, P.; Takezako, N.; Hori, M.; Leleu, X.; LeBlanc, R.; Suzuki, K.; Raab, M.S.; et al. Elotuzumab plus Pomalidomide and Dexamethasone for Multiple Myeloma. *N. Engl. J. Med.* **2018**, *379*, 1811–1822. [CrossRef] [PubMed]
36. Tai, Y.T.; Mayes, P.A.; Acharya, C.; Zhong, M.Y.; Cea, M.; Cagnetta, A.; Craigen, J.; Yates, J.; Gliddon, L.; Fieles, W.; et al. Novel anti-B-cell maturation antigen antibody-drug conjugate (GSK2857916) selectively induces killing of multiple myeloma. *Blood* **2014**, *123*, 3128–3138. [CrossRef]
37. Trudel, S.; Lendvai, N.; Popat, R.; Voorhees, P.M.; Reeves, B.; Libby, E.N.; Richardson, P.G.; Hoos, A.; Gupta, I.; Bragulat, V.; et al. Antibody-drug conjugate, GSK2857916, in relapsed/refractory multiple myeloma: An update on safety and efficacy from dose expansion phase I study. *Blood Cancer J.* **2019**, *9*, 37. [CrossRef]
38. Schönfeld, K.; Zuber, C.; Pinkas, J.; Häder, T.; Bernöster, K.; Uherek, C. Indatuximab ravtansine (BT062) combination treatment in multiple myeloma: Pre-clinical studies. *J. Hematol. Oncol.* **2017**, *10*, 13. [CrossRef]
39. Jagannath, S.; Heffner Jr, L.T.; Ailawadhi, S.; Munshi, N.C.; Zimmerman, T.M.; Rosenblatt, J.; Lonial, S.; Chanan-Khan, A.; Ruehle, M.; Rharbaoui, F.; et al. Indatuximab Ravtansine (BT062) Monotherapy in Patients With Relapsed and/or Refractory Multiple Myeloma. *Clin. Lymphoma. Myeloma. Leuk.* **2019**, *19*, 372–380. [CrossRef]
40. Ailawadhi, S.; Kelly, K.R.; Vescio, R.A.; Jagannath, S.; Wolf, J.; Gharibo, M.; Sher, T.; Bojanini, L.; Kirby, M.; Chanan-Khan, A. A Phase I Study to Assess the Safety and Pharmacokinetics of Single-agent Lorvotuzumab Mertansine (IMGN901) in Patients with Relapsed and/or Refractory CD-56-positive Multiple Myeloma. *Clin. Lymphoma. Myeloma. Leuk.* **2019**, *19*, 29–34. [CrossRef]

41. Kaufman, J.L.; Niesvizky, R.; Stadtmauer, E.A.; Chanan-Khan, A.; Siegel, D.; Horne, H.; Wegener, W.A.; Goldenberg, D.M. Phase I, multicentre, dose-escalation trial of monotherapy with milatuzumab (humanized anti-CD74 monoclonal antibody) in relapsed or refractory multiple myeloma. *Br. J. Haematol.* **2013**, *163*, 478–486. [CrossRef] [PubMed]
42. Hipp, S.; Tai, Y.T.; Blanset, D.; Deegen, P.; Wahl, J.; Thomas, O.; Rattel, B.; Adam, P.J.; Anderson, K.C.; Friedrich, M. A novel BCMA/CD3 bispecific T-cell engager for the treatment of multiple myeloma induces selective lysis in vitro and in vivo. *Leukemia* **2017**, *31*, 1743–1751. [CrossRef] [PubMed]
43. Topp, M.S.; Duell, J.; Zugmaier, G.; Attal, M.; Moreau, P.; Langer, C.; Krönke, J.; Facon, T.; Salnikov, A.V.; Lesley, R.; et al. Anti-B-Cell Maturation Antigen BiTE Molecule AMG 420 Induces Responses in Multiple Myeloma. *J. Clin. Oncol. Off. J. Am. Soc. Clin. Oncol.* **2020**, *38*, 775–783. [CrossRef] [PubMed]
44. Usmani, S.Z.; Mateos, M.V.; Nahi, H.; Krishnan, A.Y.; van de Donk, N.W.; San Miguel, J.; Oriol, A.; Rosiñol, L.; Chari, A.; Adams, H.; et al. Phase I study of teclistamab, a humanized B-cell maturation antigen (BCMA) x CD3 bispecific antibody, in relapsed/refractory multiple myeloma (R/R MM). *J. Clin. Oncol.* **2020**, *38* (Suppl. 15), 100. [CrossRef]
45. Lesokhin, A.M.; Ansell, S.M.; Armand, P.; Scott, E.C.; Halwani, A.; Gutierrez, M.; Millenson, M.M.; Cohen, A.D.; Schuster, S.J.; Lebovic, D.; et al. Nivolumab in Patients With Relapsed or Refractory Hematologic Malignancy: Preliminary Results of a Phase Ib Study. *J. Clin. Oncol. Off. J. Am. Soc. Clin. Oncol.* **2016**, *34*, 2698–2704. [CrossRef] [PubMed]
46. Mateos, M.V.; Blacklock, H.; Schjesvold, F.; Oriol, A.; Simpson, D.; George, A.; Goldschmidt, H.; Larocca, A.; Chanan-Khan, A.; Sherbenou, D.; et al. Pembrolizumab plus pomalidomide and dexamethasone for patients with relapsed or refractory multiple myeloma (KEYNOTE-183): A randomised, open-label, phase 3 trial. *Lancet Haematol.* **2019**, *6*, e459–e469. [CrossRef]
47. Brudno, J.N.; Maric, I.; Hartman, S.D.; Rose, J.J.; Wang, M.; Lam, N.; Stetler-Stevenson, M.; Salem, D.; Yuan, C.; Pavletic, S.; et al. T Cells Genetically Modified to Express an Anti-B-Cell Maturation Antigen Chimeric Antigen Receptor Cause Remissions of Poor-Prognosis Relapsed Multiple Myeloma. *J. Clin. Oncol. Off. J. Am. Soc. Clin. Oncol.* **2018**, *36*, 2267–2280. [CrossRef]
48. Cohen, A.D.; Garfall, A.L.; Stadtmauer, E.A.; Melenhorst, J.J.; Lacey, S.F.; Lancaster, E.; Vogl, D.T.; Weiss, B.M.; Dengel, K.; Nelson, A.; et al. B cell maturation antigen-specific CAR T cells are clinically active in multiple myeloma. *J. Clin. Investig.* **2019**, *129*, 2210–2221. [CrossRef]
49. Wang, B.Y.; Zhao, W.H.; Liu, J.; Chen, Y.X.; Cao, X.M.; Yang, Y.; Zhang, Y.L.; Wang, F.X.; Zhang, P.Y.; Lei, B.; et al. Long-Term Follow-up of a Phase 1, First-in-Human Open-Label Study of LCAR-B38M, a Structurally Differentiated Chimeric Antigen Receptor T (CAR-T) Cell Therapy Targeting B-Cell Maturation Antigen (BCMA), in Patients (pts) with Relapsed/Refractory Multiple Myeloma (RRMM). *Blood* **2019**, *134* (Suppl. 1), 579.
50. Zhao, W.H.; Liu, J.; Wang, B.Y.; Chen, Y.X.; Cao, X.M.; Yang, Y.; Zhang, Y.L.; Wang, F.X.; Zhang, P.Y.; Lei, B.; et al. A phase 1, open-label study of LCAR-B38M, a chimeric antigen receptor T cell therapy directed against B cell maturation antigen, in patients with relapsed or refractory multiple myeloma. *J. Hematol. Oncol.* **2018**, *11*, 141. [CrossRef]
51. Xu, J.; Chen, L.J.; Yang, S.S.; Sun, Y.; Wu, W.; Liu, Y.F.; Xu, J.; Zhuang, Y.; Zhang, W.; Weng, X.Q.; et al. Exploratory trial of a biepitopic CAR T-targeting B cell maturation antigen in relapsed/refractory multiple myeloma. *Proc. Natl. Acad. Sci. USA* **2019**, *116*, 9543–9551. [CrossRef] [PubMed]
52. Madduri, D.; Berdeja, J.G.; Usmani, S.Z.; Jakubowiak, A.; Agha, M.; Cohen, A.D. CARTITUDE-1: Phase 1b/2 Study of Ciltacabtagene Autoleucel, a B-Cell Maturation Antigen-Directed Chimeric Antigen Receptor T Cell Therapy, in Relapsed/Refractory Multiple Myeloma. *Blood* **2020**, *136* (Suppl. 1), 22–25. [CrossRef]
53. Munshi, N.C.; Anderson, L.D., Jr.; Shah, N.; Jagannath, S.; Berdeja, J.G.; Lonial, S.; Raje, N.S.; Siegel, D.S.; Lin, Y.; Oriol, A.; et al. Idecabtagene vicleucel (ide-cel; bb2121), a BCMA-targeted CAR T-cell therapy, in patients with relapsed and refractory multiple myeloma (RRMM): Initial KarMMa results. *J. Clin. Oncol.* **2020**, *38* (Suppl. 15), 8503. [CrossRef]
54. Mailankody, S.; Jakubowiak, A.J.; Htut, M.; Costa, L.J.; Lee, K.; Ganguly, S.; Kaufman, J.L.; Siegel, D.S.; Bensinger, W.; Cota, M.; et al. Orvacabtagene autoleucel (orva-cel), a B-cell maturation antigen (BCMA)-directed CAR T cell therapy for patients (pts) with relapsed/refractory multiple myeloma (RRMM): Update of the phase 1/2 EVOLVE study (NCT03430011). *J. Clin. Oncol.* **2020**, *38* (Suppl. 15), 8504. [CrossRef]
55. Rosenblatt, J.; Vasir, B.; Uhl, L.; Blotta, S.; MacNamara, C.; Somaiya, P.; Wu, Z.; Joyce, R.; Levine, J.D.; Dombagoda, D.; et al. Vaccination with dendritic cell/tumor fusion cells results in cellular and humoral antitumor immune responses in patients with multiple myeloma. *Blood* **2011**, *117*, 393–402. [CrossRef] [PubMed]
56. Rapoport, A.P.; Aqui, N.A.; Stadtmauer, E.A.; Vogl, D.T.; Fang, H.B.; Cai, L.; Janofsky, S.; Chew, A.; Storek, J.; Akpek, G.; et al. Combination immunotherapy using adoptive T-cell transfer and tumor antigen vaccination on the basis of hTERT and survivin after ASCT for myeloma. *Blood* **2011**, *117*, 788–797. [CrossRef] [PubMed]
57. Rosenblatt, J.; Avivi, I.; Vasir, B.; Uhl, L.; Munshi, N.C.; Katz, T.; Dey, B.R.; Somaiya, P.; Mills, H.; Campigotto, F.; et al. Vaccination with dendritic cell/tumor fusions following autologous stem cell transplant induces immunologic and clinical responses in multiple myeloma patients. *Clin. Cancer Res. Off. J. Am. Assoc. Cancer Res.* **2013**, *19*, 3640–3648. [CrossRef]
58. Rapoport, A.P.; Aqui, N.A.; Stadtmauer, E.A.; Vogl, D.T.; Xu, Y.Y.; Kalos, M.; Cai, L.; Fang, H.B.; Weiss, B.M.; Badros, A.; et al. Combination immunotherapy after ASCT for multiple myeloma using MAGE-A3/Poly-ICLC immunizations followed by adoptive transfer of vaccine-primed and costimulated autologous T cells. *Clin. Cancer Res. Off. J. Am. Assoc. Cancer Res.* **2014**, *20*, 1355–1365. [CrossRef]

59. Nooka, A.K.; Wang, M.L.; Yee, A.J.; Kaufman, J.L.; Bae, J.; Peterkin, D.; Richardson, P.G.; Raje, N.S. Assessment of Safety and Immunogenicity of PVX-410 Vaccine With or Without Lenalidomide in Patients With Smoldering Multiple Myeloma: A Nonrandomized Clinical Trial. *JAMA Oncol.* **2018**, *4*, e183267. [CrossRef]
60. Cohen, A.D.; Lendvai, N.; Nataraj, S.; Imai, N.; Jungbluth, A.A.; Tsakos, I.; Rahman, A.; Mei, A.H.; Singh, H.; Zarychta, K.; et al. Autologous Lymphocyte Infusion Supports Tumor Antigen Vaccine-Induced Immunity in Autologous Stem Cell Transplant for Multiple Myeloma. *Cancer Immunol. Res.* **2019**, *7*, 658–669. [CrossRef]
61. Deaglio, S.; Mehta, K.; Malavasi, F. Human CD38: A (r)evolutionary story of enzymes and receptors. *Leuk Res.* **2001**, *25*, 1–12. [CrossRef]
62. Deaglio, S.; Vaisitti, T.; Billington, R.; Bergui, L.; Omede, P.; Genazzani, A.A.; Malavasi, F. CD38/CD19: A lipid raft-dependent signaling complex in human B cells. *Blood* **2007**, *109*, 5390–5398. [CrossRef] [PubMed]
63. Malavasi, F.; Deaglio, S.; Funaro, A.; Ferrero, E.; Horenstein, A.L.; Ortolan, E.; Vaisitti, T.; Aydin, S. Evolution and function of the ADP ribosyl cyclase/CD38 gene family in physiology and pathology. *Physiol. Rev.* **2008**, *88*, 841–886. [CrossRef] [PubMed]
64. van de Donk, N.W.C.J.; Usmani, S.Z. CD38 Antibodies in Multiple Myeloma: Mechanisms of Action and Modes of Resistance. *Front. Immunol.* **2018**, *9*, 2134. [CrossRef] [PubMed]
65. Nijhof, I.S.; Groen, R.W.; Noort, W.A.; van Kessel, B.; de Jong-Korlaar, R.; Bakker, J.; Van Bueren, J.J.; Parren, P.W.; Lokhorst, H.M.; Van De Donk, N.W.; et al. Preclinical Evidence for the Therapeutic Potential of CD38-Targeted Immuno-Chemotherapy in Multiple Myeloma Patients Refractory to Lenalidomide and Bortezomib. *Clin. Cancer Res. Off. J. Am. Assoc. Cancer Res.* **2015**, *21*, 2802–2810. [CrossRef] [PubMed]
66. Moreau, P.; Attal, M.; Hulin, C.; Arnulf, B.; Belhadj, K.; Benboubker, L.; Béné, M.C.; Broijl, A.; Caillon, H.; Caillot, D.; et al. Bortezomib, thalidomide, and dexamethasone with or without daratumumab before and after autologous stem-cell transplantation for newly diagnosed multiple myeloma (CASSIOPEIA): A randomised, open-label, phase 3 study. *Lancet* **2019**, *394*, 29–38. [CrossRef]
67. Mateos, M.V.; Cavo, M.; Blade, J.; Dimopoulos, M.A.; Suzuki, K.; Jakubowiak, A.; Knop, S.; Doyen, C.; Lucio, P.; Nagy, Z.; et al. Overall survival with daratumumab, bortezomib, melphalan, and prednisone in newly diagnosed multiple myeloma (ALCYONE): A randomised, open-label, phase 3 trial. *Lancet* **2020**, *395*, 132–141. [CrossRef]
68. Facon, T.; Kumar, S.; Plesner, T.; Orlowski, R.Z.; Moreau, P.; Bahlis, N.; Basu, S.; Nahi, H.; Hulin, C.; Quach, H.; et al. Daratumumab plus Lenalidomide and Dexamethasone for Untreated Myeloma. *N. Engl. J. Med.* **2019**, *380*, 2104–2115. [CrossRef]
69. Chari, A.; Suvannasankha, A.; Fay, J.W.; Arnulf, B.; Kaufman, J.L.; Ifthikharuddin, J.J.; Weiss, B.M.; Krishnan, A.; Lentzsch, S.; Comenzo, R.; et al. Daratumumab plus pomalidomide and dexamethasone in relapsed and/or refractory multiple myeloma. *Blood* **2017**, *130*, 974–981. [CrossRef]
70. Dimopoulos, M.; Quach, H.; Mateos, M.V.; Landgren, O.; Leleu, X.; Siegel, D.; Weisel, K.; Yang, H.; Klippel, Z.; Zahlten-Kumeli, A.; et al. Carfilzomib, dexamethasone, and daratumumab versus carfilzomib and dexamethasone for patients with relapsed or refractory multiple myeloma (CANDOR): Results from a randomised, multicentre, open-label, phase 3 study. *Lancet* **2020**, *396*, 186–197. [CrossRef]
71. Attal, M.; Richardson, P.G.; Rajkumar, S.V.; San-Miguel, J.; Beksac, M.; Spicka, I.; Leleu, X.; Schjesvold, F.; Moreau, P.; Dimopoulos, M.A.; et al. Isatuximab plus pomalidomide and low-dose dexamethasone versus pomalidomide and low-dose dexamethasone in patients with relapsed and refractory multiple myeloma (ICARIA-MM): A randomised, multicentre, open-label, phase 3 study. *Lancet* **2019**, *394*, 2096–2107. [CrossRef]
72. De Weers, M.; Tai, Y.T.; Van Der Veer, M.S.; Bakker, J.M.; Vink, T.; Jacobs, D.C.; Oomen, L.A.; Peipp, M.; Valerius, T.; Slootstra, J.W.; et al. Daratumumab, a novel therapeutic human CD38 monoclonal antibody, induces killing of multiple myeloma and other hematological tumors. *J. Immunol.* **2011**, *186*, 1840–1848. [CrossRef]
73. Overdijk, M.B.; Verploegen, S.; Bögels, M.; van Egmond, M.; van Bueren, J.J.; Mutis, T.; Groen, R.W.; Breij, E.; Martens, A.C.; Bleeker, W.K.; et al. Antibody-mediated phagocytosis contributes to the anti-tumor activity of the therapeutic antibody daratumumab in lymphoma and multiple myeloma. *mAbs* **2015**, *7*, 311–321. [CrossRef] [PubMed]
74. Franssen, L.E.; Stege, C.A.M.; Zweegman, S.; van de Donk, N.W.C.J.; Nijhof, I.S. Resistance Mechanisms Towards CD38-Directed Antibody Therapy in Multiple Myeloma. *J. Clin. Med.* **2020**, *9*, 1195. [CrossRef] [PubMed]
75. Overdijk, M.B.; Jansen, J.M.; Nederend, M.; van Bueren, J.J.; Groen, R.W.; Parren, P.W.; Leusen, J.H.; Boross, P. The Therapeutic CD38 Monoclonal Antibody Daratumumab Induces Programmed Cell Death via Fcγ Receptor-Mediated Cross-Linking. *J. Immunol.* **2016**, *197*, 807–813. [CrossRef] [PubMed]
76. Krejcik, J.; Casneuf, T.; Nijhof, I.S.; Verbist, B.; Bald, J.; Plesner, T.; Syed, K.; Liu, K.; van de Donk, N.W.; Weiss, B.M.; et al. Daratumumab depletes CD38+ immune regulatory cells, promotes T-cell expansion, and skews T-cell repertoire in multiple myeloma. *Blood* **2016**, *128*, 384–394. [CrossRef] [PubMed]
77. Kitadate, A.; Kobayashi, H.; Abe, Y.; Narita, K.; Miura, D.; Takeuchi, M.; Matsue, K. Pre-treatment CD38-positive regulatory T cells affect the durable response to daratumumab in relapsed/refractory multiple myeloma patients. *Haematologica* **2020**, *105*, e37–e40. [CrossRef]
78. Nijhof, I.S.; Groen, R.W.; Lokhorst, H.M.; Van Kessel, B.; Bloem, A.C.; Van Velzen, J.; de Jong-Korlaar, R.; Yuan, H.; Noort, W.A.; Klein, S.K.; et al. Upregulation of CD38 expression on multiple myeloma cells by all-trans retinoic acid improves the efficacy of daratumumab. *Leukemia* **2015**, *29*, 2039–2049. [CrossRef]

79. Fedele, P.L.; Willis, S.N.; Liao, Y.; Low, M.S.; Rautela, J.; Segal, D.H.; Gong, J.N.; Huntington, N.D.; Shi, W.; Huang, D.; et al. IMiDs prime myeloma cells for daratumumab-mediated cytotoxicity through loss of Ikaros and Aiolos. *Blood* **2018**, *132*, 2166–2178. [CrossRef]
80. García-Guerrero, E.; Gogishvili, T.; Danhof, S.; Schreder, M.; Pallaud, C.; Pérez-Simón, J.A.; Einsele, H.; Hudecek, M. Panobinostat induces CD38 upregulation and augments the antimyeloma efficacy of daratumumab. *Blood* **2017**, *129*, 3386–3388. [CrossRef]
81. García-Guerrero, E.; Götz, R.; Doose, S.; Sauer, M.; Rodríguez-Gil, A.; Nerreter, T.; Kortüm, K.M.; Pérez-Simón, J.A.; Einsele, H.; Hudecek, M.; et al. Upregulation of CD38 expression on multiple myeloma cells by novel HDAC6 inhibitors is a class effect and augments the efficacy of daratumumab. *Leukemia* **2020**, *29*, 1–4. [CrossRef] [PubMed]
82. Zipfel, P.F.; Skerka, C. Complement regulators and inhibitory proteins. *Nat. Rev. Immunol.* **2009**, *9*, 729–740. [CrossRef] [PubMed]
83. Nijhof, I.S.; Casneuf, T.; Van Velzen, J.; van Kessel, B.; Axel, A.E.; Syed, K.; Groen, R.W.; van Duin, M.; Sonneveld, P.; Minnema, M.C.; et al. CD38 expression and complement inhibitors affect response and resistance to daratumumab therapy in myeloma. *Blood* **2016**, *128*, 959–970. [CrossRef] [PubMed]
84. Barclay, A.N.; Van den Berg, T.K. The interaction between signal regulatory protein alpha (SIRPα) and CD47: Structure, function, and therapeutic target. *Annu. Rev. Immunol.* **2014**, *32*, 25–50. [CrossRef] [PubMed]
85. Saito, Y.; Iwamura, H.; Kaneko, T.; Ohnishi, H.; Murata, Y.; Okazawa, H.; Kanazawa, Y.; Sato-Hashimoto, M.; Kobayashi, H.; Oldenborg, P.A.; et al. Regulation by SIRPα of dendritic cell homeostasis in lymphoid tissues. *Blood* **2010**, *116*, 3517–3525. [CrossRef] [PubMed]
86. Abrisqueta, P.; Sancho, J.M.; Cordoba, R.; Persky, D.O.; Andreadis, C.; Huntington, S.F.; Carpio, C.; Morillo Giles, D.; Wei, X.; Li, Y.F.; et al. Anti-CD47 Antibody, CC-90002, in Combination with Rituximab in Subjects with Relapsed and/or Refractory Non-Hodgkin Lymphoma (R/R NHL). *Blood* **2019**, *134* (Suppl. 1), 4089. [CrossRef]
87. Naicker, S.; Rigalou, A.; McEllistrim, C.; Natoni, A.; Chiu, C.; Sasser, K.; Ryan, A.; O'Dwyer, M. Patient Data Supports the Rationale of Low Dose Cyclophosphamide to Potentiate the Anti-Myeloma Activity of Daratumumab through Augmentation of Macrophage-Induced ADCP. *Blood* **2017**, *130* (Suppl. 1), 121.
88. Rigalou, A.; Ryan, A.; Natoni, A.; Chiu, C.; Sasser, K.; O'Dwyer, M.E. Potentiation of Anti-Myeloma Activity of Daratumumab with Combination of Cyclophosphamide, Lenalidomide or Bortezomib Via a Tumor Secretory Response That Greatly Augments Macrophage-Induced ADCP. *Blood* **2016**, *128*, 2101. [CrossRef]
89. Nimmerjahn, F.; Ravetch, J.V. Fcgamma receptors as regulators of immune responses. *Nat. Rev. Immunol.* **2008**, *8*, 34–47. [CrossRef]
90. van de Donk, N.W.; Casneuf, T.; Di Cara, A.; Parren, P.W.; Zweegman, S.; van Kessel, B.; Lokhorst, H.M.; Usmani, S.Z.; Lonial, S.; Richardson, P.G.; et al. Impact of Fc gamma receptor polymorphisms on efficacy and safety of daratumumab in relapsed/refractory multiple myeloma. *Br. J. Haematol.* **2019**, *184*, 475–479. [CrossRef]
91. Sanne, J.; van de Donk, N.W.; Minnema, M.C.; Huang, J.H.; Aarts-Riemens, T.; Bovenschen, N.; Yuan, H.; Groen, R.W.; McMillin, D.W.; Jakubikova, J.; et al. Accessory cells of the microenvironment protect multiple myeloma from T-cell cytotoxicity through cell adhesion-mediated immune resistance. *Clin. Cancer Res. Off. J. Am. Assoc. Cancer Res.* **2013**, *19*, 5591–5601.
92. Van Der Veer, M.S.; de Weers, M.; van Kessel, B.; Bakker, J.M.; Wittebol, S.; Parren, P.W.; Lokhorst, H.M.; Mutis, T. Towards effective immunotherapy of myeloma: Enhanced elimination of myeloma cells by combination of lenalidomide with the human CD38 monoclonal antibody daratumumab. *Haematologica* **2011**, *96*, 284–290. [CrossRef] [PubMed]
93. Nijhof, I.S.; van Bueren, J.J.; van Kessel, B.; Andre, P.; Morel, Y.; Lokhorst, H.M.; van de Donk, N.W.; Parren, P.W.; Mutis, T. Daratumumab-mediated lysis of primary multiple myeloma cells is enhanced in combination with the human anti-KIR antibody IPH2102 and lenalidomide. *Haematologica* **2015**, *100*, 263–268. [CrossRef] [PubMed]
94. Wang, Y.; Zhang, Y.; Hughes, T.; Zhang, J.; Caligiuri, M.A.; Benson, D.M.; Yu, J. Fratricide of NK Cells in Daratumumab Therapy for Multiple Myeloma Overcome by Ex Vivo-Expanded Autologous NK Cells. *Clin. Cancer Res. Off. J. Am. Assoc. Cancer Res.* **2018**, *24*, 4006–4017. [CrossRef] [PubMed]
95. Cannons, J.L.; Tangye, S.G.; Schwartzberg, P.L. SLAM family receptors and SAP adaptors in immunity. *Annu. Rev. Immunol.* **2011**, *29*, 665–705. [CrossRef]
96. Collins, S.M.; Bakan, C.E.; Swartzel, G.D.; Hofmeister, C.C.; Efebera, Y.A.; Kwon, H.; Starling, G.C.; Ciarlariello, D.; Bhaskar, S.; Briercheck, E.L.; et al. Elotuzumab directly enhances NK cell cytotoxicity against myeloma via CS1 ligation: Evidence for augmented NK cell function complementing ADCC. *Cancer Immunol. Immunother.* **2013**, *62*, 1841–1849. [CrossRef]
97. Hartmut, G.; Mai, E.K.; Hans, S.; Uta, B.; Kaya, H.; Christina, K. Bortezomib, Lenalidomide and Dexamethasone with or Without Elotuzumab as Induction Therapy for Newly-Diagnosed, Transplant-Eligible Multiple Myeloma. 2020. Available online: https://library.ehaweb.org/eha/2020/eha25th/295023/hartmut.goldschmidt.bortezomib.lenalidomide.and.dexamethasone.with.or.without (accessed on 14 December 2020).
98. Usmani, S.Z.; Ailawadhi, S.; Sexton, R.; Hoering, A.; Lipe, B.; Hita, S.; Durie, B.G.; Zonder, J.A.; Dhodapkar, M.V.; Callander, N.S.; et al. Primary analysis of the randomized phase II trial of bortezomib, lenalidomide, dexamthasone with/without elotuzumab for newly diagnosed, high-risk multiple myeloma (SWOG-1211). *J. Clin. Oncol.* **2020**, *38* (Suppl. 15), 8507. [CrossRef]

99. Bristol Myers Squibb Reports Primary Results of ELOQUENT-1 Study Evaluating Empliciti (Elotuzumab) Plus Revlimid (lenalidomide) and Dexamethasone in Patients with Newly Diagnosed, Untreated Multiple Myeloma. Available online: https://news.bms.com/news/corporate-financial/2020/Bristol-Myers-Squibb-Reports-Primary-Results-of-ELOQUENT-1-Study-Evaluating-Empliciti-elotuzumab-Plus-Revlimid-lenalidomide-and-Dexamethasone-in-Patients-with-Newly-Diagnosed-Untreated-Multiple-Myeloma/default.aspx (accessed on 14 December 2020).
100. Lonial, S.; Lee, H.C.; Badros, A.; Trudel, S.; Nooka, A.K.; Chari, A.; Abdallah, A.O.; Callander, N.; Lendvai, N.; Sborov, D. Belantamab mafodotin for relapsed or refractory multiple myeloma (DREAMM-2): A two-arm, randomised, open-label, phase 2 study. *Lancet Oncol.* **2020**, *21*, 207–221. [CrossRef]
101. Farooq, A.V.; Degli Esposti, S.; Popat, R.; Thulasi, P.; Lonial, S.; Nooka, A.K.; Jakubowiak, A.; Sborov, D.; Zaugg, B.E.; Badros, A.Z.; et al. Corneal Epithelial Findings in Patients with Multiple Myeloma Treated with Antibody-Drug Conjugate Belantamab Mafodotin in the Pivotal, Randomized, DREAMM-2 Study. *Ophthalmol. Ther.* **2020**, *9*, 889–911. [CrossRef]
102. Sanderson, R.D.; Lalor, P.; Bernfield, M. B lymphocytes express and lose syndecan at specific stages of differentiation. *Cell Regul.* **1989**, *1*, 27–35. [CrossRef]
103. Ishitsuka, K.; Jimi, S.; Goldmacher, V.S.; Ab, O.; Tamura, K. Targeting CD56 by the maytansinoid immunoconjugate IMGN901 (huN901-DM1): A potential therapeutic modality implication against natural killer/T cell malignancy. *Br. J. Haematol.* **2008**, *141*, 129–131. [CrossRef] [PubMed]
104. Stein, R.; Mattes, M.J.; Cardillo, T.M.; Hansen, H.J.; Chang, C.H.; Burton, J.; Govindan, S.; Goldenberg, D.M. CD74: A new candidate target for the immunotherapy of B-cell neoplasms. *Clin. Cancer Res. Off. J. Am. Assoc. Cancer Res.* **2007**, *13 Pt 2*, 5556s–5563s. [CrossRef]
105. Zanwar, S.; Nandakumar, B.; Kumar, S. Immune-based therapies in the management of multiple myeloma. *Blood Cancer. J.* **2020**, *10*, 84. [CrossRef] [PubMed]
106. Baeuerle, P.A.; Kufer, P.; Bargou, R. BiTE: Teaching antibodies to engage T-cells for cancer therapy. *Curr. Opin. Mol. Ther.* **2009**, *11*, 22–30. [PubMed]
107. Velasquez, M.P.; Bonifant, C.L.; Gottschalk SRedirecting, T. cells to hematological malignancies with bispecific antibodies. *Blood* **2018**, *131*, 30–38. [CrossRef] [PubMed]
108. Kadowaki, N. Cancer therapy using bispecific antibodies. *Rinsho Ketsueki.* **2018**, *59*, 1942–1947.
109. Loffler, A.; Kufer, P.; Lutterbuse, R.; Zettl, F.; Daniel, P.T.; Schwenkenbecher, J.M.; Riethmuller, G.; Dorken, B.; Bargou, R.C. A recombinant bispecific single-chain antibody, CD19 x CD3, induces rapid and high lymphoma-directed cytotoxicity by unstimulated T lymphocytes. *Blood* **2000**, *95*, 2098–2103. [CrossRef]
110. Gökbuget, N.; Dombret, H.; Bonifacio, M.; Reichle, A.; Graux, C.; Faul, C.; Diedrich, H.; Topp, M.S.; Brüggemann, M.; Horst, H.A.; et al. Blinatumomab for minimal residual disease in adults with B-cell precursor acute lymphoblastic leukemia. *Blood* **2018**, *131*, 1522–1531. [CrossRef]
111. Goyos, A.; Li, C.M.; Deegen, P.; Bogner, P.; Thomas, O.; Wahl, J.; Goldstein, R.; Friedrich, M.; Coxon, A.; Balazs, M.; et al. Abstract LB-299: Cynomolgus monkey plasma cell gene signature to quantify the in vivo activity of a half-life extended anti-BCMA BiTE®for the treatment of multiple myeloma. *Cancer Res.* **2018**, *78* (Suppl. 13). [CrossRef]
112. Cho, S.F.; Lin, L.; Xing, L.; Liu, J.; Yu, T.; Wen, K.; Hsieh, P.; Munshi, N.; Anderson, K.; Tai, Y.T. Anti-BCMA BiTE® AMG 701 Potently Induces Specific T Cell Lysis of Human Multiple Myeloma (MM) Cells and Immunomodulation in the Bone Marrow Microenvironment. *Blood* **2018**, *132* (Suppl. 1), 592. [CrossRef]
113. Pillarisetti, K.; Powers, G.; Luistro, L.; Babich, A.; Baldwin, E.; Li, Y.; Zhang, X.; Mendonça, M.; Majewski, N.; Nanjunda, R.; et al. Teclistamab is an active T cell-redirecting bispecific antibody against B-cell maturation antigen for multiple myeloma. *Blood Adv.* **2020**, *4*, 4538–4549. [CrossRef] [PubMed]
114. Costa, L.J.; Wong, S.W.; Bermúdez, A.; de la Rubia, J.; Mateos, M.V.; Ocio, E.M.; Rodríguez-Otero, P.; San-Miguel, J.; Li, S.; Sarmiento, R.; et al. Interim Results from the First Phase 1 Clinical Study of the B-cell Maturation Antigen (BCMA) 2+1 T Cell Engager (TCE) CC-93269 in Patients (PTS) with Relapsed/Refractory Multiple Myeloma (RRMM). Available online: https://library.ehaweb.org/eha/2020/eha25th/295025/luciano.j.costa.interim.results.from.the.first.phase.1.clinical.study.of.the (accessed on 14 December 2020).
115. Richter, J.R.; Landgren, C.O.; Kauh, J.S.; Back, J.; Salhi, Y.; Reddy, V.; Bayever, E.; Berdej, A. Phase 1, multicenter, open-label study of single-agent bispecific antibody t-cell engager GBR 1342 in relapsed/refractory multiple myeloma. *J. Clin. Oncol.* **2018**, *36* (Suppl. 15), TPS3132. [CrossRef]
116. Cohen, A.D.; Harrison, S.J.; Krishnan, A.; Fonseca, R.; Forsberg, P.A.; Spencer, A. Initial Clinical Activity and Safety of BFCR4350A, a FcRH5/CD3 T-Cell-Engaging Bispecific Antibody, in Relapsed/Refractory Multiple Myeloma. *Blood* **2020**, *136* (Suppl. 1), 42–43. [CrossRef]
117. Chari, A.; Berdeja, J.G.; Oriol, A.; van de Donk, N.W.C.J.; Rodriguez, P.; Askari, E. A Phase 1, First-in-Human Study of Talquetamab, a G Protein-Coupled Receptor Family C Group 5 Member D (GPRC5D) x CD3 Bispecific Antibody, in Patients with Relapsed and/or Refractory Multiple Myeloma (RRMM). *Blood* **2020**, *136* (Suppl. 1), 40–41. [CrossRef]
118. Wu, L.; Seung, E.; Xu, L.; Rao, E.; Lord, D.M.; Wei, R.R.; Cortez-Retamozo, V.; Ospina, B.; Posternak, V.; Ulinski, G.; et al. Trispecific antibodies enhance the therapeutic efficacy of tumor-directed T cells through T cell receptor co-stimulation. *Nat. Cancer* **2020**, *1*, 86–98. [CrossRef]

119. Lancman, G.; Richter, J.; Chari, A. Bispecifics, trispecifics, and other novel immune treatments in myeloma. *Hematology* **2020**, *2020*, 264–271. [CrossRef]
120. Dunn, G.P.; Bruce, A.T.; Ikeda, H.; Old, L.J.; Schreiber, R.D. Cancer immunoediting: From immunosurveillance to tumor escape. *Nat. Immunol.* **2002**, *3*, 991–998. [CrossRef]
121. Vesely, M.D.; Kershaw, M.H.; Schreiber, R.D.; Smyth, M.J. Natural innate and adaptive immunity to cancer. *Annu. Rev. Immunol.* **2011**, *29*, 235–271. [CrossRef]
122. Salmaninejad, A.; Valilou, S.F.; Shabgah, A.G.; Aslani, S.; Alimardani, M.; Pasdar, A.; Sahebkar, A. PD-1/PD-L1 pathway: Basic biology and role in cancer immunotherapy. *J. Cell Physiol.* **2019**, *234*, 16824–16837. [CrossRef]
123. Costa, F.; Das, R.; Kini Bailur, J.; Dhodapkar, K.; Dhodapkar, M.V. Checkpoint Inhibition in Myeloma: Opportunities and Challenges. *Front. Immunol.* **2018**, *9*, 2204. [CrossRef]
124. Dyck, L.; Mills, K.H.G. Immune checkpoints and their inhibition in cancer and infectious diseases. *Eur. J. Immunol.* **2017**, *47*, 765–779. [CrossRef] [PubMed]
125. Pardoll, D.M. The blockade of immune checkpoints in cancer immunotherapy. *Nat. Rev. Cancer* **2012**, *12*, 252–264. [CrossRef] [PubMed]
126. Gong, J.; Chehrazi-Raffle, A.; Reddi, S.; Salgia, R. Development of PD-1 and PD-L1 inhibitors as a form of cancer immunotherapy: A comprehensive review of registration trials and future considerations. *J Immunother. Cancer* **2018**, *6*, 8. [CrossRef] [PubMed]
127. Pratt, G.; Goodyear, O.; Moss, P. Immunodeficiency and immunotherapy in multiple myeloma. *Br. J. Haematol.* **2007**, *138*, 563–579. [CrossRef] [PubMed]
128. Ratta, M.; Fagnoni, F.; Curti, A.; Vescovini, R.; Sansoni, P.; Oliviero, B.; Fogli, M.; Ferri, E.; Della Cuna, G.R.; Tura, S.; et al. cells are functionally defective in multiple myeloma: The role of interleukin-6. *Blood* **2002**, *100*, 230–237. [CrossRef]
129. Bahlis, N.J.; King, A.M.; Kolonias, D.; Carlson, L.M.; Liu, H.Y.; Hussein, M.A.; Terebelo, H.R.; Byrne, G.E.; Levine, B.L.; Boise, L.H.; et al. CD28-mediated regulation of multiple myeloma cell proliferation and survival. *Blood* **2007**, *109*, 5002–5010. [CrossRef]
130. Rosenblatt, J.; Avigan, D. Targeting the PD-1/PD-L1 axis in multiple myeloma: A dream or a reality? *Blood* **2017**, *129*, 275–279. [CrossRef]
131. Paiva, B.; Azpilikueta, A.; Puig, N.; Ocio, E.M.; Sharma, R.; Oyajobi, B.O.; Labiano, S.; San-Segundo, L.; Rodriguez, A.; Aires-Mejia, I.; et al. PD-L1/PD-1 presence in the tumor microenvironment and activity of PD-1 blockade in multiple myeloma. *Leukemia* **2015**, *29*, 2110–2113. [CrossRef]
132. Lozano, E.; Díaz, T.; Mena, M.P.; Suñe, G.; Calvo, X.; Calderón, M.; Pérez-Amill, L.; Rodríguez, V.; Pérez-Galán, P.; Roué, G.; et al. Loss of the Immune Checkpoint CD85j/LILRB1 on Malignant Plasma Cells Contributes to Immune Escape in Multiple Myeloma. *J. Immunol.* **2018**, *200*, 2581–2591. [CrossRef]
133. Guillerey, C.; Harjunpää, H.; Carrié, N.; Kassem, S.; Teo, T.; Miles, K.; Krumeich, S.; Weulersse, M.; Cuisinier, M.; Stannard, K.; et al. TIGIT immune checkpoint blockade restores CD8+ T-cell immunity against multiple myeloma. *Blood* **2018**, *132*, 1689–1694. [CrossRef]
134. Ribrag, V.; Avigan, D.E.; Green, D.J.; Wise-Draper, T.; Posada, J.G.; Vij, R.; Zhu, Y.; Farooqui, M.Z.; Marinello, P.; Siegel, D.S. Phase 1b trial of pembrolizumab monotherapy for relapsed/refractory multiple myeloma: KEYNOTE-013. *Br. J. Haematol.* **2019**, *186*, e41–e44. [CrossRef] [PubMed]
135. Usmani, S.Z.; Schjesvold, F.; Oriol, A.; Karlin, L.; Cavo, M.; Rifkin, R.M.; Yimer, H.A.; LeBlanc, R.; Takezako, N.; McCroskey, R.D.; et al. Pembrolizumab plus lenalidomide and dexamethasone for patients with treatment-naive multiple myeloma (KEYNOTE-185): A randomised, open-label, phase 3 trial. *Lancet Haematol.* **2019**, *6*, e448–e458. [CrossRef]
136. Schumacher, T.N.; Schreiber, R.D. Neoantigens in cancer immunotherapy. *Science* **2015**, *348*, 69–74. [CrossRef] [PubMed]
137. Jelinek, T.; Paiva, B.; Hajek, R. Update on PD-1/PD-L1 Inhibitors in Multiple Myeloma. *Front. Immunol.* **2018**, *9*, 2431. [CrossRef] [PubMed]
138. Sadelain, M.; Brentjens, R.; Rivière, I. The basic principles of chimeric antigen receptor design. *Cancer Discov.* **2013**, *3*, 388–398. [CrossRef]
139. Sadelain, M.; Rivière, I.; Riddell, S. Therapeutic T cell engineering. *Nature* **2017**, *545*, 423–431. [CrossRef]
140. June, C.H.; Sadelain, M. Chimeric Antigen Receptor Therapy. *N. Engl. J. Med.* **2018**. [CrossRef]
141. Maude, S.L.; Laetsch, T.W.; Buechner, J.; Rives, S.; Boyer, M.; Bittencourt, H.; Bader, P.; Verneris, M.R.; Stefanski, H.E.; Myers, G.D.; et al. Tisagenlecleucel in Children and Young Adults with B-Cell Lymphoblastic Leukemia. *N. Engl. J. Med.* **2018**, *378*, 439–448. [CrossRef]
142. Schuster, S.J.; Svoboda, J.; Chong, E.A.; Nasta, S.D.; Mato, A.R.; Anak, Ö.; Brogdon, J.L.; Pruteanu-Malinici, I.; Bhoj, V.; Landsburg, D.; et al. Chimeric Antigen Receptor T Cells in Refractory B-Cell Lymphomas. *N. Engl. J. Med.* **2017**, *377*, 2545–2554. [CrossRef]
143. Neelapu, S.S.; Locke, F.L.; Bartlett, N.L.; Lekakis, L.J.; Miklos, D.B.; Jacobson, C.A.; Braunschweig, I.; Oluwole, O.O.; Siddiqi, T.; Lin, Y.; et al. Axicabtagene Ciloleucel CAR T-Cell Therapy in Refractory Large B-Cell Lymphoma. *N. Engl. J. Med.* **2017**, *377*, 2531–2544. [CrossRef]
144. Park, J.H.; Rivière, I.; Gonen, M.; Wang, X.; Sénéchal, B.; Curran, K.J.; Sauter, C.; Wang, Y.; Santomasso, B.; Mead, E.; et al. Long-Term Follow-up of CD19 CAR Therapy in Acute Lymphoblastic Leukemia. *N. Engl. J. Med.* **2018**, *378*, 449–459. [CrossRef] [PubMed]
145. Anonymous. Yescarta. European Medicines Agency. 2018. Available online: https://www.ema.europa.eu/en/medicines/human/EPAR/yescarta (accessed on 22 July 2020).

146. FDA. Research C for BE and YESCARTA (Axicabtagene Ciloleucel). Available online: https://www.fda.gov/vaccines-blood-biologics/cellular-gene-therapy-products/yescarta-axicabtagene-ciloleucel (accessed on 22 July 2020).
147. Anonymous. Kymriah. European Medicines Agency. 2018. Available online: https://www.ema.europa.eu/en/medicines/human/EPAR/kymriah (accessed on 22 July 2020).
148. FDA. Research C for BE and KYMRIAH (Tisagenlecleucel). Available online: https://www.fda.gov/vaccines-blood-biologics/cellular-gene-therapy-products/kymriah-tisagenlecleucel (accessed on 22 July 2020).
149. Gagelmann, N.; Riecken, K.; Wolschke, C.; Berger, C.; Ayuk, F.A.; Fehse, B.; Kröger, N. Development of CAR-T cell therapies for multiple myeloma. *Leukemia* **2020**. [CrossRef] [PubMed]
150. Sellner, L.; Fan, F.; Giesen, N.; Schubert, M.L.; Goldschmidt, H.; Müller-Tidow, C.; Dreger, P.; Raab, M.S.; Schmitt, M. B-cell maturation antigen-specific chimeric antigen receptor T cells for multiple myeloma: Clinical experience and future perspectives. *Int. J. Cancer* **2020**. [CrossRef] [PubMed]
151. Sidana, S.; Shah, N. CAR T-cell therapy: Is it prime time in myeloma? *Hematol. Am. Soc. Hematol. Educ. Program* **2019**, *2019*, 260–265. [CrossRef] [PubMed]
152. D'Agostino, M.; Raje, N. Anti-BCMA CAR T-cell therapy in multiple myeloma: Can we do better? *Leukemia* **2020**, *34*, 21–34. [CrossRef]
153. Rodríguez-Lobato, L.G.; Ganzetti, M.; Fernández de Larrea, C.; Hudecek, M.; Einsele, H.; Danhof, S. CAR T-Cells in Multiple Myeloma: State of the Art and Future Directions. *Front. Oncol.* Available online: https://www.frontiersin.org/articles/10.3389/fonc.2020.01243/full (accessed on 30 July 2020).
154. Carpenter, R.O.; Evbuomwan, M.O.; Pittaluga, S.; Rose, J.J.; Raffeld, M.; Yang, S.; Gress, R.E.; Hakim, F.T.; Kochenderfer, J.N. B-cell maturation antigen is a promising target for adoptive T-cell therapy of multiple myeloma. *Clin. Cancer Res. Off. J. Am. Assoc. Cancer Res.* **2013**, *19*, 2048–2060. [CrossRef]
155. Madry, C.; Laabi, Y.; Callebaut, I.; Roussel, J.; Hatzoglou, A.; Le Coniat, M.; Mornon, J.P.; Berger, R.; Tsapis, A. The characterization of murine BCMA gene defines it as a new member of the tumor necrosis factor receptor superfamily. *Int. Immunol.* **1998**, *10*, 1693–1702. [CrossRef]
156. Ng, L.G.; Mackay, C.R.; Mackay, F. The BAFF/APRIL system: Life beyond B lymphocytes. *Mol. Immunol.* **2005**, *42*, 763–772. [CrossRef]
157. Moreaux, J.; Legouffe, E.; Jourdan, E.; Quittet, P.; Rème, T.; Lugagne, C.; Moine, P.; Rossi, J.F.; Klein, B.; Tarte, K. BAFF and APRIL protect myeloma cells from apoptosis induced by interleukin 6 deprivation and dexamethasone. *Blood* **2004**, *103*, 3148–3157. [CrossRef]
158. Tai, Y.T.; Acharya, C.; An, G.; Moschetta, M.; Zhong, M.Y.; Feng, X.; Cea, M.; Cagnetta, A.; Wen, K.; van Eenennaam, H.; et al. APRIL and BCMA promote human multiple myeloma growth and immunosuppression in the bone marrow microenvironment. *Blood* **2016**, *127*, 3225–3236. [CrossRef]
159. Novak, A.J.; Darce, J.R.; Arendt, B.K.; Harder, B.; Henderson, K.; Kindsvogel, W.; Gross, J.A.; Greipp, P.R.; Jelinek, D.F. Expression of BCMA, TACI, and BAFF-R in multiple myeloma: A mechanism for growth and survival. *Blood* **2004**, *103*, 689–694. [CrossRef] [PubMed]
160. Friedman, K.M.; Garrett, T.E.; Evans, J.W.; Horton, H.M.; Latimer, H.J.; Seidel, S.L.; Horvath, C.J.; Morgan, R.A. Effective Targeting of Multiple B-Cell Maturation Antigen-Expressing Hematological Malignances by Anti-B-Cell Maturation Antigen Chimeric Antigen Receptor T Cells. *Hum. Gene Ther.* **2018**, *29*, 585–601. [CrossRef] [PubMed]
161. Berdeja, J.G.; Alsina, M.; Shah, N.D.; Siegel, D.S.; Jagannath, S.; Madduri, D.; Kaufman, J.L.; Munshi, N.C.; Rosenblatt, J.; Jasielec, J.K.; et al. Updated Results from an Ongoing Phase 1 Clinical Study of bb21217 Anti-Bcma CAR T Cell Therapy. *Blood* **2019**, *134* (Suppl. 1), 927. [CrossRef]
162. Mailankody, S.; Htut, M.; Lee, K.P.; Bensinger, W.; Devries, T.; Piasecki, J.; Ziyad, S.; Blake, M.; Byon, J.; Jakubowiak, A. JCARH125, Anti-BCMA CAR T-cell Therapy for Relapsed/Refractory Multiple Myeloma: Initial Proof of Concept Results from a Phase 1/2 Multicenter Study (EVOLVE). *Blood* **2018**, *132* (Suppl. 1), 957. [CrossRef]
163. Costello, C.L.; Gregory, T.K.; Ali, S.A.; Berdeja, J.G.; Patel, K.K.; Shah, N.D.; Ostertag, E.; Martin, C.; Ghoddusi, M.; Shedlock, D.J.; et al. Phase 2 Study of the Response and Safety of P-Bcma-101 CAR-T Cells in Patients with Relapsed/Refractory (r/r) Multiple Myeloma (MM) (PRIME). *Blood* **2019**, *134* (Suppl. 1), 3184. [CrossRef]
164. Green, D.J.; Pont, M.; Sather, B.D.; Cowan, A.J.; Turtle, C.J.; Till, B.G.; Nagengast, A.M.; Libby, E.N.; Becker, P.S.; Coffey, D.G.; et al. Fully Human Bcma Targeted Chimeric Antigen Receptor T Cells Administered in a Defined Composition Demonstrate Potency at Low Doses in Advanced Stage High Risk Multiple Myeloma. *Blood* **2018**, *132* (Suppl. 1), 1011. [CrossRef]
165. Mailankody, S.; Ghosh, A.; Staehr, M.; Purdon, T.J.; Roshal, M.; Halton, E.; Diamonte, C.; Pineda, J.; Anant, P.; Bernal, Y.; et al. Clinical Responses and Pharmacokinetics of MCARH171, a Human-Derived Bcma Targeted CAR T Cell Therapy in Relapsed/Refractory Multiple Myeloma: Final Results of a Phase I Clinical Trial. *Blood* **2018**, *132* (Suppl. 1), 959. [CrossRef]
166. Gagelmann, N.; Ayuk, F.; Atanackovic, D.; Kröger, N. B cell maturation antigen-specific chimeric antigen receptor T cells for relapsed or refractory multiple myeloma: A meta-analysis. *Eur. J. Haematol.* **2020**, *104*, 318–327. [CrossRef]
167. Schuster, S.J.; Bishop, M.R.; Tam, C.S.; Waller, E.K.; Borchmann, P.; McGuirk, J.P.; Jäger, U.; Jaglowski, S.; Andreadis, C.; Westin, J.R.; et al. Tisagenlecleucel in Adult Relapsed or Refractory Diffuse Large B-Cell Lymphoma. *N. Engl. J. Med.* **2019**, *380*, 45–56. [CrossRef]

168. Locke, F.L.; Ghobadi, A.; Jacobson, C.A.; Miklos, D.B.; Lekakis, L.J.; Oluwole, O.O.; Lin, Y.; Braunschweig, I.; Hill, B.T.; Timmerman, J.M.; et al. Long-term safety and activity of axicabtagene ciloleucel in refractory large B-cell lymphoma (ZUMA-1): A single-arm, multicentre, phase 1-2 trial. *Lancet Oncol.* **2019**, *20*, 31–42. [CrossRef]
169. Cao, J.; Wang, G.; Cheng, H.; Wei, C.; Qi, K.; Sang, W.; Zhenyu, L.; Shi, M.; Li, H.; Qiao, J.; et al. Potent anti-leukemia activities of humanized CD19-targeted Chimeric antigen receptor T (CAR-T) cells in patients with relapsed/refractory acute lymphoblastic leukemia. *Am. J. Hematol.* **2018**, *93*, 851–858. [CrossRef] [PubMed]
170. Lam, N.; Trinklein, N.D.; Buelow, B.; Patterson, G.H.; Ojha, N.; Kochenderfer, J.N. Anti-BCMA chimeric antigen receptors with fully human heavy-chain-only antigen recognition domains. *Nat. Commun.* **2020**, *11*, 283. [CrossRef] [PubMed]
171. Li, C.; Wang, J.; Wang, D.; Hu, G.; Yang, Y.; Zhou, X.; Meng, L.; Hong, Z.; Chen, L.; Mao, X.; et al. Efficacy and Safety of Fully Human Bcma Targeting CAR T Cell Therapy in Relapsed/Refractory Multiple Myeloma. *Blood* **2019**, *134* (Suppl. 1), 929. [CrossRef]
172. Jie, J.; Hao, S.; Jiang, S.; Li, Z.; Yang, M.; Zhang, W.; Yu, K.; Xiao, J.; Meng, H.; Ma, L.; et al. Phase 1 Trial of the Safety and Efficacy of Fully Human Anti-Bcma CAR T Cells in Relapsed/Refractory Multiple Myeloma. *Blood* **2019**, *134* (Suppl. 1), 4435. [CrossRef]
173. Guedan, S.; Posey, A.D., Jr.; Shaw, C.; Wing, A.; Da, T.; Patel, P.R.; McGettigan, S.E.; Casado-Medrano, V.; Kawalekar, O.U.; Uribe-Herranz, M.; et al. Enhancing CAR T cell persistence through ICOS and 4-1BB costimulation. *JCI Insight.* **2018**, *11*, 3. [CrossRef]
174. Brocker, T.; Karjalainen, K. Signals through T cell receptor-zeta chain alone are insufficient to prime resting T lymphocytes. *J. Exp. Med.* **1995**, *181*, 1653–1659. [CrossRef]
175. Maher, J.; Brentjens, R.J.; Gunset, G.; Rivière, I.; Sadelain, M. Human T-lymphocyte cytotoxicity and proliferation directed by a single chimeric TCRzeta/CD28 receptor. *Nat. Biotechnol.* **2002**, *20*, 70–75. [CrossRef]
176. Kawalekar, O.U.; O'Connor, R.S.; Fraietta, J.A.; Guo, L.; McGettigan, S.E.; Posey, A.D., Jr.; Patel, P.R.; Guedan, S.; Scholler, J.; Keith, B.; et al. Distinct Signaling of Coreceptors Regulates Specific Metabolism Pathways and Impacts Memory Development in CAR T Cells. *Immunity* **2016**, *44*, 712. [CrossRef]
177. Zhao, Z.; Condomines, M.; van der Stegen, S.J.; Perna, F.; Kloss, C.C.; Gunset, G.; Plotkin, J.; Sadelain, M. Structural Design of Engineered Costimulation Determines Tumor Rejection Kinetics and Persistence of CAR T Cells. *Cancer Cell* **2015**, *28*, 415–428. [CrossRef]
178. Park, J.H.; Palomba, M.L.; Batlevi, C.L.; Riviere, I.; Wang, X.; Senechal, B.; Furman, R.R.; Bernal, Y.; Hall, M.; Pineda, J.; et al. A Phase I First-in-Human Clinical Trial of CD19-Targeted 19-28z/4-1BBL Armored CAR T Cells in Patients with Relapsed or Refractory NHL and CLL Including Richter's Transformation. *Blood* **2018**, *132* (Suppl.1), 224. [CrossRef]
179. Boucher, J.C.; Li, G.; Shrestha, B.; Zhang, Y.; Vishwasrao, P.; Cabral, M.L.; Guan, L.; Davila, M.L. Mutation of the CD28 costimulatory domain confers increased CAR T cell persistence and decreased exhaustion. *J. Immunol.* **2018**, *200* (Suppl. 1), 57.28.
180. Feucht, J.; Sun, J.; Eyquem, J.; Ho, Y.J.; Zhao, Z.; Leibold, J.; Dobrin, A.; Cabriolu, A.; Hamieh, M.; Sadelain, M. Calibration of CAR activation potential directs alternative T cell fates and therapeutic potency. *Nat. Med.* **2019**, *25*, 82–88. [CrossRef] [PubMed]
181. Guedan, S.; Madar, A.; Casado-Medrano, V.; Shaw, C.; Wing, A.; Liu, F.; Young, R.M.; June, C.H.; Posey, A.D. Single residue in CD28-costimulated CAR-T cells limits long-term persistence and antitumor durability. *J. Clin. Investig.* **2020**, *130*, 3087–3097. [CrossRef] [PubMed]
182. Song, D.-G.; Ye, Q.; Poussin, M.; Harms, G.M.; Figini, M.; Powell, D.J. CD27 costimulation augments the survival and antitumor activity of redirected human T cells in vivo. *Blood* **2012**, *119*, 696–706. [CrossRef]
183. Guedan, S.; Chen, X.; Madar, A.; Carpenito, C.; McGettigan, S.E.; Frigault, M.J.; Lee, J.; Posey, A.D.; Scholler, J.; Scholler, N.; et al. ICOS-based chimeric antigen receptors program bipolar TH17/TH1 cells. *Blood* **2014**, *124*, 1070–1080. [CrossRef]
184. Wang, M.; Pruteanu, I.; Cohen, A.D.; Garfall, A.L.; Milone, M.C.; Tian, L.; Gonzalez, V.E.; Gill, S.; Frey, N.V.; Barrett, D.M.; et al. Identification and Validation of Predictive Biomarkers to CD19- and BCMA-Specific CAR T-Cell Responses in CAR T-Cell Precursors. *Blood* **2019**, *134* (Suppl. 1), 622. [CrossRef]
185. Busch, D.H.; Fräßle, S.P.; Sommermeyer, D.; Buchholz, V.R.; Riddell, S.R. Role of memory T cell subsets for adoptive immunotherapy. *Semin Immunol.* **2016**, *28*, 28–34. [CrossRef]
186. Kotani, H.; Li, G.; Yao, J.; Mesa, T.E.; Chen, J.; Boucher, J.C.; Yoder, S.J.; Zhou, J.; Davila, M.L. Aged CAR T Cells Exhibit Enhanced Cytotoxicity and Effector Function but Shorter Persistence and Less Memory-like Phenotypes. *Blood* **2018**, *132* (Suppl. 1), 2047. [CrossRef]
187. Fraietta, J.A.; Beckwith, K.A.; Patel, P.R.; Ruella, M.; Zheng, Z.; Barrett, D.M.; Lacey, S.F.; Melenhorst, J.J.; McGettigan, S.E.; Cook, D.R.; et al. Ibrutinib enhances chimeric antigen receptor T-cell engraftment and efficacy in leukemia. *Blood* **2016**, *127*, 1117–1127. [CrossRef]
188. Singh, N.; Perazzelli, J.; Grupp, S.A.; Barrett, D.M. Early memory phenotypes drive T cell proliferation in patients with pediatric malignancies. *Sci. Transl. Med.* **2016**, *8*, 320ra3. [CrossRef]
189. Schubert, M.-L.; Hoffmann, J.-M.; Dreger, P.; Müller-Tidow, C.; Schmitt, M. Chimeric antigen receptor transduced T cells: Tuning up for the next generation. *Int. J. Cancer* **2018**, *142*, 1738–1747. [CrossRef] [PubMed]
190. Suen, H.; Brown, R.; Yang, S.; Weatherburn, C.; Ho, P.J.; Woodland, N.; Nassif, N.; Barbaro, P.; Bryant, C.; Hart, D.; et al. Multiple myeloma causes clonal T-cell immunosenescence: Identification of potential novel targets for promoting tumour immunity and implications for checkpoint blockade. *Leukemia* **2016**, *30*, 1716–1724. [CrossRef] [PubMed]

191. Garfall, A.L.; Dancy, E.K.; Cohen, A.D.; Hwang, W.T.; Fraietta, J.A.; Davis, M.M.; Levine, B.L.; Siegel, D.L.; Stadtmauer, E.A.; Vogl, D.T.; et al. T-cell phenotypes associated with effective CAR T-cell therapy in postinduction vs relapsed multiple myeloma. *Blood Adv.* **2019**, *3*, 2812–2815. [CrossRef] [PubMed]
192. Sommermeyer, D.; Hudecek, M.; Kosasih, P.L.; Gogishvili, T.; Maloney, D.G.; Turtle, C.J.; Riddell, S.R. Chimeric antigen receptor-modified T cells derived from defined CD8+ and CD4+ subsets confer superior antitumor reactivity in vivo. *Leukemia* **2016**, *30*, 492–500. [CrossRef]
193. Zheng, W.; Carol, E.O.; Alli, R.; Basham, J.H.; Abdelsamed, H.A.; Palmer, L.E.; Jones, L.L.; Youngblood, B.; Geiger, T.L. PI3K orchestration of the in vivo persistence of chimeric antigen receptor-modified T cells. *Leukemia* **2018**, *32*, 1157–1167. [CrossRef]
194. Zhou, J.; Jin, L.; Wang, F.; Zhang, Y.; Liu, B.; Zhao, T. Chimeric antigen receptor T (CAR-T) cells expanded with IL-7/IL-15 mediate superior antitumor effects. *Protein Cell* **2019**, *10*, 764–769. [CrossRef]
195. Ajina, A.; Maher, J. Strategies to Address Chimeric Antigen Receptor Tonic Signaling. *Mol. Cancer Ther.* **2018**, *17*, 1795–1815. [CrossRef]
196. Calderon, H.; Mamonkin, M.; Guedan, S. Analysis of CAR-Mediated Tonic Signaling. In *Chimeric Antigen Receptor T Cells*; Humana: New York, NY, USA, 2020.
197. Hermanson, D.L.; Barnett, B.E.; Rengarajan, S.; Codde, R.; Wang, X.; Tan, Y.; Martin, C.E.; Smith, J.B.; He, J.; Mathur, R.; et al. A Novel Bcma-Specific, Centyrin-Based CAR-T Product for the Treatment of Multiple Myeloma. *Blood* **2016**, *128*, 2127. [CrossRef]
198. Watanabe, N.; Bajgain, P.; Sukumaran, S.; Ansari, S.; Heslop, H.E.; Rooney, C.M.; Brenner, M.K.; Leen, A.M.; Vera, J.F. Fine-tuning the CAR spacer improves T-cell potency. *Oncoimmunology* **2016**, *5*, e1253656. [CrossRef]
199. Hudecek, M.; Sommermeyer, D.; Kosasih, P.L.; Silva-Benedict, A.; Liu, L.; Rader, C.; Jensen, M.C.; Riddell, S.R. The nonsignaling extracellular spacer domain of chimeric antigen receptors is decisive for in vivo antitumor activity. *Cancer Immunol. Res.* **2015**, *3*, 125–135. [CrossRef]
200. Smith, E.L.; Staehr, M.; Masakayan, R.; Tatake, I.J.; Purdon, T.J.; Wang, X.; Wang, P.; Liu, H.; Xu, Y.; Garrett-Thomson, S.C.; et al. Development and Evaluation of an Optimal Human Single-Chain Variable Fragment-Derived BCMA-Targeted CAR T Cell Vector. *Mol. Ther. J. Am. Soc. Gene Ther.* **2018**, *26*, 1447–1456. [CrossRef] [PubMed]
201. Eyquem, J.; Mansilla-Soto, J.; Giavridis, T.; van der Stegen, S.J.; Hamieh, M.; Cunanan, K.M.; Odak, A.; Gönen, M.; Sadelain, M. Targeting a CAR to the TRAC locus with CRISPR/Cas9 enhances tumour rejection. *Nature* **2017**, *543*, 113–117. [CrossRef] [PubMed]
202. Wherry, E.J.; Kurachi, M. Molecular and cellular insights into T cell exhaustion. *Nat. Rev. Immunol.* **2015**, *15*, 486–499. [CrossRef] [PubMed]
203. Blank, C.U.; Haining, W.N.; Held, W.; Hogan, P.G.; Kallies, A.; Lugli, E.; Lynn, R.C.; Philip, M.; Rao, A.; Restifo, N.P.; et al. Defining "T cell exhaustion". *Nat. Rev. Immunol.* **2019**, *19*, 665–674. [CrossRef]
204. Zhang, Z.; Liu, S.; Zhang, B.; Qiao, L.; Zhang, Y.; Zhang, Y. T Cell Dysfunction and Exhaustion in Cancer. *Front. Cell Dev. Biol.* **2020**, *8*, 17. [CrossRef]
205. Yoon, D.H.; Osborn, M.J.; Tolar, J.; Kim, C.J. Incorporation of Immune Checkpoint Blockade into Chimeric Antigen Receptor T Cells (CAR-Ts): Combination or Built-In CAR-T. *Int. J. Mol. Sci.* **2018**, *19*, 340. [CrossRef]
206. Maude, S.L.; Hucks, G.E.; Seif, A.E.; Talekar, M.K.; Teachey, D.T.; Baniewicz, D.; Callahan, C.; Gonzalez, V.; Nazimuddin, F.; Gupta, M.; et al. The effect of pembrolizumab in combination with CD19-targeted chimeric antigen receptor (CAR) T cells in relapsed acute lymphoblastic leukemia (ALL). *J. Clin. Oncol.* **2017**, *35* (Suppl. 15), 103. [CrossRef]
207. Li, A.M.; Hucks, G.E.; Dinofia, A.M.; Seif, A.E.; Teachey, D.T.; Baniewicz, D.; Callahan, C.; Fasano, C.; McBride, B.; Gonzalez, V.; et al. Checkpoint Inhibitors Augment CD19-Directed Chimeric Antigen Receptor (CAR) T Cell Therapy in Relapsed B-Cell Acute Lymphoblastic. *Leuk. Blood* **2018**, *132* (Suppl. 1), 556. [CrossRef]
208. Cherkassky, L.; Morello, A.; Villena-Vargas, J.; Feng, Y.; Dimitrov, D.S.; Jones, D.R.; Sadelain, M.; Adusumilli, P.S. Human CAR T cells with cell-intrinsic PD-1 checkpoint blockade resist tumor-mediated inhibition. *J. Clin. Investig.* **2016**, *126*, 3130–3144. [CrossRef]
209. Rupp, L.J.; Schumann, K.; Roybal, K.T.; Gate, R.E.; Chun, J.Y.; Lim, W.A.; Marson, A. CRISPR/Cas9-mediated PD-1 disruption enhances anti-tumor efficacy of human chimeric antigen receptor T cells. *Sci. Rep.* **2017**, *7*, 737. [CrossRef]
210. Rafiq, S.; Yeku, O.O.; Jackson, H.J.; Purdon, T.J.; van Leeuwen, D.G.; Drakes, D.J.; Song, M.; Miele, M.M.; Li, Z.; Wang, P.; et al. Targeted delivery of a PD-1-blocking scFv by CAR-T cells enhances anti-tumor efficacy in vivo. *Nat. Biotechnol.* **2018**, *36*, 847–856. [CrossRef] [PubMed]
211. Li, S.; Siriwon, N.; Zhang, X.; Yang, S.; Jin, T.; He, F.; Kim, Y.J.; Mac, J.; Lu, Z.; Wang, S.; et al. Enhanced Cancer Immunotherapy by Chimeric Antigen Receptor-Modified T Cells Engineered to Secrete Checkpoint Inhibitors. *Clin. Cancer Res. Off. J. Am. Assoc. Cancer Res.* **2017**, *23*, 6982–6992. [CrossRef] [PubMed]
212. Prosser, M.E.; Brown, C.E.; Shami, A.F.; Forman, S.J.; Jensen, M.C. Tumor PD-L1 co-stimulates primary human CD8(+) cytotoxic T cells modified to express a PD1:CD28 chimeric receptor. *Mol. Immunol.* **2012**, *51*, 263–272. [CrossRef]
213. Liu, X.; Ranganathan, R.; Jiang, S.; Fang, C.; Sun, J.; Kim, S.; Newick, K.; Lo, A.; June, C.H.; Zhao, Y.; et al. A Chimeric Switch-Receptor Targeting PD1 Augments the Efficacy of Second-Generation CAR T Cells in Advanced Solid Tumors. *Cancer Res.* **2016**, *76*, 1578–1590. [CrossRef] [PubMed]
214. Wei, J.; Luo, C.; Wang, Y.; Guo, Y.; Dai, H.; Tong, C.; Ti, D.; Wu, Z.; Han, W. PD-1 silencing impairs the anti-tumor function of chimeric antigen receptor modified T cells by inhibiting proliferation activity. *J Immunother. Cancer* **2019**, *7*, 209. [CrossRef]

215. Zah, E.; Nam, E.; Bhuvan, V.; Tran, U.; Ji, B.Y.; Gosliner, S.B.; Wang, X.; Brown, C.E.; Chen, Y.Y. Systematically optimized BCMA/CS1 bispecific CAR-T cells robustly control heterogeneous multiple myeloma. *Nat. Commun.* **2020**, *11*, 2283. [CrossRef]
216. Minnie, S.A.; Hill, G.R. Immunotherapy of multiple myeloma. *J. Clin. Investig.* **2020**, *130*, 1565–1575. [CrossRef]
217. García-Guerrero, E.; Sierro-Martínez, B.; Pérez-Simón, J.A. Overcoming Chimeric Antigen Receptor (CAR) Modified T-Cell Therapy Limitations in Multiple Myeloma. *Front. Immunol.* **2020**, *11*, 1128. [CrossRef]
218. Laurent, S.A.; Hoffmann, F.S.; Kuhn, P.H.; Cheng, Q.; Chu, Y.; Schmidt-Supprian, M.; Hauck, S.M.; Schuh, E.; Krumbholz, M.; Rübsamen, H.; et al. γ-Secretase directly sheds the survival receptor BCMA from plasma cells. *Nat. Commun.* **2015**, *6*, 7333. [CrossRef]
219. Sanchez, E.; Li, M.; Kitto, A.; Li, J.; Wang, C.S.; Kirk, D.T.; Yellin, O.; Nichols, C.M.; Dreyer, M.P.; Ahles, C.P.; et al. B-cell maturation antigen is elevated in multiple myeloma and correlates with disease status and survival. *Br. J. Haematol.* **2012**, *158*, 727–738. [CrossRef]
220. Ghermezi, M.; Li, M.; Vardanyan, S.; Harutyunyan, N.M.; Gottlieb, J.; Berenson, A.; Spektor, T.M.; Andreu-Vieyra, C.; Petraki, S.; Sanchez, E.; et al. Serum B-cell maturation antigen: A novel biomarker to predict outcomes for multiple myeloma patients. *Haematologica* **2017**, *102*, 785–795. [CrossRef] [PubMed]
221. Bujarski, S.; Soof, C.; Chen, H.; Li, M.; Sanchez, E.; Wang, C.S.; Emamy-Sadr, M.; Swift, R.A.; Rahbari, K.J.; Patil, S.; et al. Serum b-cell maturation antigen levels to predict progression free survival and responses among relapsed or refractory multiple myeloma patients treated on the phase I IRUX trial. *J. Clin. Oncol.* **2018**, *36* (Suppl. 15), e24313. [CrossRef]
222. Pont, M.J.; Hill, T.; Cole, G.O.; Abbott, J.J.; Kelliher, J.; Salter, A.I.; Hudecek, M.; Comstock, M.L.; Rajan, A.; Patel, B.K.; et al. γ-Secretase inhibition increases efficacy of BCMA-specific chimeric antigen receptor T cells in multiple myeloma. *Blood* **2019**, *134*, 1585–1597. [CrossRef] [PubMed]
223. Holthof, L.C.; Mutis, T. Challenges for Immunotherapy in Multiple Myeloma: Bone Marrow Microenvironment-Mediated Immune Suppression and Immune Resistance. *Cancers* **2020**, *12*, 988. [CrossRef] [PubMed]
224. Rodriguez-Garcia, A.; Palazon, A.; Noguera-Ortega, E.; Powell, D.J.; Guedan, S. CAR-T Cells Hit the Tumor Microenvironment: Strategies to Overcome Tumor Escape. *Front. Immunol.* **2020**, *11*, 1109. [CrossRef] [PubMed]
225. Lo, A.S.Y.; Taylor, J.R.; Farzaneh, F.; Kemeny, D.M.; Dibb, N.J.; Maher, J. Harnessing the tumour-derived cytokine, CSF-1, to co-stimulate T-cell growth and activation. *Mol. Immunol.* **2008**, *45*, 1276–1287. [CrossRef]
226. Di Stasi, A.; De Angelis, B.; Rooney, C.M.; Zhang, L.; Mahendravada, A.; Foster, A.E.; Heslop, H.E.; Brenner, M.K.; Dotti, G.; Savoldo, B. T lymphocytes coexpressing CCR4 and a chimeric antigen receptor targeting CD30 have improved homing and antitumor activity in a Hodgkin tumor model. *Blood* **2009**, *113*, 6392–6402. [CrossRef]
227. Craddock, J.A.; Lu, A.; Bear, A.; Pule, M.; Brenner, M.K.; Rooney, C.M.; Foster, A.E. Enhanced tumor trafficking of GD2 chimeric antigen receptor T cells by expression of the chemokine receptor CCR2b. *J. Immunother.* **2010**, *33*, 780–788. [CrossRef]
228. Tran, E.; Chinnasamy, D.; Yu, Z.; Morgan, R.A.; Lee, C.C.; Restifo, N.P.; Rosenberg, S.A. Immune targeting of fibroblast activation protein triggers recognition of multipotent bone marrow stromal cells and cachexia. *J. Exp. Med.* **2013**, *210*, 1125–1135. [CrossRef]
229. Wang, L.C.; Lo, A.; Scholler, J.; Sun, J.; Majumdar, R.S.; Kapoor, V.; Antzis, M.; Cotner, C.E.; Johnson, L.A.; Durham, A.C.; et al. Targeting fibroblast activation protein in tumor stroma with chimeric antigen receptor T cells can inhibit tumor growth and augment host immunity without severe toxicity. *Cancer Immunol. Res.* **2014**, *2*, 154–166. [CrossRef]
230. Caruana, I.; Savoldo, B.; Hoyos, V.; Weber, G.; Liu, H.; Kim, E.S.; Ittmann, M.M.; Marchetti, D.; Dotti, G. Heparanase promotes tumor infiltration and antitumor activity of CAR-redirected T lymphocytes. *Nat. Med.* **2015**, *21*, 524–529. [CrossRef] [PubMed]
231. Leen, A.M.; Sukumaran, S.; Watanabe, N.; Mohammed, S.; Keirnan, J.; Yanagisawa, R.; Anurathapan, U.; Rendon, D.; Heslop, H.E.; Rooney, C.M.; et al. Reversal of tumor immune inhibition using a chimeric cytokine receptor. *Mol. Ther. J. Am. Soc. Gene Ther.* **2014**, *22*, 1211–1220. [CrossRef] [PubMed]
232. Wilkie, S.; Burbridge, S.E.; Chiapero-Stanke, L.; Pereira, A.C.; Cleary, S.; van der Stegen, S.J.; Spicer, J.F.; Davies, D.M.; Maher, J. Selective expansion of chimeric antigen receptor-targeted T-cells with potent effector function using interleukin-4. *J. Biol. Chem.* **2010**, *285*, 25538–25544. [CrossRef] [PubMed]
233. Mohammed, S.; Sukumaran, S.; Bajgain, P.; Watanabe, N.; Heslop, H.E.; Rooney, C.M.; Brenner, M.K.; Fisher, W.E.; Leen, A.M.; Vera, J.F. Improving Chimeric Antigen Receptor-Modified T Cell Function by Reversing the Immunosuppressive Tumor Microenvironment of Pancreatic Cancer. *Mol. Ther. J. Am. Soc. Gene Ther.* **2017**, *25*, 249–258. [CrossRef] [PubMed]
234. Yamamoto, T.N.; Lee, P.H.; Vodnala, S.K.; Gurusamy, D.; Kishton, R.J.; Yu, Z.; Eidizadeh, A.; Eil, R.; Fioravanti, J.; Gattinoni, L.; et al. T cells genetically engineered to overcome death signaling enhance adoptive cancer immunotherapy. *J. Clin. Investig.* **2019**, *129*, 1551–1565. [CrossRef] [PubMed]
235. Ruella, M.; Klichinsky, M.; Kenderian, S.S.; Shestova, O.; Ziober, A.; Kraft, D.O.; Feldman, M.; Wasik, M.A.; June, C.H.; Gill, S. Overcoming the Immunosuppressive Tumor Microenvironment of Hodgkin Lymphoma Using Chimeric Antigen Receptor T Cells. *Cancer Discov.* **2017**, *7*, 1154–1167. [CrossRef]
236. Parihar, R.; Rivas, C.; Huynh, M.; Omer, B.; Lapteva, N.; Metelitsa, L.S.; Gottschalk, S.M.; Rooney, C.M. NK Cells Expressing a Chimeric Activating Receptor Eliminate MDSCs and Rescue Impaired CAR-T Cell Activity against Solid Tumors. *Cancer Immunol. Res.* **2019**, *7*, 363–375. [CrossRef]
237. Hoyos, V.; Savoldo, B.; Quintarelli, C.; Mahendravada, A.; Zhang, M.; Vera, J.; Heslop, H.E.; Rooney, C.M.; Brenner, M.K.; Dotti, G. Engineering CD19-specific T lymphocytes with interleukin-15 and a suicide gene to enhance their anti-lymphoma/leukemia effects and safety. *Leukemia* **2010**, *24*, 1160–1170. [CrossRef]

238. Yeku, O.O.; Purdon, T.J.; Koneru, M.; Spriggs, D.; Brentjens, R.J. Armored CAR T cells enhance antitumor efficacy and overcome the tumor microenvironment. *Sci. Rep.* **2017**, *7*, 10541. [CrossRef]
239. Chmielewski, M.; Abken, H. CAR T Cells Releasing IL-18 Convert to T-Bethigh FoxO1low Effectors that Exhibit Augmented Activity against Advanced Solid Tumors. *Cell Rep.* **2017**, *21*, 3205–3219. [CrossRef]
240. Hu, B.; Ren, J.; Luo, Y.; Keith, B.; Young, R.M.; Scholler, J.; Zhao, Y.; June, C.H. Augmentation of Antitumor Immunity by Human and Mouse CAR T Cells Secreting IL-18. *Cell Rep.* **2017**, *20*, 3025–3033. [CrossRef] [PubMed]
241. Chmielewski, M.; Hombach, A.A.; Abken, H. Of CARs and TRUCKs: Chimeric antigen receptor (CAR) T cells engineered with an inducible cytokine to modulate the tumor stroma. *Immunol. Rev.* **2014**, *257*, 83–90. [CrossRef] [PubMed]
242. Wu, L.; Wei, Q.; Brzostek, J.; Gascoigne, N.R.J. Signaling from T cell receptors (TCRs) and chimeric antigen receptors (CARs) on T cells. *Cell Mol. Immunol.* **2020**, *17*, 600–612. [CrossRef] [PubMed]
243. Etxeberria, I.; Olivera, I.; Bolaños, E.; Cirella, A.; Teijeira, Á.; Berraondo, P.; Melero, I. Engineering bionic T cells: Signal 1, signal 2, signal 3, reprogramming and the removal of inhibitory mechanisms. *Cell Mol. Immunol.* **2020**, *17*, 576–586. [CrossRef]
244. Gattinoni, L.; Finkelstein, S.E.; Klebanoff, C.A.; Antony, P.A.; Palmer, D.C.; Spiess, P.J.; Hwang, L.N.; Yu, Z.; Wrzesinski, C.; Heimann, D.M.; et al. Removal of homeostatic cytokine sinks by lymphodepletion enhances the efficacy of adoptively transferred tumor-specific CD8+ T cells. *J. Exp. Med.* **2005**, *202*, 907–912. [CrossRef]
245. Corrigan-Curay, J.; Kiem, H.P.; Baltimore, D.; O'reilly, M.; Brentjens, R.J.; Cooper, L.; Forman, S.; Gottschalk, S.; Greenberg, P.; Junghans, R.; et al. T-cell immunotherapy: Looking forward. *Mol. Ther. J. Am. Soc. Gene Ther.* **2014**, *22*, 1564–1574. [CrossRef]
246. Antony, P.A.; Piccirillo, C.A.; Akpinarli, A.; Finkelstein, S.E.; Speiss, P.J.; Surman, D.R.; Palmer, D.C.; Chan, C.C.; Klebanoff, C.A.; Overwijk, W.W.; et al. CD8+ T cell immunity against a tumor/self-antigen is augmented by CD4+ T helper cells and hindered by naturally occurring T regulatory cells. *J. Immunol.* **2005**, *174*, 2591–2601. [CrossRef]
247. Neelapu, S.S. CAR-T efficacy: Is conditioning the key? *Blood* **2019**, *133*, 1799–1800. [CrossRef]
248. Hirayama, A.V.; Gauthier, J.; Hay, K.A.; Voutsinas, J.M.; Wu, Q.; Gooley, T.; Li, D.; Cherian, S.; Chen, X.; Pender, B.S.; et al. The response to lymphodepletion impacts PFS in patients with aggressive non-Hodgkin lymphoma treated with CD19 CAR T cells. *Blood* **2019**, *133*, 1876–1887. [CrossRef]
249. Park, J.H.; Geyer, M.B.; Brentjens, R.J. CD19-targeted CAR T-cell therapeutics for hematologic malignancies: Interpreting clinical outcomes to date. *Blood* **2016**, *127*, 3312–3320. [CrossRef]
250. Zhang, T.; Cao, L.; Xie, J.; Shi, N.; Zhang, Z.; Luo, Z.; Yue, D.; Zhang, Z.; Wang, L.; Han, W.; et al. Efficiency of CD19 chimeric antigen receptor-modified T cells for treatment of B cell malignancies in phase I clinical trials: A meta-analysis. *Oncotarget* **2015**, *6*, 33961–33971. [CrossRef] [PubMed]
251. Turtle, C.J.; Hanafi, L.A.; Berger, C.; Gooley, T.A.; Cherian, S.; Hudecek, M.; Sommermeyer, D.; Melville, K.; Pender, B.; Budiarto, T.M.; et al. CD19 CAR-T cells of defined CD4+:CD8+ composition in adult B cell ALL patients. *J. Clin. Investig.* **2016**, *126*, 2123–2138. [CrossRef] [PubMed]
252. Shah, N.N.; Fry, T.J. Mechanisms of resistance to CAR T cell therapy. *Nat. Rev. Clin. Oncol.* **2019**, *16*, 372–385. [CrossRef] [PubMed]
253. Fry, T.J.; Shah, N.N.; Orentas, R.J.; Stetler-Stevenson, M.; Yuan, C.M.; Ramakrishna, S.; Wolters, P.; Martin, S.; Delbrook, C.; Yates, B.; et al. CD22-targeted CAR T cells induce remission in B-ALL that is naive or resistant to CD19-targeted CAR immunotherapy. *Nat. Med.* **2018**, *24*, 20–28. [CrossRef]
254. Martin, N.; Thompson, E.; Dell'Aringa, J.; Paiva, B.; Munshi, N.; San Miguel, J. Correlation of Tumor BCMA Expression with Response and Acquired Resistance to Idecabtagene Vicleucel in the KarMMa Study in Relapsed and Refractory Multiple Myeloma. 2020. Available online: https://library.ehaweb.org/eha/2020/eha25th/294902/nathan.martin.correlation.of.tumor.bcma.expression.with.response.and.acquired.html?f=listing%3D3%2Abrowseby%3D8%2Asortby%3D1%2Amedia%3D1 (accessed on 8 August 2020).
255. Da Via, M.C.; Dietrich, O.; Truger, M.; Arampatzi, P.; Duell, J.; Zhou, X.; Tabares, P.; Danhof, S.; Kraus, S.; Meggendorfer, M. Biallelic Deletion of Chromosome 16p Encompassing the BCMA Locus as a Tumor-Intrinsic Resistance Mechanism to BCMA-Directed CAR T in Multiple Myeloma. 2020. Available online: https://library.ehaweb.org/eha/2020/eha25th/294800/leo.rasche.biallelic.deletion.of.chromosome.16p.encompassing.the.bcma.locus.as.html?f=listing%3D0%2Abrowseby%3D8%2Asortby%3D2%2Asearch%3Dcar-t (accessed on 8 August 2020).
256. Grupp, S.A.; Kalos, M.; Barrett, D.; Aplenc, R.; Porter, D.L.; Rheingold, S.R.; Teachey, D.T.; Chew, A.; Hauck, B.; Wright, J.F.; et al. Chimeric antigen receptor-modified T cells for acute lymphoid leukemia. *N. Engl. J. Med.* **2013**, *368*, 1509–1518. [CrossRef]
257. Rosenthal, J.; Naqvi, A.S.; Luo, M.; Wertheim, G.; Paessler, M.; Thomas-Tikhonenko, A.; Rheingold, S.R.; Pillai, V. Heterogeneity of surface CD19 and CD22 expression in B lymphoblastic leukemia. *Am. J. Hematol.* **2018**, *93*, E352–E355. [CrossRef]
258. Schürch, C.M.; Rasche, L.; Frauenfeld, L.; Weinhold, N.; Fend, F. A review on tumor heterogeneity and evolution in multiple myeloma: Pathological, radiological, molecular genetics, and clinical integration. *Virchows Arch. Int. J. Pathol.* **2020**, *476*, 337–351. [CrossRef]
259. Sotillo, E.; Barrett, D.M.; Black, K.L.; Bagashev, A.; Oldridge, D.; Wu, G.; Sussman, R.; Lanauze, C.; Ruella, M.; Gazzara, M.R.; et al. Convergence of Acquired Mutations and Alternative Splicing of CD19 Enables Resistance to CART-19 Immunotherapy. *Cancer Discov.* **2015**, *5*, 1282–1295. [CrossRef]
260. Orlando, E.J.; Han, X.; Tribouley, C.; Wood, P.A.; Leary, R.J.; Riester, M.; Levine, J.E.; Qayed, M.; Grupp, S.A.; Boyer, M.; et al. Genetic mechanisms of target antigen loss in CAR19 therapy of acute lymphoblastic leukemia. *Nat. Med.* **2018**, *24*, 1504–1506. [CrossRef]

261. Fischer, J.; Paret, C.; El Malki, K.; Alt, F.; Wingerter, A.; Neu, M.A.; Kron, B.; Russo, A.; Lehmann, N.; Roth, L.; et al. CD19 Isoforms Enabling Resistance to CART-19 Immunotherapy Are Expressed in B-ALL Patients at Initial Diagnosis. *J. Immunother.* **2017**, *40*, 187–195. [CrossRef]
262. Gardner, R.; Wu, D.; Cherian, S.; Fang, M.; Hanafi, L.A.; Finney, O.; Smithers, H.; Jensen, M.C.; Riddell, S.R.; Maloney, D.G.; et al. Acquisition of a CD19-negative myeloid phenotype allows immune escape of MLL-rearranged B-ALL from CD19 CAR-T-cell therapy. *Blood* **2016**, *127*, 2406–2410. [CrossRef] [PubMed]
263. Jacoby, E.; Nguyen, S.M.; Fountaine, T.J.; Welp, K.; Gryder, B.; Qin, H.; Yang, Y.; Chien, C.D.; Seif, A.E.; Lei, H.; et al. CD19 CAR immune pressure induces B-precursor acute lymphoblastic leukaemia lineage switch exposing inherent leukaemic plasticity. *Nat. Commun.* **2016**, *7*, 12320. [CrossRef] [PubMed]
264. Hamieh, M.; Dobrin, A.; Cabriolu, A.; van der Stegen, S.J.; Giavridis, T.; Mansilla-Soto, J.; Eyquem, J.; Zhao, Z.; Whitlock, B.M.; Miele, M.M.; et al. CAR T cell trogocytosis and cooperative killing regulate tumour antigen escape. *Nature* **2019**, *568*, 112–116. [CrossRef]
265. Perez-Amill, L.; Suñe, G.; Antoñana-Vildosola, A.; Castella, M.; Najjar, A.; Bonet, J.; Fernández-Fuentes, N.; Inogés, S.; López, A.; Bueno, C.; et al. Preclinical development of a humanized chimeric antigen receptor against B cell maturation antigen for multiple myeloma. *Haematologica* **2020**. [CrossRef] [PubMed]
266. Ruella, M.; Xu, J.; Barrett, D.M.; Fraietta, J.A.; Reich, T.J.; Ambrose, D.E.; Klichinsky, M.; Shestova, O.; Patel, P.R.; Kulikovskaya, I.; et al. Induction of resistance to chimeric antigen receptor T cell therapy by transduction of a single leukemic B cell. *Nat. Med.* **2018**, *24*, 1499–1503. [CrossRef] [PubMed]
267. Johnson, L.A.; Morgan, R.A.; Dudley, M.E.; Cassard, L.; Yang, J.C.; Hughes, M.S.; Kammula, U.S.; Royal, R.E.; Sherry, R.M.; Wunderlich, J.R.; et al. Gene therapy with human and mouse T-cell receptors mediates cancer regression and targets normal tissues expressing cognate antigen. *Blood* **2009**, *114*, 535–546. [CrossRef]
268. Maude, S.; Barrett, D.M. Current status of chimeric antigen receptor therapy for haematological malignancies. *Br. J. Haematol.* **2016**, *172*, 11–22. [CrossRef]
269. Tamura, H.; Ishibashi, M.; Sunakawa, M.; Inokuchi, K. Immunotherapy for Multiple Myeloma. *Cancers* **2019**, *11*, 2009. [CrossRef]
270. Abbott, R.C.; Cross, R.S.; Jenkins, M.R. Finding the Keys to the CAR: Identifying Novel Target Antigens for T Cell Redirection Immunotherapies. *Int. J. Mol. Sci.* **2020**, *21*, 515. [CrossRef]
271. Hosen, N. Chimeric Antigen Receptor T-Cell Therapy for Multiple Myeloma. *Cancers* **2019**, *11*, 2024. [CrossRef]
272. Guedan, S.; Calderon, H.; Posey, A.D.; Maus, M.V. Engineering and Design of Chimeric Antigen Receptors. *Mol. Ther. Methods Clin. Dev.* **2019**, *12*, 145–156. [CrossRef] [PubMed]
273. Rafiq, S.; Hackett, C.S.; Brentjens, R.J. Engineering strategies to overcome the current roadblocks in CAR T cell therapy. *Nat. Rev. Clin. Oncol.* **2020**, *17*, 147–167. [CrossRef] [PubMed]
274. Kang, L.; Zhang, J.; Li, M.; Xu, N.; Qi, W.; Tan, J.; Lou, X.; Yu, Z.; Sun, J.; Wang, Z.; et al. Characterization of novel dual tandem CD19/BCMA chimeric antigen receptor T cells to potentially treat multiple myeloma. *Biomark Res.* **2020**, *8*, 14. [CrossRef] [PubMed]
275. Chen, K.H.; Wada, M.; Pinz, K.G.; Liu, H.; Shuai, X.; Chen, X.; Yan, L.E.; Petrov, J.C.; Salman, H.; Senzel, L.; et al. A compound chimeric antigen receptor strategy for targeting multiple myeloma. *Leukemia* **2018**, *32*, 402–412. [CrossRef] [PubMed]
276. de Larrea, C.F.; Staehr, M.; Lopez, A.V.; Ng, K.Y.; Chen, Y.; Godfrey, W.D.; Purdon, T.J.; Ponomarev, V.; Wendel, H.G.; Brentjens, R.J.; et al. Defining an Optimal Dual-Targeted CAR T-cell Therapy Approach Simultaneously Targeting BCMA and GPRC5D to Prevent BCMA Escape–Driven Relapse in Multiple Myeloma. *Blood Cancer Discov.* **2020**. Available online: https://bloodcancerdiscov.aacrjournals.org/content/early/2020/06/30/2643-3230.BCD-20-0020 (accessed on 9 August 2020).
277. Popat, R.; Zweegman, S.; Cavet, J.; Yong, K.; Lee, L.; Faulkner, J.; Kotsopoulou, E.; Al-Hajj, M.; Thomas, S.; Cordoba, S.P.; et al. Phase 1 First-in-Human Study of AUTO2, the First Chimeric Antigen Receptor (CAR) T Cell Targeting APRIL for Patients with Relapsed/Refractory Multiple Myeloma (RRMM). *Blood* **2019**, *134* (Suppl. 1), 3112. [CrossRef]
278. Li, C.; Mei, H.; Hu, Y.; Guo, T.; Liu, L.; Jiang, H.; Tang, L.; Wu, Y.; Ai, L.; Deng, J.; et al. A Bispecific CAR-T Cell Therapy Targeting Bcma and CD38 for Relapsed/Refractory Multiple Myeloma: Updated Results from a Phase 1 Dose-Climbing Trial. *Blood* **2019**, *134* (Suppl. 1), 930. [CrossRef]
279. Zhang, H.; Gao, L.; Liu, L.; Wang, J.; Wang, S.; Gao, L.; Zhang, C.; Liu, Y.; Kong, P.; Liu, J.; et al. A Bcma and CD19 Bispecific CAR-T for Relapsed and Refractory Multiple Myeloma. *Blood* **2019**, *134* (Suppl. 1), 3147. [CrossRef]
280. Yan, L.; Yan, Z.; Shang, J.; Shi, X.; Jin, S.; Kang, L.; Qu, S.; Zhou, J.; Kang, H.; Wang, R.; et al. Sequential CD19- and Bcma-Specific Chimeric Antigen Receptor T Cell Treatment for RRMM: Report from a Single Center Study. *Blood* **2019**, *134* (Suppl. 1), 578. [CrossRef]
281. Garcia-Guerrero, E.; Rodríguez-Lobato, L.G.; Danhof, S.; Sierro-Martínez, B.; Goetz, R.; Sauer, M. ATRA Augments BCMA Expression on Myeloma Cells and Enhances Recognition By BCMA-CAR T-Cells. *Blood* **2020**, *136* (Suppl. 1), 13–14. [CrossRef]
282. Cowan, A.J.; Pont, M.; Sather, B.D.; Turtle, C.J.; Till, B.G.; Nagengast, A.M.; Libby, I.I.I.E.N.; Becker, P.S.; Coffey, D.G.; Tuazon, S.A.; et al. Efficacy and Safety of Fully Human Bcma CAR T Cells in Combination with a Gamma Secretase Inhibitor to Increase Bcma Surface Expression in Patients with Relapsed or Refractory Multiple Myeloma. *Blood* **2019**, *134* (Suppl. 1), 204. [CrossRef]
283. Pinto, V.; Bergantim, R.; Caires, H.R.; Seca, H.; Guimarães, J.E.; Vasconcelos, M.H. Multiple Myeloma: Available Therapies and Causes of Drug Resistance. *Cancers* **2020**, *12*, 407. [CrossRef] [PubMed]

284. Basak, G.W.; Carrier, E. The Search for Multiple Myeloma Stem Cells: The Long and Winding Road. *Biol Blood Marrow Transpl.* **2010**, *16*, 587–594. [CrossRef] [PubMed]
285. Matsui, W.; Wang, Q.; Barber, J.P.; Brennan, S.; Smith, B.D.; Borrello, I.; McNiece, I.; Lin, L.; Ambinder, R.F.; Peacock, C.; et al. Clonogenic multiple myeloma progenitors, stem cell properties, and drug resistance. *Cancer Res.* **2008**, *68*, 190–197. [CrossRef] [PubMed]
286. Paiva, B.; Puig, N.; Cedena, M.T.; de Jong, B.G.; Ruiz, Y.; Rapado, I.; Martinez-Lopez, J.; Cordon, L.; Alignani, D.; Delgado, J.A.; et al. Differentiation stage of myeloma plasma cells: Biological and clinical significance. *Leukemia* **2017**, *31*, 382–392. [CrossRef] [PubMed]
287. Olson, M.; Radhakrishnan, S.V.; Luetkens, T.; Atanackovic, D. The role of surface molecule CD229 in Multiple Myeloma. *Clin. Immunol.* **2019**, *204*, 69–73. [CrossRef] [PubMed]
288. Garfall, A.L.; Stadtmauer, E.A.; Hwang, W.T.; Lacey, S.F.; Melenhorst, J.J.; Krevvata, M.; Carroll, M.P.; Matsui, W.H.; Wang, Q.; Dhodapkar, M.V.; et al. Anti-CD19 CAR T cells with high-dose melphalan and autologous stem cell transplantation for refractory multiple myeloma. *JCI Insight* **2019**, *21*, 4. [CrossRef]
289. Atanackovic, D.; Panse, J.; Hildebrandt, Y.; Jadczak, A.; Kobold, S.; Cao, Y.; Templin, J.; Meyer, S.; Reinhard, H.; Bartels, K.; et al. Surface molecule CD229 as a novel target for the diagnosis and treatment of multiple myeloma. *Haematologica* **2011**, *96*, 1512–1520. [CrossRef] [PubMed]
290. Nerreter, T.; Letschert, S.; Götz, R.; Doose, S.; Danhof, S.; Einsele, H.; Sauer, M.; Hudecek, M. Super-resolution microscopy reveals ultra-low CD19 expression on myeloma cells that triggers elimination by CD19 CAR-T. *Nat. Commun.* **2019**, *10*, 3137. [CrossRef] [PubMed]
291. Bonifant, C.L.; Jackson, H.J.; Brentjens, R.J.; Curran, K.J. Toxicity and management in CAR T-cell therapy. *Mol. Ther. Oncolytics* **2016**, *3*, 16011. [CrossRef]
292. Neelapu, S.S.; Tummala, S.; Kebriaei, P.; Wierda, W.; Gutierrez, C.; Locke, F.L.; Komanduri, K.V.; Lin, Y.; Jain, N.; Daver, N.; et al. Chimeric antigen receptor T-cell therapy—Assessment and management of toxicities. *Nat. Rev. Clin. Oncol.* **2018**, *15*, 47–62. [CrossRef]
293. Shimabukuro-Vornhagen, A.; Gödel, P.; Subklewe, M.; Stemmler, H.J.; Schlößer, H.A.; Schlaak, M.; Kochanek, M.; Böll, B.; von Bergwelt-Baildon, M.S. Cytokine release syndrome. *J. Immunother. Cancer* **2018**, *6*, 56. [CrossRef] [PubMed]
294. Neelapu, S.S. Managing the toxicities of CAR T-cell therapy. *Hematol. Oncol.* **2019**, *37* (Suppl. 1), 48–52. [CrossRef] [PubMed]
295. Yáñez, L.; Sánchez-Escamilla, M.; Perales, M.-A. CAR T Cell Toxicity: Current Management and Future Directions. *HemaSphere* **2019**, *3*, e186. [CrossRef] [PubMed]
296. Gust, J.; Hay, K.A.; Hanafi, L.A.; Li, D.; Myerson, D.; Gonzalez-Cuyar, L.F.; Yeung, C.; Liles, W.C.; Wurfel, M.; Lopez, J.A.; et al. Endothelial Activation and Blood-Brain Barrier Disruption in Neurotoxicity after Adoptive Immunotherapy with CD19 CAR-T Cells. *Cancer Discov.* **2017**, *7*, 1404–1419. [CrossRef]
297. Taraseviciute, A.; Tkachev, V.; Ponce, R.; Turtle, C.J.; Snyder, J.M.; Liggitt, H.D.; Myerson, D.; Gonzalez-Cuyar, L.; Baldessari, A.; English, C.; et al. Chimeric Antigen Receptor T Cell-Mediated Neurotoxicity in Nonhuman Primates. *Cancer Discov.* **2018**, *8*, 750–763. [CrossRef]
298. Lee, D.W.; Santomasso, B.D.; Locke, F.L.; Ghobadi, A.; Turtle, C.J.; Brudno, J.N.; Maus, M.V.; Park, J.H.; Mead, E.; Pavletic, S.; et al. ASTCT Consensus Grading for Cytokine Release Syndrome and Neurologic Toxicity Associated with Immune Effector Cells. *Biol. Blood Marrow Transpl.* **2019**, *25*, 625–638. [CrossRef]
299. Mahadeo, K.M.; Khazal, S.J.; Abdel-Azim, H.; Fitzgerald, J.C.; Taraseviciute, A.; Bollard, C.M.; Tewari, P.; Duncan, C.; Traube, C.; McCall, D.; et al. Management guidelines for paediatric patients receiving chimeric antigen receptor T cell therapy. *Nat. Rev. Clin. Oncol.* **2019**, *16*, 45–63. [CrossRef]
300. Yakoub-Agha, I.; Chabannon, C.; Bader, P.; Basak, G.W.; Bonig, H.; Ciceri, F.; Corbacioglu, S.; Duarte, R.F.; Einsele, H.; Hudecek, M.; et al. Management of adults and children undergoing chimeric antigen receptor T-cell therapy: Best practice recommendations of the European Society for Blood and Marrow Transplantation (EBMT) and the Joint Accreditation Committee of ISCT and EBMT (JACIE). *Haematologica* **2020**, *105*, 297–316. [CrossRef]
301. Lamers, C.H.; Sleijfer, S.; Van Steenbergen, S.; Van Elzakker, P.; Van Krimpen, B.; Groot, C.; Vulto, A.; Den Bakker, M.; Oosterwijk, E.; Debets, R.; et al. Treatment of metastatic renal cell carcinoma with CAIX CAR-engineered T cells: Clinical evaluation and management of on-target toxicity. *Mol. Ther. J. Am. Soc. Gene Ther.* **2013**, *21*, 904–912. [CrossRef]
302. Morgan, R.A.; Yang, J.C.; Kitano, M.; Dudley, M.E.; Laurencot, C.M.; Rosenberg, S.A. Case report of a serious adverse event following the administration of T cells transduced with a chimeric antigen receptor recognizing ERBB2. *Mol. Ther. J. Am. Soc. Gene Ther.* **2010**, *18*, 843–851. [CrossRef]
303. Thistlethwaite, F.C.; Gilham, D.E.; Guest, R.D.; Rothwell, D.G.; Pillai, M.; Burt, D.J.; Byatte, A.J.; Kirillova, N.; Valle, J.W.; Sharma, S.K.; et al. The clinical efficacy of first-generation carcinoembryonic antigen (CEACAM5)-specific CAR T cells is limited by poor persistence and transient pre-conditioning-dependent respiratory toxicity. *Cancer Immunol. Immunother.* **2017**, *66*, 1425–1436. [CrossRef] [PubMed]
304. Berdeja, J.G.; Madduri, D.; Usmani, S.Z.; Singh, I.; Zudaire, E.; Yeh, T.M.; Allred, A.J.; Olyslager, Y.; Banerjee, A.; Goldberg, J.D.; et al. Update of CARTITUDE-1: A phase Ib/II study of JNJ-4528, a B-cell maturation antigen (BCMA)-directed CAR-T-cell therapy, in relapsed/refractory multiple myeloma. *J. Clin. Oncol.* **2020**, *38* (Suppl. 15), 8505. [CrossRef]

305. Salter, A.I.; Ivey, R.G.; Kennedy, J.J.; Voillet, V.; Rajan, A.; Alderman, E.J.; Voytovich, U.J.; Lin, C.; Sommermeyer, D.; Liu, L.; et al. Phosphoproteomic analysis of chimeric antigen receptor signaling reveals kinetic and quantitative differences that affect cell function. *Sci. Signal.* **2018**, *11*, eaat6753. [CrossRef] [PubMed]
306. Di Stasi, A.; Tey, S.K.; Dotti, G.; Fujita, Y.; Kennedy-Nasser, A.; Martinez, C.; Straathof, K.; Liu, E.; Durett, A.G.; Grilley, B.; et al. Inducible apoptosis as a safety switch for adoptive cell therapy. *N. Engl. J. Med.* **2011**, *365*, 1673–1683. [CrossRef] [PubMed]
307. Wang, X.; Chang, W.C.; Wong, C.W.; Colcher, D.; Sherman, M.; Ostberg, J.R.; Forman, S.J.; Riddell, S.R.; Jensen, M.C. A transgene-encoded cell surface polypeptide for selection, in vivo tracking, and ablation of engineered cells. *Blood* **2011**, *118*, 1255–1263. [CrossRef]
308. Mestermann, K.; Giavridis, T.; Weber, J.; Rydzek, J.; Frenz, S.; Nerreter, T.; Mades, A.; Sadelain, M.; Einsele, H.; Hudecek, M. The tyrosine kinase inhibitor dasatinib acts as a pharmacologic on/off switch for CAR T cells. *Sci. Transl. Med.* **2019**, *11*, eaau5907. [CrossRef]
309. Caruso, H.G.; Hurton, L.V.; Najjar, A.; Rushworth, D.; Ang, S.; Olivares, S.; Mi, T.; Switzer, K.; Singh, H.; Huls, H.; et al. Tuning Sensitivity of CAR to EGFR Density Limits Recognition of Normal Tissue While Maintaining Potent Antitumor Activity. *Cancer Res.* **2015**, *75*, 3505–3518. [CrossRef]
310. Arcangeli, S.; Rotiroti, M.C.; Bardelli, M.; Simonelli, L.; Magnani, C.F.; Biondi, A.; Biagi, E.; Tettamanti, S.; Varani, L. Balance of Anti-CD123 Chimeric Antigen Receptor Binding Affinity and Density for the Targeting of Acute Myeloid Leukemia. *Mol. Ther. J. Am. Soc. Gene Ther.* **2017**, *25*, 1933–1945. [CrossRef]
311. Han, C.; Sim, S.J.; Kim, S.H.; Singh, R.; Hwang, S.; Kim, Y.I.; Park, S.H.; Kim, K.H.; Lee, D.G.; Oh, H.S.; et al. Desensitized chimeric antigen receptor T cells selectively recognize target cells with enhanced antigen expression. *Nat. Commun.* **2018**, *9*, 468. [CrossRef]
312. Roybal, K.T.; Rupp, L.J.; Morsut, L.; Walker, W.J.; McNally, K.A.; Park, J.S.; Lim, W.A. Precision Tumor Recognition by T Cells With Combinatorial Antigen-Sensing Circuits. *Cell* **2016**, *164*, 770–779. [CrossRef]
313. Wu, C.-Y.; Roybal, K.T.; Puchner, E.M.; Onuffer, J.; Lim, W.A. Remote control of therapeutic T cells through a small molecule-gated chimeric receptor. *Science* **2015**, *350*, aab4077. [CrossRef] [PubMed]
314. Lanitis, E.; Poussin, M.; Klattenhoff, A.W.; Song, D.; Sandaltzopoulos, R.; June, C.H.; Powell, D.J. Chimeric antigen receptor T Cells with dissociated signaling domains exhibit focused antitumor activity with reduced potential for toxicity in vivo. *Cancer Immunol. Res.* **2013**, *1*, 43–53. [CrossRef] [PubMed]
315. Kloss, C.C.; Condomines, M.; Cartellieri, M.; Bachmann, M.; Sadelain, M. Combinatorial antigen recognition with balanced signaling promotes selective tumor eradication by engineered T cells. *Nat. Biotechnol.* **2013**, *31*, 71–75. [CrossRef] [PubMed]
316. He, X.; Feng, Z.; Ma, J.; Ling, S.; Cao, Y.; Gurung, B.; Wu, Y.; Katona, B.W.; O'Dwyer, K.P.; Siegel, D.L.; et al. Bispecific and split CAR T cells targeting CD13 and TIM3 eradicate acute myeloid leukemia. *Blood* **2020**, *135*, 713–723. [CrossRef] [PubMed]
317. Fedorov, V.D.; Themeli, M.; Sadelain, M. PD-1- and CTLA-4-based inhibitory chimeric antigen receptors (iCARs) divert off-target immunotherapy responses. *Sci. Transl. Med.* **2013**, *5*, 215ra172. [CrossRef] [PubMed]
318. Depil, S.; Duchateau, P.; Grupp, S.A.; Mufti, G.; Poirot, L. "Off-the-shelf" allogeneic CAR T cells: Development and challenges. *Nat. Rev. Drug Discov.* **2020**, *19*, 185–199. [CrossRef] [PubMed]
319. Brudno, J.N.; Somerville, R.P.; Shi, V.; Rose, J.J.; Halverson, D.C.; Fowler, D.H.; Gea-Banacloche, J.C.; Pavletic, S.Z.; Hickstein, D.D.; Lu, T.L.; et al. Allogeneic T Cells That Express an Anti-CD19 Chimeric Antigen Receptor Induce Remissions of B-Cell Malignancies That Progress After Allogeneic Hematopoietic Stem-Cell Transplantation Without Causing Graft-Versus-Host Disease. *J. Clin. Oncol. Off. J. Am. Soc. Clin. Oncol.* **2016**, *34*, 1112–1121. [CrossRef]
320. Kochenderfer, J.N.; Dudley, M.E.; Carpenter, R.O.; Kassim, S.H.; Rose, J.J.; Telford, W.G.; Hakim, F.T.; Halverson, D.C.; Fowler, D.H.; Hardy, N.M.; et al. Donor-derived CD19-targeted T cells cause regression of malignancy persisting after allogeneic hematopoietic stem cell transplantation. *Blood* **2013**, *122*, 4129–4139. [CrossRef]
321. Chu, J.; Deng, Y.; Benson, D.M.; He, S.; Hughes, T.; Zhang, J.; Peng, Y.; Mao, H.; Yi, L.; Ghoshal, K.; et al. CS1-specific chimeric antigen receptor (CAR)-engineered natural killer cells enhance in vitro and in vivo antitumor activity against human multiple myeloma. *Leukemia* **2014**, *28*, 917–927. [CrossRef]
322. Liu, E.; Tong, Y.; Dotti, G.; Shaim, H.; Savoldo, B.; Mukherjee, M.; Orange, J.; Wan, X.; Lu, X.; Reynolds, A.; et al. Cord blood NK cells engineered to express IL-15 and a CD19-targeted CAR show long-term persistence and potent antitumor activity. *Leukemia* **2018**, *32*, 520–531. [CrossRef]
323. Torikai, H.; Reik, A.; Liu, P.Q.; Zhou, Y.; Zhang, L.; Maiti, S.; Huls, H.; Miller, J.C.; Kebriaei, P.; Rabinovitch, B.; et al. A foundation for universal T-cell based immunotherapy: T cells engineered to express a CD19-specific chimeric-antigen-receptor and eliminate expression of endogenous TCR. *Blood* **2012**, *119*, 5697–5705. [CrossRef] [PubMed]
324. Poirot, L.; Philip, B.; Schiffer-Mannioui, C.; Le Clerre, D.; Chion-Sotinel, I.; Derniame, S.; Potrel, P.; Bas, C.; Lemaire, L.; Galetto, R.; et al. Multiplex Genome-Edited T-cell Manufacturing Platform for "Off-the-Shelf" Adoptive T-cell Immunotherapies. *Cancer Res.* **2015**, *75*, 3853–3864. [CrossRef] [PubMed]
325. Taylor, C.J.; Peacock, S.; Chaudhry, A.N.; Bradley, J.A.; Bolton, E.M. Generating an iPSC bank for HLA-matched tissue transplantation based on known donor and recipient HLA types. *Cell Stem Cell* **2012**, *11*, 147–152. [CrossRef] [PubMed]
326. Wang, D.; Quan, Y.; Yan, Q.; Morales, J.E.; Wetsel, R.A. Targeted Disruption of the β2-Microglobulin Gene Minimizes the Immunogenicity of Human Embryonic Stem Cells. *Stem Cells Transl. Med.* **2015**, *4*, 1234–1245. [CrossRef]

327. Sommer, C.; Boldajipour, B.; Valton, J.; Galetto, R.; Bentley, T.; Sutton, J.; Ni, Y.; Leonard, M.; Van Blarcom, T.; Smith, J.; et al. ALLO-715, an Allogeneic BCMA CAR T Therapy Possessing an Off-Switch for the Treatment of Multiple Myeloma. *Blood* **2018**, *132* (Suppl. 1), 591. [CrossRef]
328. Cranert, S.A.; Richter, M.; Tong, M.; Weiss, L.; Tan, Y.; Ostertag, E.M.; Coronella, J.; Shedlock, D.J. Manufacture of an Allogeneic CAR-T Stem Cell Memory Product Candidate for Multiple Myeloma, P-Bcma-ALLO1, Is Robust, Reproducible and Highly Scalable. *Blood* **2019**, *134* (Suppl. 1), 4445. [CrossRef]
329. Mathur, R.; Zhang, Z.; He, J.; Galetto, R.; Gouble, A.; Chion-Sotinel, I.; Filipe, S.; Gariboldi, A.; Veeramachaneni, T.; Manasanch, E.E.; et al. Universal SLAMF7-Specific CAR T-Cells As Treatment for Multiple Myeloma. *Blood* **2017**, *130* (Suppl. 1), 502.
330. Mailankody, S.; Matous, J.V.; Liedtke, M.; Sidana, S.; Malik, S.; Nath, R. Universal: An Allogeneic First-in-Human Study of the Anti-Bcma ALLO-715 and the Anti-CD52 ALLO-647 in Relapsed/Refractory Multiple Myeloma. *Blood* **2020**, *136* (Suppl. 1), 24–25. [CrossRef]
331. Santomasso, B.; Bachier, C.; Westin, J.; Rezvani, K.; Shpall, E.J. The Other Side of CAR T-Cell Therapy: Cytokine Release Syndrome, Neurologic Toxicity, and Financial Burden. *Am. Soc. Clin. Oncol. Educ. Book* **2019**, *39*, 433–444. [CrossRef]
332. Nam, S.; Smith, J.; Yang, G. Driving the next wave of innovation in CAR T-cell Therapies | McKinsey. 2019. Available online: https://www.mckinsey.com/industries/pharmaceuticals-and-medical-products/our-insights/driving-the-next-wave-of-innovation-in-car-t-cell-therapies (accessed on 15 August 2020).
333. ICER (Institute for Clinical and Economic Review); CTAF (California Technology Assessment Forum). Chimeric Antigen Receptor T-Cell Therapy for B-Cell Cancers: Effectiveness and Value. In *Final Evidence Report*; ICER: Boston, MA, USA, 2018.
334. Lin, J.K.; Lerman, B.J.; Barnes, J.I.; Boursiquot, B.C.; Tan, Y.J.; Robinson, A.Q.; Davis, K.L.; Owens, D.K.; Goldhaber-Fiebert, J.D. Cost Effectiveness of Chimeric Antigen Receptor T-Cell Therapy in Relapsed or Refractory Pediatric B-Cell Acute Lymphoblastic. *Leuk. J. Clin. Oncol. Off. J. Am. Soc. Clin. Oncol.* **2018**, *13*, JCO2018790642. [CrossRef]
335. Kebriaei, P.; Izsvák, Z.; Narayanavari, S.A.; Singh, H.; Ivics, Z. Gene Therapy with the Sleeping Beauty Transposon System. *Trends Genet TIG* **2017**, *33*, 852–870. [CrossRef] [PubMed]
336. Ramanayake, S.; Bilmon, I.; Bishop, D.; Dubosq, M.C.; Blyth, E.; Clancy, L.; Gottlieb, D.; Micklethwaite, K. Low-cost generation of Good Manufacturing Practice-grade CD19-specific chimeric antigen receptor-expressing T cells using piggyBac gene transfer and patient-derived materials. *Cytotherapy* **2015**, *17*, 1251–1267. [CrossRef] [PubMed]
337. Rosenblatt, J.; Avivi, I.; Binyamini, N.; Uhl, L.; Somaiya, P.; Stroopinsky, D.; Palmer, K.A.; Coll, M.D.; Katz, T.; Bisharat, L.; et al. Blockade of PD-1 in Combination with Dendritic Cell/Myeloma Fusion Cell Vaccination Following Autologous Stem Cell Transplantation Is Well Tolerated, Induces Anti-Tumor Immunity and May Lead to Eradication of Measureable Disease. *Blood* **2015**, *126*, 4218. [CrossRef]
338. Yang, Y. Cancer immunotherapy: Harnessing the immune system to battle cancer. *J. Clin. Investig.* **2015**, *125*, 3335–3337. [CrossRef]
339. Ventola, C.L. Cancer Immunotherapy, Part 3: Challenges and Future Trends. *Pharm. Ther.* **2017**, *42*, 514–521.
340. Pardoll, D. Cancer and the Immune System: Basic Concepts and Targets for Intervention. *Semin Oncol.* **2015**, *42*, 523–538. [CrossRef]
341. Zugazagoitia, J.; Guedes, C.; Ponce, S.; Ferrer, I.; Molina-Pinelo, S.; Paz-Ares, L. Current Challenges in Cancer Treatment. *Clin. Ther.* **2016**, *38*, 1551–1566. [CrossRef]
342. Pawlyn, C.; Davies, F.E. Toward personalized treatment in multiple myeloma based on molecular characteristics. *Blood* **2019**, *133*, 660–675. [CrossRef]
343. Krzyszczyk, P.; Acevedo, A.; Davidoff, E.J.; Timmins, L.M.; Marrero-Berrios, I.; Patel, M.; White, C.; Lowe, C.; Sherba, J.J.; Hartmanshenn, C.; et al. The growing role of precision and personalized medicine for cancer treatment. *Technology* **2018**, *6*, 79–100. [CrossRef]
344. Le Tourneau, C.; Borcoman, E.; Kamal, M. Molecular profiling in precision medicine oncology. *Nat. Med.* **2019**, *25*, 711–712. [CrossRef]
345. Rothwell, D.G.; Ayub, M.; Cook, N.; Thistlethwaite, F.; Carter, L.; Dean, E.; Smith, N.; Villa, S.; Dransfield, J.; Clipson, A.; et al. Utility of ctDNA to support patient selection for early phase clinical trials: The TARGET study. *Nat. Med.* **2019**, *25*, 738–743. [CrossRef] [PubMed]
346. Sicklick, J.K.; Kato, S.; Okamura, R.; Schwaederle, M.; Hahn, M.E.; Williams, C.B.; De, P.; Krie, A.; Piccioni, D.E.; Miller, V.A.; et al. Molecular profiling of cancer patients enables personalized combination therapy: The I-PREDICT study. *Nat. Med.* **2019**, *25*, 744–750. [CrossRef] [PubMed]
347. Rodon, J.; Soria, J.C.; Berger, R.; Miller, W.H.; Rubin, E.; Kugel, A.; Tsimberidou, A.; Saintigny, P.; Ackerstein, A.; Braña, I.; et al. Genomic and transcriptomic profiling expands precision cancer medicine: The WINTHER trial. *Nat. Med.* **2019**, *25*, 751–758. [CrossRef] [PubMed]
348. Marquart, J.; Chen, E.Y.; Prasad, V. Estimation of the Percentage of US Patients with Cancer Who Benefit From Genome-Driven Oncology. *JAMA Oncol.* **2018**, *4*, 1093–1098. [CrossRef]
349. Hoos, A.; Eggermont, A.M.; Janetzki, S.; Hodi, F.S.; Ibrahim, R.; Anderson, A.; Humphrey, R.; Blumenstein, B.; Old, L.; Wolchok, J. Improved endpoints for cancer immunotherapy trials. *J. Natl. Cancer Inst.* **2010**, *102*, 1388–1397. [CrossRef]
350. Park, J.J.H.; Hsu, G.; Siden, E.G.; Thorlund, K.; Mills, E.J. An overview of precision oncology basket and umbrella trials for clinicians. *CA Cancer J. Clin.* **2020**, *70*, 125–137. [CrossRef]

351. Jørgensen, J.; Hanna, E.; Kefalas, P. Outcomes-based reimbursement for gene therapies in practice: The experience of recently launched CAR-T cell therapies in major European countries. *J. Mark Access Health Policy* **2020**, *8*, 1715536. [CrossRef]
352. Gandhi, U.H.; Cornell, R.F.; Lakshman, A.; Gahvari, Z.J.; McGehee, E.; Jagosky, M.H.; Gupta, R.; Varnado, W.; Fiala, M.A.; Chhabra, S.; et al. Outcomes of Patients with Multiple Myeloma Refractory to CD38-Targeted Monoclonal Antibody Therapy. *Leukemia* **2019**, *33*, 2266–2275. [CrossRef]

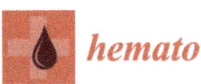

Review

Current Status of CAR-T Cell Therapy in Multiple Myeloma

Juan Luis Reguera-Ortega, Estefanía García-Guerrero and Jose Antonio Pérez-Simón *

Department of Hematology, Instituto de Biomedicina de Sevilla (IBIS/CSIC/CIBERONC), University Hospital Virgen del Rocio, Universidad de Sevilla, 41013 Sevilla, Spain; juanlu_jlr@hotmail.com (J.L.R.-O.); egarcia-ibis@us.es (E.G.-G.)
* Correspondence: Josea.perez.simon.sspa@juntadeandalucia.es

Abstract: Current data on CAR-T cell-based therapy is really promising in multiple myeloma, especially in terms of response. In heavily pretreated patients, who have already received proteasome inhibitors, immunomodulatory drugs and monoclonal antibodies, current trials report an overall response rate ranging from 81 to 97% and 45 to 67% of complete remission rates. Data are less encouraging in terms of duration of response, although most recent trials have shown significant improvements in terms of event-free survival, with medians ranging from 8 to 14 months and up to 77% progression-free survival at 12 months with an acceptable toxicity profile. These data will be consolidated in future years and will provide new evidence on the best timing for CAR-T cell therapy. Moreover, new CAR-T designs are underway and will challenge the current results.

Keywords: myeloma; CAR T-cells; target antigen

1. Introduction

The introduction of proteasome inhibitors (PI) and immunomodulatory drugs (IMIDs) in the early 2000 has improved survival in patients with multiple myeloma (MM).

Currently, the standard treatment of MM is based on a combination of drugs with different mechanisms of action and synergistic effects, including proteasome inhibitors (bortezomib, carfilzomib, ixazomib), immunomodulatory drugs (thalidomide, lenalidomide, pomalidomide), alkylating agents (melphalan, cyclophosphamide, bendamustine), steroids and, recently, anti-CD38 monoclonal antibodies (daratumumab, isatuximab) and anti-SLAMF7 monoclonal antibody (elotuzumab). Furthermore, the addition of immunotherapy with conjugated antibodies (belantamab mafadotin) represents a therapeutic approach for refractory patients, improving survival expectations among this patient population.

Although all these drugs have improved the outcome of MM, most patients still die due to disease progression [1]. Patients who are refractory to PI, IMIDs and alkylating agents have a median overall survival of less than a year [2,3].

Therapy with genetically modified T-cells expressing a chimeric antigen receptor (CAR) represents a cutting-edge approach. Results reported in acute lymphoblastic leukaemia (ALL) [4] and non-Hodgkin lymphoma (NHL) [5–7] with CD19 CAR-T cells has led to the search for other targets and to expand this treatment to other diseases, such as MM. Therefore, the identification of new antigens in plasma cells which can be used as a potential target has become a priority in the development of new therapeutic approaches based on immunotherapy. Thus, extensive efforts are being put into the development of new CAR therapies to treat MM as well as novel bispecific T cell engagers/antibodies (teclistamab, talquetamab). Unlike CAR-T cell products, bispecific antibodies do not require long production times or adequate lymphocyte counts. By contrast, CAR-T cells require only one dose instead of continuous therapy with bispecific antibodies [8].

Selection of an adequate antigen is a key factor for the development of an optimal CAR-T cell product. As antigen recognition does not depend on the human leukocyte antigen (HLA) system, a tumour target should be present on the cellular surface.

One of these antigens is B-cell maturation antigen (BCMA), which is highly expressed on the surface of malignant plasma cells but not on normal tissues, except for a low expression on mature B-cells [9].

Different antigens are currently being evaluated as possible targets for CAR therapy, including CD138, CD19, kappa light chain and BCMA. Some trials using these antigens have shown promising results, mainly in terms of response rate. However, no plateau has been observed in overall survival and disease-free survival curves, which translates the lack of durable remissions. Therefore, it will be necessary to overcome potential limitations hindering the efficacy of CAR-T cells in MM, such as lack of effectiveness, off-tumour toxicities, loss of antigen or interference with soluble protein present in patients' plasma [10].

2. Results

Clinical trials of CAR-T cell therapy against MM have demonstrated promising clinical activity, providing unprecedented response rates in these heavily pretreated patients, the most commonly explored target being BCMA. There are more than 50 clinical trials ongoing using BCMA as a target. As mentioned previously, BCMA is a very specific antigen of plasma cells and mature B-cells, avoiding off-tumour toxicities following infusion [11,12].

The first clinical trial with BCMA-specific CAR was published in 2018 by Brudno et al. [13]. Sixteen patients received 9×10^6 CAR-BCMA T cells/kg. The patients had a median of 9.5 prior lines of therapy. The overall response rate was 81%, with 63% very good partial response or complete response. The median event-free survival was 31 weeks. Twelve patients (82%) developed CRS, including 6 (38%) with grade $\geq$ 3 CRS. Neurotoxicity was reported in 3 (19%) patients.

Idecabtagene vicleucel (ide-cel), initially known as bb2121, was developed by Bluebirdbio by transducing autologous T lymphocytes with a lentiviral vector to incorporate a second-generation CAR composed of an anti-BCMA single-variable chain domain, 41BB costimulatory domain and CD3-zeta as a signalling domain [14,15]. Lymphodepletion chemotherapy consisted of fludarabine and cyclophosphamide. In the dose escalating phase, the following doses were analysed: 50×10^6, 150×10^6, 450×10^6 and 800×10^6 CAR-positive (CAR+) T cells, with a 20% variation allowed. The expansion phase was achieved with 150×10^6 to 450×10^6 CAR+ T cells. A phase 1 trial using ide-cel included 33 patients who received multiple lines of treatment. The overall response rate was 85% with 45% of complete remission. Cytokine release syndrome (CRS) incidence was 76%, although only 2 patients developed CRS grade $\geq$ 3. Results of the phase 2 trial (KarMMa) have been published by Munshi et al. [16,17]. Of 140 patients enrolled, 128 received ide-cel. Patients had a median of 6 prior lines of therapy, 84% were refractory to at least one PI, one IMID and one anti-CD38. Eighty-eight percent received bridging therapy during the manufacturing process, but only 4% had some degree of response. With a median follow-up of 13.3 months, 94 of 128 (73%) patients had a response, and 42 of 128 (33%) achieved a complete remission (CR) or better. Thirty-three of 128 (26%) had CR with minimal residual disease (MRD)-negative status. Median progression-free survival (PFS) was 8.8 months and median overall survival was 19.4 months. The most common side effects among the 128 infused patients included neutropenia in 117 (91%) patients, anaemia in 89 (70%) and thrombocytopenia in 81 (63%). One hundred and seven (84%) developed CRS, including 7 (5%) with grade $\geq$ 3 CRS. Neurotoxicity was reported in 23 (18%) patients and were of grade 3 in 4 (3%) patients. Persistence of CAR+ T cells was documented in 59% of patients at 6 months and in 36% at 12 months following the infusion.

In addition to ide-cel, Wang B.-Y. et al. have developed a bispecific CAR with two BCMA binding sites (ciltacabtagene autoleucel or cilta-cel) [18,19]. A phase 1 study enrolled 57 patients, and lymphodepletion chemotherapy was based on single-agent cyclophosphamide. Fifty-one of 57 (90%) patients developed CRS, although only 7% had grade $\geq$ 3 CRS. Only one patient suffered from neurotoxicity. The overall response rate (ORR) was

88% with 47% of CR. Median PFS was 20 months. CAR+ T cells were not detectable in peripheral blood in 71% of patients at 4 months following infusion.

Similar results were reported in a phase 1b/2 study (CARTITUDE-1) performed in the United States [20]. Ninety-seven patients were enrolled; all of them had previously been exposed to PI, IMIDs and anti-CD38, and median lines of prior treatment was 6. Lymphodepletion included fludarabine and cyclophosphamide. The last update was presented at the European Hematology Association (EHA) congress in June 2021 [21]. The overall response rate was 97%, and 67% achieved CR. The median time to complete remission or better was 2 months (range, 1–15 months). Among 57 evaluable patients for MRD, 93% achieved MRD-negative status at 10^{-5}. At 12 months, PFS was 77%, and overall survival (OS) was 89%. Median PFS has not been reached yet. The most common grade 3/4 toxicities were neutropenia in 95% of patients, anaemia in 68% and thrombocytopenia in 60%. Cytokine release syndrome was reported in 95% of the patients, 4% were grade 3/4, median time to onset was 7 days and median duration was 4 days. One patient died due to grade 5 CRS and hemophagocytic lymphohistiocytosis (HLH). Neurotoxicity occurred in 21% of the patients, and 10% were grade 3/4.

Cohen et al. [22] conducted a phase I study (NCT02546167) to evaluate autologous T cells lentivirally-transduced with a fully-human, BCMA-specific CAR containing CD3ζ and 4-1BB signalling domains (CART-BCMA). Twenty-five subjects were treated in 3 cohorts: (1) $1-5 \times 10^8$ CART-BCMA cells alone; (2) cyclophosphamide 1.5 g/m^2 + $1-5 \times 10^7$ CART-BCMA cells; and (3) cyclophosphamide 1.5 g/m^2 + $1-5 \times 10^8$ CART-BCMA cells. Toxicities included CRS 22/25 patients (88%) (32% g3-4) and neurotoxicity 8/25 patients (32%) (12% G3-4). The following responses were seen: 44% in cohort 1, 20% in cohort 2 and 64% in cohort 3 (including 5PR, 5 VGPR and 2CR)

Finally, the Memorial Sloan Kettering Cancer Centre group has developed a fully human anti-BCMA CAR-T cell (JCARH125, orvacabtagene-autoleucel, orva-cel) [23]. Infusion ratio CD4:CD8 is 1:1 to enhance memory T cell expansion [24]. Phase 1/2 trial (EVOLVE study) [25] still has a follow-up of only 6 months, but ORR of patients who received doses between 300 and 600×10^6 CAR+ T cells was 92% and 35% were CR. Ninety-four percent of patients were refractory to one PI, one IMID and one anti-CD38, and median number of prior regimens was 6. Incidence of CRS was 89%, only 3% developed grade $\geq$ 3. Neurotoxicity occurred in 13%, 3% were grade $\geq$ 3. There were no data on PFS in this study at the time of writing this manuscript.

These encouraging results need to be confirmed in phase 3 studies. There are two ongoing phase 3 trials (KarMMa-3 and CARTITUDE-4) comparing the efficacy and safety of BCMA CAR-T cell versus other anti-MM therapies treatments, both given in early stages of the disease.

All these studies are summarized in Table 1.

Table 1. Summary of clinical trials on MM using CAR-T.

Study	n	Phase	Vector	Product	Costimulatory Domain	LD Chemo Therapy	CAR_T Cell Dose	Previous Lines Median	CRS ≥ Grade 3	ICANS ≥ Grade 3	ORR %	CR %	MDR neg %	Median PFS (Months)	Median OS (Months)
CRB-401[1]	33	1	Lenti	Ide-Cel (bb2121)	4-1BB	FluCy	50/150/450/800 × 10^6 cells	7	6	3	85	45	94	11.8	NA
KArMMA[2,3]	128	2	Lenti	Ide-Cel (bb2121)	4-1BB	FluCy	150/300/450 × 10^6 cells	6	6	3	73	53	33	8.8	19.4
LEGEND-2[3]	57/74	1	Lenti	Ciltacabtagene Autoleucel LCAR-B38M (JNJ68284528)	4-1BB	Cy	0.5×10^6 cells/kg	3	7	0	89	74	68	19.9	36.1
CARTITUDE-1[4,5]	97	1b/2	Lenti	Ciltacabtagene Autoleucel LCAR-B38M (JNJ68284528)	4-1BB	Flu/Cy	0.75×10^6 cells/kg	6	4	10	97	67	93	Not reached	NA
EVOLVE[6]	44	1	Lenti	Orvacabtagene autocel (JCARH125)	4-1BB	Flu/Cy	50/150/450 × 10^6 cells	7	9	7	82	27	67	NA	NA
EVOLVE[7]	62	1	Lenti	Orvacabtagene autocel (JCARH125)	4-1BB	Flu/Cy	300/450/600 × 10^6 cells	6	3	3	92	35	96	NA	NA
NCI[8]	16	1	Retro	NA	CD28	Flu/Cy	9×10^6 cells/kg	9	38	19	81	63	100	31 wks	NA
UPENN[9]	25	1	Lenti	NA	4-1BB	None or Cy	10/50/100/500 × 10^6 cells	7	32	12	63	28	33	65-125 d	502 d
CT053[10]	24	1	Retro	CT053	4-1BB	Flu/Cy	150×10^6 cells	4.5	0	4	88	83	85	NA	NA
Dual CD19-BCMA[11]	10	1	Lenti	Sequential CART-CD19/CART-BCMA	CD28	Flu/Cy	CD19: 1×10^7 cells BCMA: $3/5/6.5 \times 10^7$ cells	4	10	0	90	40	30	5	NA
FHVH-BCMA-T[12]	21	1	Retro	FHVH-BCMA-T	4-1BB	Flu/Cy	0.75/1.5/3/6/12 × 10^6 cells	6	19	10	90	NA	NA	NA	NA

Adapted from Wudhikarn ASH 2020: [1]. Raje NEJM 2019; [2]. Munshi 2020; [3]. Berdeja Blood 2019; 34 Wang Blood 2019, 134 (supl 1): 579; [4]. Maduri Blood 2019, 134 (supl 1): 577; [5] Berdeja JCO 2020, 38 (supl 15): 8505; [6]. Stadtmauer Science 2020; [7]. Mailankody JCO 2020, 38 (supl 15): 8504; [8]. Brudno JCO 2018; [9]. Cohen JCO 2019; [10]. Jie Blood 2019, 134 (supl 1): 4435; [11]. Yan Cancer Medicine 2021. [12]. Mikkilineni Blood 2020, 136 (supl 1): 50–51.

An important issue which will lead to discussion will be to define the place of new alternative approaches, such as conjugated antibodies or bispecific antibodies in the MM treatment algorithm, and whether, due to their safety profile, there will be a patient profile who will benefit more from these approaches than from CAR-T cell treatment.

Unfortunately, although most anti-BCMA CAR-T cell studies have described remarkable efficacy in terms of responses, event-free survival curves did not show a plateau, and most patients eventually relapse. Mechanisms related to CAR-T cell failure or resistance are multifactorial, including patient's characteristics and disease biological features [26]. Loss of antigen at the time of relapse is one of the main mechanisms of resistance. In this regard, a selection of a clone with homozygous deletion of BCMA has been recently reported as the underlying mechanism of immune escape after anti-BCMA CAR-T cell therapy [27].

There are three ways to overcome this obstacle, namely CAR-T cells directed towards other antigens, dual CAR-T cells and antigen overexpression strategies [28,29].

Regarding the development of dual CAR-T cells, one potential approach is the elaboration through a bicistronic vector of two different CARs on the same T cell [30,31], another approach is the administration of two CAR-T cells produced independently and infused together or sequentially. Fernandez de Larrea et al. [30] demonstrated that expressing two CARs on a single cell enhanced the strength of CAR-T cell/target cell interactions. Also, developing a single product significantly reduces cost resources and time.

There are different ongoing clinical trials evaluating the efficacy and safety of anti-CD38 CAR-T cells alone or in combination with other CARs. The phase 1 study NCT03464916 evaluates an anti-CD38 CAR-T cell in relapse/refractory (R/R) MM patients. No results have been published yet. A phase 1/2 study, NCT03767751, is testing a dual anti-CD38 and BCMA CAR-T cells [32], and the phase 1/2 study NCT03125577 is assessing the combination of an anti-CD19 CAR-T cell plus an anti-CD38 CAR-T cell.

Regarding antigen overexpression strategies, the administration of an oral gamma secretase inhibitor to increase BCMA expression on the plasma cell surface has been assessed in a clinical trial (NCT03502577), and preliminary results in 6 patients showed an ORR of 100% [33–35]. In this sense, various approaches are being evaluated at the pre-clinical level, such as the case of trans retinoic acid (ATRA) (García-Guerrero et al.) [36]. It has recently been reported that BCMA expression in myeloma cells can be increased by epigenetic modulation with ATRA. After ATRA treatment, MM cells have an increased susceptibility to anti-BCMA CAR-T cell treatment in vitro and in vivo preclinical models, which can be further increased by combined treatment of ATRA and g-secretase inhibitors. Some other relevant pre-clinical data has been recently published. In this sense, GPRC5D has been reported as a novel target antigen for the immunotherapy of MM. GPRC5D is a human orphan family C G protein-coupled receptor recently described to be expressed on 98% of CD138-positive cells [37,38]. The restricted expression pattern of GPRC5D makes it an ideal target for immunotherapy. Consequently, GPRC5D CAR-T cells were generated by Smith et al. [38], showing anti-tumour efficacy against myeloma cells both in vitro and in vivo. Of note, GPRC5D CAR-T cells were also effective in eradication of myeloma cells after BCMA CAR-T cell treatment in a mouse model, which might be an option to overcome BCMA antigen escape.

Preclinical studies have also shown that CD138 is an effective target for the treatment of MM [39]. There is only one published study with an anti-CD138 CAR-T cells for R/R MM patients treated with chemotherapy and autologous stem cell transplant (ASCT). The CAR gene was detectable in peripheral blood of all patients and persisted for at least 4 weeks after the infusion. Four patients responded, but none of them achieved a CR; response lasted from 3 to 7 months. The remaining patients progressed despite having detectable CAR in marrow samples until day +90.

Although CD19 expression is uncommon on plasma cells, there is a small population of CD19+ myeloma cells which could constitute a reservoir of myeloma-initiating stem cells. The presence of CD19+ myeloma cells has been associated with a higher relapse rate and poor overall survival [40]. Therefore, targeting CD19 represents an interesting strategy to eliminate this subset of CD19+ cells. In the NCT02135406 study, ten patients with refractory MM received anti-CD19 CAR-T cells following an ASCT [41]. All patients received a previous ASCT, which resulted in a poor response with a PFS of less than one year. CD19 expression on myeloma cells was assessed by flow cytometry. As expected, the predominant myeloma population was CD19- in all patients. However, 7 out of 9 evaluable patients had subpopulations of CD19+ cells, ranging from 0.04% to 1.6%. In 10 of 11 subjects, the maximum planned dose of CTL019, 5×10^7 cells, was manufactured. In one subject, manufacturing was unsuccessful due to failure of autologous T cells to proliferate in culture. The median transduction efficiency was 10.1% (range 1.2–23.2), and the median total T cell dose was 4.4×10^8 (range 1.1×10^8 to 6.0×10^8). An ORR was achieved in 8 patients at 100 days after ASCT (including 1sCR, 4 VGPR, and 2 PR). This might be due to the fact that a significant fraction of myeloma cells expresses CD19 at molecular density, which is detectable by direct stochastic optical reconstruction microscopy (dSTORM) but not by flow cytometry [42]. Interestingly, less than 100 CD19 molecules are required for myeloma cell detection by CD19 CAR-T cells. In addition, evidence of a less differentiated MM subclone (CD19+ CD138−) with drug-resistance and disease propagating properties has emerged [40]. These results highlight antigen recognition by CAR even when it is present in very low density or not detectable by flow cytometry. Despite these encouraging findings, the use of CD19 CAR-T cells as a potential treatment for MM needs to be further explored. To determine whether CTL019 infusion improved PFS after ASCT, the authors compared each subject's PFS after ASCT versus ASCT followed by CTL019. Two patients had significantly increased PFS after CTL019 (479 versus 181 days, 249 versus 127 days).

Yan L et al., a cooperative group from China, have published a phase 1 trial with 10 patients treated with sequential infusions of an anti-CD19 CAR-T cell followed by an anti-BCMA CAR-T cell [43,44]. Patients received lymphodepletion chemotherapy with fludarabine and cyclophosphamide on days -5, -4 and -3. Patients were infused on day 0 with a fixed dose of 1×10^7/kg antiCD19 CAR-T, on day 1 with 40% of anti-BCMA-CART and on day 2 with the remaining dose. Three dose levels were assessed for anti-BCMA CAR-T (3×10^7/kg, 5×10^7/kg and 6.5×10^7/kg). Median follow-up was 20 months. Ninety percent of patients developed CRS grade 1-2. Overall response rate was 90% with 40% of strict CR. Three out of 4 patients in strict RC maintained PFS at 2 years of follow-up.

A host immune response against a murine CAR is another potential limitation to CAR T cell persistence. Thus, developing a fully human CAR construct is an area of active research for several groups.

Jie J et al. developed the first fully human anti-BCMA CAR-T cell called CT053 [45]. Twenty-four patients with a median age of 60.1 years were included in the phase 1 trial. The subjects had a median of 4.5 prior regimens of therapy. They enrolled a high-risk population with extramedullary involvement (45.8%), ECOG score 2–3 (33.3%) and ISS grade 3 (37.5%). Overall response rate was 87.5% with 79.2% of CR. Among 20 subjects who underwent the evaluation of minimal residual disease (MRD) status, 17 achieved MRD-negative status. Median duration of response was 21.8 months. They demonstrated a good safety profile. The most common grade 3 or higher toxicities were neutropenia (66.7%), decreased lymphocyte count (79.2%) and thrombocytopenia (25%). In view of these results, a phase 1b/2 study (LUMMICAR-2) with CT053 is ongoing [46]. Patients received fludarabine and cyclophosphamide on days -5, -4 and -3. CT053 dose was $1.5–3.0 \times 10^8$, and it was administered in a single infusion. Median age was 59 years, and median number of prior lines of treatment was 6. Sixty-four percent of patients were refractory to 5 lines of treatment, and all received bridging therapy. Results published so far included 10 evaluable patients with a median follow-up of 4.5 months. Overall response rate was 100%, and 40% achieved at least a CR. Responses have been independent of BCMA expression in bone marrow. Peak CAR-T cell expansion was observed between 7 and 14 days after infusion. No grade 3 or higher CRS or neurotoxicity was observed.

Also, at the American Society of Hematology (ASH) meeting in 2020, the Kochenderfer group reported the results of a phase 1 trial with a fully human CAR-T cell which has a

BCMA heavy chain single binding domain (FHVH-CD8BBZ) [47]. The FHVH33 binding domain lacks the light chain, artificial linker sequence and 2 associated junctions of a scFv, which can be immunogenic leading to CAR rejection. FHVH33-CD8BBZ was encoded by a γ-retroviral vector and incorporated FHVH33, CD8α hinge and transmembrane domains, a 4-1BB costimulatory domain and a CD3ζ domain. Twenty-one patients were enrolled, median number of prior lines of treatment was 6 and median age was 64 years. Lymphodepletion consisted of fludarabine and cyclophosphamide on days -5, -4 and -3. The maximum tolerated dose was $6 \times 10^{[6]}$ CAR+ T cells /kg. The overall response rate was 90%. At the last cut-off, 10 patients maintained the response with a range of 0–80 weeks of follow-up. Ten patients discontinued the study, 9 due to disease progression and 1 due to death because of virus influenzae infection. Cytokine release syndrome occurred in 95% of patients, 20% were grade 3 and there were no grade 4 CRS. Thirty-eight percent developed neurotoxicity, but only 9% were grade 3.

Tumour microenvironment plays a crucial role in CAR-T cell resistance through immunological escape [48–51]. Some studies have shown that a high number of immunosuppressant cells, regulatory T cells, helper-2 T cells, cancer associated fibroblasts or osteoclasts contribute to decrease effector T cell activation and impair their function [51]. So, developing CAR-T cells against programmed death 1 and programmed death-ligand 1 (PD1/PDL1) might decrease the relapse risk related to the effect of microenvironment [52,53], but off-target toxicities might also increase.

Finally, and probably the most promising long-term strategy to overcome current limitations is the development of allogeneic CAR-T cells. There are already several phase 1 clinical trials assessing allogeneic CAR-T cells in R/R MM patients (UNIVERSAL trial, NCT04093596; MELANI-01 trial, NCT04142619; ALLO-605-201, NCT05000450; BCMA-UCART, NCT03752541; CTX120, NCT04244656; CYAD-211, NCT04613557). The reduction in time to infusion may be critical for life expectancy in a MM patient with refractory disease. Products from patients with fewer prior lines of treatment have a higher proportion of memory T cells and better ratio of CD4 T cell/CD8 T cells, which might improve the duration and depth of response 53. This statement must be confirmed in further studies since Yan et al. [44] describe 3 patients infused with alloCAR products who had early relapses. In this sense, Shah et al. designed a clinical trial with a next-generation CAR-T cell (bb21217) [54]. bb21217 is an anti-BCMA CAR-T cell therapy that uses the same CAR molecule as idecabtagene vicleucel (bb2121) but adds the PI3K inhibitor bb007 during ex vivo culture to enrich the cell product for memory-like T cells, thereby reducing the proportion of highly differentiated or senescent T cells. In the update presented at the American Society of Hematology Annual Meeting 2020, response was assessed per investigator for 44 patients with ≥2 months of follow up or PD/death within 2 months. Twenty-four (55%) patients had confirmed response per IMWG criteria, including 8 (18%) with ≥CR and 13 (30%) with VGPR. CRS occurred in 67% of patients and neurotoxicity in 22% [55]. In the context of allogeneic CAR-T cells, to decrease the risk of graft-versus-host disease (GvHD) several bioengineering methods have been planned to regulate the expression of T cell receptor (TCR) and major histocompatibility complex (MHC) [56,57].

Another field under development is the use of CARs in natural killer cells (NK) as NK cells reduce the risk of GvHD and CRS [58,59]. There is an ongoing phase 1/2 study with anti-BCMA CAR NK cells (NCT03940833).

3. Conclusions

Exciting times are ahead of us, with this wide variety of options for improvement. Soon, the CARs we will be administering will differ greatly from the ones we have available now, including those not approved yet in Europe for commercial use. Furthermore, defining the profile of patients who will benefit from these treatments in an early stage of the disease remains an unsolved challenge.

Author Contributions: J.L.R.-O. wrote and revised the manuscript and references and supervised the table. E.G.-G. wrote the manuscript and table, assisted in the elaboration of the references list.

J.A.P.-S. supervised the manuscript, figures and references. All authors have read and agreed to the published version of the manuscript.

Funding: The authors would like to thank the CIBERONC (CB16/12/00480) and Red TerCel, and ISCIII (RD16/0011/0015, RD16/0011/0035).

Institutional Review Board Statement: Not applicable.

Informed Consent Statement: Not applicable.

Conflicts of Interest: Jose A Perez Simon participated in advisory boards and/or educational sessions and/or research projects from Novartis, BMS/Celgene, Kyte, JANSSEN. All other authors declare no conflict of interest.

References

1. Gandhi, U.H.; Cornell, R.F.; Lakshman, A.; Gahvari, Z.J.; McGehee, E.; Jagosky, M.H.; Gupta, R.; Varnado, W.; Fiala, M.A.; Chhabra, S.; et al. Outcomes of patients with multiple myeloma refractory to CD38-targeted monoclonal antibody therapy. *Leukemia* **2019**, *33*, 2266–2275. [CrossRef]
2. Schinke, C.; Hoering, A.; Wang, H.; Carlton, V.; Thanandrarajan, S.; Deshpande, S.; Patel, P.; Molnar, G.; Susanibar, S.; Mohan, M.; et al. The prognostic value of the depth of response in multiple myeloma depends on the time of assessment, risk status and molecular subtype. *Haematologica* **2017**, *102*, e313–e316. [CrossRef] [PubMed]
3. Kumar, S.; Paiva, B.; Anderson, K.C.; Durie, B.; Landgren, O.; Moreau, P.; Munshi, N.; Lonial, S.; Bladé, J.; Mateos, M.-V.; et al. International Myeloma Working Group consensus criteria for response and minimal residual disease assessment in multiple myeloma. *Lancet Oncol.* **2016**, *17*, e328–e346. [CrossRef]
4. Maude, S.L.; Laetsch, T.W.; Buechner, J.; Rives, S.; Boyer, M.; Bittencourt, H.; Bader, P.; Verneris, M.R.; Stefanski, H.E.; Myers, G.D.; et al. Tisagenlecleucel in Children and Young Adults with B-Cell Lymphoblastic Leukemia. *N. Engl. J. Med.* **2018**, *378*, 439–448. [CrossRef]
5. Schuster, S.J.; Bishop, M.R.; Tam, C.S.; Waller, E.K.; Borchmann, P.; McGuirk, J.P.; Jäger, U.; Jaglowski, S.; Andreadis, C.; Westin, J.R.; et al. Tisagenlecleucel in Adult Relapsed or Refractory Diffuse Large B-Cell Lymphoma. *N. Engl. J. Med.* **2019**, *380*, 45–56. [CrossRef]
6. Neelapu, S.S.; Locke, F.L.; Bartlett, N.L.; Lekakis, L.J.; Miklos, D.B.; Jacobson, C.A.; Braunschweig, I.; Oluwole, O.O.; Siddiqi, T.; Lin, Y.; et al. Axicabtagene Ciloleucel CAR T-Cell Therapy in Refractory Large B-Cell Lymphoma. *N. Engl. J. Med.* **2017**, *377*, 2531–2544. [CrossRef] [PubMed]
7. Abramson, J.S.; Palomba, M.L.; Gordon, L.I.; Lunning, M.A.; Wang, M.; Arnason, J.; Mehta, A.; Purev, E.; Maloney, D.G.; Andreadis, C.; et al. Lisocabtagene maraleucel for patients with relapsed or refractory large B-cell lymphomas (TRANSCEND NHL 001): A multicentre seamless design study. *Lancet* **2020**, *396*, 839–852. [CrossRef]
8. Barilà, G.; Rizzi, R.; Zambello, R.; Musto, P. Drug Conjugated and Bispecific Antibodies for Multiple Myeloma: Improving Immunotherapies off the Shelf. *Pharmaceuticals* **2021**, *14*, 40. [CrossRef]
9. Carpenter, R.O.; Evbuomwan, M.O.; Pittaluga, S.; Rose, J.J.; Raffeld, M.; Yang, S.; Gress, R.E.; Hakim, F.T.; Kochenderfer, J.N. B-cell maturation antigen is a promising target for adoptive T-cell therapy of multiple myeloma. *Clin. Cancer Res.* **2013**, *19*, 2048–2060. [CrossRef]
10. Kravets, V.G.; Zhang, Y.; Sun, H. Chimeric-Antigen-Receptor (CAR) T Cells and the Factors Influencing their Therapeutic Efficacy. *J. Immunol. Res. Ther.* **2017**, *2*, 100–113. [PubMed]
11. Green, D.J.; Pont, M.; Sather, B.D.; Cowan, A.J.; Turtle, C.J.; Till, B.G.; Nagengast, A.M.; Libby, E.N., III; Becker, P.S.; Coffey, D.G.; et al. Fully Human Bcma Targeted Chimeric Antigen Receptor T Cells Administered in a Defined Composition Demonstrate Potency at Low Doses in Advanced Stage High Risk Multiple Myeloma. *Blood* **2018**, *132*, 1011. [CrossRef]
12. Timmers, M.; Roex, G.; Wang, Y.; Campillo-Davo, D.; Van Tendeloo, V.F.I.; Chu, Y.; Berneman, Z.; Luo, F.; Van Acker, H.H.; Anguille, S. Chimeric Antigen Receptor-Modified T Cell Therapy in Multiple Myeloma: Beyond B Cell Maturation Antigen. *Front. Immunol.* **2019**, *10*, 1613. [CrossRef] [PubMed]
13. Brudno, J.N.; Maric, I.; Hartman, S.D.; Rose, J.J.; Wang, M.; Lam, N.; Stetler-Stevenson, M.; Salem, D.; Yuan, C.; Pavletic, S.; et al. T Cells Genetically Modified to Express an Anti–B-Cell Maturation Antigen Chimeric Antigen Receptor Cause Remissions of Poor-Prognosis Relapsed Multiple Myeloma. *J. Clin. Oncol.* **2018**, *36*, 2267–2280. [CrossRef]
14. Raje, N.; Berdeja, J.; Lin, Y.; Siegel, D.; Jagannath, S.; Madduri, D.; Liedtke, M.; Rosenblatt, J.; Maus, M.V.; Turka, A.; et al. Anti-BCMA CAR T-Cell Therapy bb2121 in Relapsed or Refractory Multiple Myeloma. *N. Engl. J. Med.* **2019**, *380*, 1726–1737. [CrossRef]
15. Berdeja, J.G.; Alsina, M.; Shah, N.D.; Siegel, D.S.; Jagannath, S.; Madduri, D.; Kaufman, J.L.; Munshi, N.C.; Rosenblatt, J.; Jasielec, J.K.; et al. Updated Results from an Ongoing Phase 1 Clinical Study of bb21217 Anti-Bcma CAR T Cell Therapy. *Blood* **2019**, *134*, 927. [CrossRef]
16. Munshi, N.C.; Anderson, J.L.D., Jr.; Shah, N.; Jagannath, S.; Berdeja, J.G.; Lonial, S.; Raje, N.S.; Siegel, D.S.D.; Lin, Y.; Oriol, A.; et al. Idecabtagene vicleucel (ide-cel; bb2121), a BCMA-targeted CAR T-cell therapy, in patients with relapsed and refractory multiple myeloma (RRMM): Initial KarMMa results. *J. Clin. Oncol.* **2020**, *38*, 8503. [CrossRef]

17. Oriol, A.; Abril, L.; Torrent, A.; Ibarra, G.; Ribera, J.-M. The role of idecabtagene vicleucel in patients with heavily pretreated refractory multiple myeloma. *Ther. Adv. Hematol.* **2021**, *12*. [CrossRef]
18. Wang, B.-Y.; Zhao, W.-H.; Liu, J.; Chen, Y.-X.; Cao, X.-M.; Yang, Y.; Zhang, Y.-L.; Wang, F.-X.; Zhang, P.-Y.; Lei, B.; et al. Long-Term Follow-up of a Phase 1, First-in-Human Open-Label Study of LCAR-B38M, a Structurally Differentiated Chimeric Antigen Receptor T (CAR-T) Cell Therapy Targeting B-Cell Maturation Antigen (BCMA), in Patients (pts) with Relapsed/Refractory Multiple Myeloma (RRMM). *Blood* **2019**, *134*, 579. [CrossRef]
19. Zhao, W.-H.; Liu, J.; Wang, B.-Y.; Chen, Y.-X.; Cao, X.-M.; Yang, Y.; Zhang, Y.-L.; Wang, F.-X.; Zhang, P.-Y.; Lei, B.; et al. A phase 1, open-label study of LCAR-B38M, a chimeric antigen receptor T cell therapy directed against B cell maturation antigen, in patients with relapsed or refractory multiple myeloma. *J. Hematol. Oncol.* **2018**, *11*, 141. [CrossRef]
20. Madduri, D.; Usmani, S.Z.; Jagannath, S.; Singh, I.; Zudaire, E.; Yeh, T.-M.; Allred, A.J.; Banerjee, A.; Goldberg, J.D.; Schecter, J.M.; et al. Results from CARTITUDE-1: A Phase 1b/2 Study of JNJ-4528, a CAR-T Cell Therapy Directed Against B-Cell Maturation Antigen (BCMA), in Patients with Relapsed and/or Refractory Multiple Myeloma (R/R MM). *Blood* **2019**, *134*, 577. [CrossRef]
21. Usmani, S.Z.; Berdeja, J.G.; Madduri, D.; Jakubowiak, A.J.; Agha, M.E.; Cohen, A.D.; Hari, P.; Yeh, T.-M.; Olyslager, Y.; Banerjee, A.; et al. Ciltacabtagene autoleucel, a B-cell maturation antigen (BCMA)-directed chimeric antigen receptor T-cell (CAR-T) therapy, in relapsed/refractory multiple myeloma (R/R MM): Updated results from CARTITUDE-1. *J. Clin. Oncol.* **2021**, *39*, 8005. [CrossRef]
22. Cohen, A.D.; Garfall, A.L.; Stadtmauer, E.A.; Melenhorst, J.J.; Lacey, S.F.; Lancaster, E.; Vogl, D.T.; Weiss, B.M.; Dengel, K.; Nelson, A.; et al. B cell maturation antigen–specific CAR T cells are clinically active in multiple myeloma. *J. Clin. Investig.* **2019**, *129*, 2210–2221. [CrossRef] [PubMed]
23. Mailankody, S.; Htut, M.; Lee, K.P.; Bensinger, W.; Devries, T.; Piasecki, J.; Ziyad, S.; Blake, M.; Byon, J.; Jakubowiak, A. JCARH125, anti-BCMA CAR T-cell therapy for relapsed/refractory multiple myeloma: Initial proof of concept results from a phase 1/2 multicenter study (EVOLVE). *Blood* **2018**, *132*, 957. [CrossRef]
24. Sommermeyer, D.; Hudecek, M.; Kosasih, P.L.; Gogishvili, T.; Maloney, D.G.; Turtle, C.J.; Riddell, S.R. Chimeric antigen receptor-modified T cells derived from defined CD8+ and CD4+ subsets confer superior antitumor reactivity in vivo. *Leukemia* **2016**, *30*, 492–500. [CrossRef] [PubMed]
25. Mailankody, S.; Jakubowiak, A.J.; Htut, M.; Costa, L.J.; Lee, K.; Ganguly, S.; Kaufman, J.L.; Siegel, D.S.D.; Bensinger, W.; Cota, M. Orvacabtagene autoleucel (orva-cel), a B- cellmaturation antigen (BCMA)-directed CAR T cell therapy for patients (pts) with relapsed/refractory multiple myeloma (RRMM): Update of the phase 1/2 EVOLVE study (NCT03430011). *J. Clin. Oncol.* **2020**, *38*, 8504. [CrossRef]
26. Fraietta, J.A.; Lacey, S.F.; Orlando, E.J.; Pruteanu-Malinici, I.; Gohil, M.; Lundh, S.; Boesteanu, A.C.; Wang, Y.; O'Connor, R.S.; Hwang, W.-T.; et al. Determinants of response and resistance to CD19 chimeric antigen receptor (CAR) T cell therapy of chronic lymphocytic leukemia. *Nat. Med.* **2018**, *24*, 563–571. [CrossRef]
27. Da Vià, M.C.; Dietrich, O.; Truger, M.; Arampatzi, P.; Duell, J.; Heidemeier, A.; Zhou, X.; Danhof, S.; Kraus, S.; Chatterjee, M.; et al. Homozygous BCMA gene deletion in response to anti-BCMA CAR T cells in a patient with multiple myeloma. *Nat. Med.* **2021**, *27*, 616–619. [CrossRef]
28. Works, M.; Soni, N.; Hauskins, C.; Sierra, C.; Baturevych, A.; Jones, J.C.; Curtis, W.; Carlson, P.; Johnstone, T.G.; Kugler, D.; et al. Anti-B-cell maturation antigen chimeric antigen receptor T cell function against multiple myeloma is enhanced in the presence of lenalidomide. *Mol. Cancer Ther.* **2019**, *18*, 2246–2257. [CrossRef]
29. Wang, X.; Walter, M.; Urak, R.; Weng, L.; Huynh, C.; Lim, L.; Wong, C.W.; Chang, W.-C.; Thomas, S.; Sanchez, J.F.; et al. Lenalidomide Enhances the Function of CS1 Chimeric Antigen Receptor–Redirected T Cells Against Multiple Myeloma. *Clin. Cancer Res.* **2018**, *24*, 106–119. [CrossRef]
30. de Larrea, C.F.; Staehr, M.; Lopez, A.V.; Ng, K.Y.; Chen, Y.; Godfrey, W.D.; Purdon, T.J.; Ponomarev, V.; Wendel, H.-G.; Brentjens, R.J.; et al. Defining an optimal dualtargeted CAR T- cell therapy approach simultaneously targeting BCMA and GPRC5D to prevent BCMA escape– driven relapse in multiple myeloma. *Blood Cancer Discov.* **2020**, *1*, 146–154. [CrossRef]
31. Zah, E.; Nam, E.; Bhuvan, V.; Tran, U.; Ji, B.Y.; Gosliner, S.B.; Wang, X.; Brown, C.E.; Chen, Y.Y. Systematically optimized BCMA/CS1 bispecific CAR-T cells robustly control heterogeneous multiple myeloma. *Nat. Commun.* **2020**, *11*, 2283. [CrossRef] [PubMed]
32. Li, C.; Mei, H.; Hu, Y.; Guo, T.; Liu, L.; Jiang, H.; Tang, L.; Wu, Y.; Ai, L.; Deng, J. A bispecific CAR-T cell therapy targeting BCMA and CD38 for relapsed/refractory multiple myeloma: Updated results from a phase 1 dose-climbing trial. *Blood* **2019**, *134*, 930. [CrossRef]
33. Pont, M.J.; Hill, T.; Cole, G.O.; Abbott, J.J.; Kelliher, J.; Salter, A.I.; Hudecek, M.; Comstock, M.L.; Rajan, A.; Patel, B.K.R.; et al. γ-Secretase inhibition increases efficacy of BCMA-specific chimeric antigen receptor T cells in multiple myeloma. *Blood* **2019**, *134*, 1585–1597. [CrossRef] [PubMed]
34. Laurent, S.A.; Hoffmann, F.S.; Kuhn, P.-H.; Cheng, Q.; Chu, Y.; Schmidt-Supprian, M.; Hauck, S.; Schuh, E.; Krumbholz, M.; Rübsamen, H.; et al. γ-secretase directly sheds the survival receptor BCMA from plasma cells. *Nat. Commun.* **2015**, *6*, 7333. [CrossRef]
35. Cowan, A.J.; Pont, M.; Sather, B.D.; Turtle, M.C.J.; Till, B.G.; Nagengast, R.A.M.; Libby, I.E.N.; Becker, P.S.; Coffey, D.G.; Tuazon, S.A.; et al. Efficacy and Safety of Fully Human Bcma CAR T Cells in Combination with a Gamma Secretase Inhibitor to Increase Bcma Surface Expression in Patients with Relapsed or Refractory Multiple Myeloma. *Blood* **2019**, *134*, 204. [CrossRef]

36. Garcia-Guerrero, G.; Rodríguez-Lobato, L.G.; Danhof, S.; Sierro-Martínez, B.; Goetz, R.; Sauer, M.; Perez-Simon, J.A.; Einsele, H.; Hudecek, M.; Prommersbe, S. ATRA Augments BCMA Expression on Myeloma Cells and Enhances Recognition By BCMA-CAR T-Cells. *Blood* **2020**, *136*, 13–14. [CrossRef]
37. Bräuner-Osborne, H.; Jensen, A.A.; Sheppard, P.O.; Brodin, B.; Krogsgaard-Larsen, P.; O'Hara, P. Cloning and characterization of a human orphan family C G-protein coupled receptor GPRC5D. *Biochim. Et Biophys. Acta (BBA)-Gene Struct. Expr.* **2001**, *1518*, 237–248. [CrossRef]
38. Smith, E.L.; Harrington, K.; Staehr, M.; Masakayan, R.; Jones, J.; Long, T.J.; Ng, K.Y.; Ghoddusi, M.; Purdon, T.J.; Wang, X.; et al. GPRC5D is a target for the immunotherapy of multiple myeloma with rationally designed CAR T cells. *Sci. Transl. Med.* **2019**, *11*, eaau7746. [CrossRef] [PubMed]
39. Sun, C.; Mahendravada, A.; Ballard, B.; Kale, B.; Ramos, C.; West, J.; Maguire, T.; McKay, K.; Lichtman, E.; Tuchman, S.; et al. Safety and efficacy of targeting CD138 with a chimeric antigen receptor for the treatment of multiple myeloma. *Oncotarget* **2019**, *10*, 2369–2383. [CrossRef]
40. Matsui, W.; Wang, Q.; Barber, J.P.; Brennan, S.; Smith, B.D.; Borrello, I.; McNiece, I.; Lin, L.; Ambinder, R.F.; Peacock, C.; et al. Clonogenic Multiple Myeloma Progenitors, Stem Cell Properties, and Drug Resistance. *Cancer Res.* **2008**, *68*, 190–197. [CrossRef] [PubMed]
41. Garfall, A.; Stadtmauer, E.; Hwang, W.; Lacey, S.F.; Melenhorst, J.J.; Krevvata, M.; Carroll, M.P.; Matsui, M.H.; Wang, Q.; Dhodapkar, M.V.; et al. Anti-CD19 CAR T cells with high-dose melphalan and autologous stem cell transplantation for refractory multiple myeloma. *JCI Insight* **2018**, *3*, e120505. [CrossRef] [PubMed]
42. Nerreter, T.; Letschert, S.; Götz, R.; Doose, S.; Danhof, S.; Einsele, H.; Sauer, M.; Hudecek, M. Super-resolution microscopy reveals ultra-low CD19 expression on myeloma cells that triggers elimination by CD19 CAR-T. *Nat. Commun.* **2019**, *10*, 3137. [CrossRef] [PubMed]
43. Yan, Z.; Cao, J.; Cheng, H.; Qiao, J.; Zhang, H.; Wang, Y.; Shi, M.; Lan, J.; Fei, X.; Jin, L.; et al. A combination of humanised anti-CD19 and anti-BCMA CAR T cells in patients with relapsed or refractory multiple myeloma: A single-arm, phase 2 trial. *Lancet Haematol.* **2019**, *6*, e521–e529. [CrossRef]
44. Yan, L.; Qu, S.; Shang, J.; Shi, X.; Kang, L.; Xu, N.; Zhu, H.; Zhou, J.; Jin, S.; Yao, W.; et al. Sequential CD19 and BCMA-specific CAR T-cell treatment elicits sustained remission of relapsed and/or refractory myeloma. *Cancer Med.* **2021**, *10*, 563–574. [CrossRef] [PubMed]
45. Jie, J.; Hao, S.; Jiang, S.; Li, Z.; Yang, M.; Zhang, W.; Yu, K.; Xiao, J.; Meng, H.; Ma, L.; et al. Phase 1 Trial of the Safety and Efficacy of Fully Human Anti-Bcma CAR T Cells in Relapsed/Refractory Multiple Myeloma. *Blood* **2019**, *134*, 4435. [CrossRef]
46. Kumar, S.; Baz, R.; Orlowski, R.; Larry, D.A., Jr.; Ma, H.; Shrewsbury, A.; Croghan, K.A.; Bilgi, M.; Kansagra, A.; Kapoor, P.; et al. Results from Lummicar-2: A Phase 1b/2 Study of Fully Human B-Cell Maturation Antigen-Specific CAR T Cells (CT053) in Patients with Relapsed and/or Refractory Multiple Myeloma. *Blood* **2020**, *136*, 28–29. [CrossRef]
47. Mikkilineni, L.; Manasanch, E.; Vanasse, D.; Brudno, J.N.; Mann, J.; Sherry, R.; Goff, S.L.; Yang, J.C.; Lam, N.; Maric, I.; et al. Deep and Durable Remissions of Relapsed Multiple Myeloma on a First-in-Humans Clinical Trial of T Cells Expressing an Anti-B-Cell Maturation Antigen (BCMA) Chimeric Antigen Receptor (CAR) with a Fully-Human Heavy-Chain-Only Antigen Recognition Domain. *Blood* **2020**, *136*, 50–51. [CrossRef]
48. Kawano, Y.; Moschetta, M.; Manier, S.; Glavey, S.; Görgün, G.T.; Roccaro, A.M.; Anderson, K.C.; Ghobrial, I.M. Targeting the bone marrow microenvironment in multiple myeloma. *Immunol. Rev.* **2015**, *263*, 160–172. [CrossRef] [PubMed]
49. Yeku, O.O.; Purdon, T.J.; Koneru, M.; Spriggs, D.; Brentjens, R.J. Armored CAR T cells enhance antitumor efficacy and overcome the tumor microenvironment. *Sci. Rep.* **2017**, *7*, 10541. [CrossRef] [PubMed]
50. Zhang, C.; Peng, Y.; Hublitz, P.; Zhang, H.; Dong, T. Genetic abrogation of immune checkpoints in antigen-specific cytotoxic T-lymphocyte as a potential alternative to blockade immunotherapy. *Sci. Rep.* **2018**, *8*, 5549. [CrossRef] [PubMed]
51. Sakemura, R.; Cox, M.J.; Hansen, M.J.; Hefazi, M.; Roman, C.M.; Schick, K.J.; Tapper, E.E.; Moreno, P.R.; Ruff, M.W.; Walters, D.K.; et al. Targeting Cancer Associated Fibroblasts in the Bone Marrow Prevents Resistance to Chimeric Antigen Receptor T Cell Therapy in Multiple Myeloma. *Blood* **2019**, *134*, 865. [CrossRef]
52. Rafiq, S.; Yeku, O.O.; Jackson, H.J.; Purdon, T.J.; Van Leeuwen, D.G.; Drakes, D.J.; Song, M.; Miele, M.M.; Li, Z.; Wang, P.; et al. Targeted delivery of a PD-1-blocking scFv by CAR-T cells enhances anti-tumor efficacy in vivo. *Nat. Biotechnol.* **2018**, *36*, 847–856. [CrossRef]
53. Suarez, E.; Chang, D.-K.; Sun, J.; Sui, J.; Freeman, G.J.; Signoretti, S.; Zhu, Q.; Marasco, W.A. Chimeric antigen receptor T cells secreting anti-PD-L1 antibodies more effectively regress renal cell carcinoma in a humanized mouse model. *Oncotarget* **2016**, *7*, 34341–34355. [CrossRef]
54. Shah, N.; Alsina, M.; Siegel, D.S.; Jagannath, S.; Madduri, D.; Kaufman, J.L.; Turka, A.; Lam, L.P.; Massaro, M.M.; Hege, K.; et al. Initial Results from a Phase 1 Clinical Study of bb21217, a Next-Generation Anti Bcma CAR T Therapy. *Blood* **2018**, *132*, 488. [CrossRef]
55. Alsina, M.; Shah, N.; Raje, N.S.; Jagannath, S.; Madduri, D.; Kaufman, J.L.; Siegel, D.S.; Munshi, N.C.; Rosenblatt, J.; Lin, Y.; et al. Updated Results from the Phase I CRB-402 Study of Anti-Bcma CAR-T Cell Therapy bb21217 in Patients with Relapsed and Refractory Multiple Myeloma: Correlation of Expansion and Duration of Response with T Cell Phenotypes. *Blood* **2020**, *136*, 25–26. [CrossRef]

56. Garfall, A.L.; Dancy, E.K.; Cohen, A.D.; Hwang, W.-T.; Fraietta, J.A.; Davis, M.M.; Levine, B.L.; Siegel, D.L.; Stadtmauer, E.A.; Vogl, D.T.; et al. T-cell phenotypes associated with effective CAR T-cell therapy in postinduction vs relapsed multiple myeloma. *Blood Adv.* **2019**, *3*, 2812–2815. [CrossRef]
57. Sadelain, M.; Rivière, M.S.I.; Riddell, S. Therapeutic T cell engineering. *Nat. Cell Biol.* **2017**, *545*, 423–431. [CrossRef]
58. Themeli, M.; Kloss, C.C.; Ciriello, G.; Fedorov, V.D.; Perna, F.; Gonen, M.; Sadelain, M. Generation of tumor-targeted human T lymphocytes from induced pluripotent stem cells for cancer therapy. *Nat. Biotechnol.* **2013**, *31*, 928–933. [CrossRef] [PubMed]
59. Bjordahl, R.; Gaidarova, S.; Goodridge, J.P.; Mahmood, S.; Bonello, G.; Robinson, M.; Ruller, C.; Pribadi, M.; Lee, T.; Abujarour, R.; et al. FT576: A novel multiplexed engineered off-the- shelf natural killer cell immunotherapy for the dualtargeting of CD38 and Bcma for the treatment of multiple myeloma. *Blood* **2019**, *134*, 3214. [CrossRef]

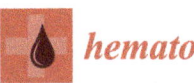

Review

Donor Lymphocyte Infusion to Enhance the Graft-versus-Myeloma Effect

Nico Gagelmann and Nicolaus Kröger *

Department of Stem Cell Transplantation, University Medical Center Hamburg-Eppendorf, 20246 Hamburg, Germany; n.gagelmann@uke.de
* Correspondence: nkroeger@uke.uni-hamburg.de; Tel.: +49-40-7410-54851

Abstract: Donor lymphocyte infusion (DLI) has the potential to significantly deepen the response after allogeneic stem cell transplantation (ASCT) in multiple myeloma (MM). Subsequently, DLI offers the opportunity for long-term progression-free and, most importantly, overall survival for patients with MM. DLI application is a complex procedure, whereby many factors need to be considered (e.g., patient-oriented factors prior to application, disease-specific factors, as well as possible combinations with further therapies during and after DLI). There are two settings in which DLI can be given, they are as follows: as a salvage option in progressive disease or in the prophylactic setting for MM patients with resolved disease to further deepen the response. While the first studies used DLI in the salvage setting, results for prophylactic DLI appear to be associated with better and prolonged outcomes. Furthermore, DLI (both prophylactic and salvage) given earlier after ASCT (3–6 months) appear to be associated with better outcomes. The incorporation of novel agents showed similar responses and survival after DLI. However, updated and larger evaluations are urgently needed to determine the specific role of multiple variables in such a complex treatment environment of ASCT in an ever-evolving field of MM. This review underlines the rationale for DLI after ASCT, results in the salvage and prophylactic settings, patterns of disease progression after DLI, as well as avenues to further enhance the graft-versus-myeloma effect exerted by DLI.

Keywords: graft-versus-myeloma; donor lymphocyte infusion; myeloma; allogeneic stem cell transplantation; prophylaxis; salvage; relapse

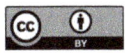

1. Introduction

Multiple myeloma (MM) is a yet incurable hematologic malignancy that has benefited from the advent of novel agents over the last decade. Despite major advances in treating MM throughout the disease course, allogeneic stem cell transplantation (alloSCT) remains a potentially curative treatment option [1,2]. However, the application of alloSCT is increasingly challenged by new therapies and its inherent association with treatment-associated morbidity and mortality [3,4]. Therefore, the proper incorporation of alloSCT within a whole (immune-) therapeutic environment, which improves outcome of specific subgroups of patients, needs yet to be identified, especially in the advent of ever-improving outcomes using novel agents [5–7].

Alloreactive immune effector cells originating from an MM-free graft may exert graft-versus-myeloma (GVM) effects, which can lead to the long-term control of disease [8]. One immunotherapeutic approach post-alloSCT is donor lymphocyte infusion (DLI), which is believed to augment these GVM effects supporting MM control, by deepening responses [9,10]. On the other hand, DLI may cause graft-versus-host disease (GVHD), which could become life threatening if it is acute, whereas even chronic GVHD may be important for the exertion of GVM effects [11]. Here, we present a comprehensive review of the role and the potential benefits and risks of DLI in post-alloSCT therapy for MM.

2. Prophylactic Setting

Although DLI was mostly given in the context of refractory or progressive disease posttransplant (see above), this modality of immunotherapy has also been adopted for and incorporated into the prophylactic post-alloSCT setting for patients with resolved disease. These prophylactic applications of DLI using a prespecified schedule or planned escalated incremental doses during T-cell reconstitution may enhance donor-derived T-cell reconstitution and further support the GVM effect.

One early single-center analysis of 24 patients undergoing CD6 T-cell-depleted alloSCT from HLA-identical sibling donors between 1996 and 1999 evaluated prophylactic CD4+ DLI 6 to 9 months after alloSCT [12]. All patients, including patients with complete remission after alloSCT, were eligible to receive DLI if there was no evidence of GVHD and if they were not receiving medication for GVHD. The first 11 patients received a single infusion of 3×10^7 cells/kg, and 3 patients received a single infusion of 1×10^7 cells/kg. After DLI, no other immune-modulating therapy nor prophylaxis for GVHD was given. Fourteen patients received DLI, 3 in complete response and 11 with persistent disease after BMT. Significant GVM responses were noted, resulting in 6 complete responses and 4 partial responses in patients with previous persistent disease. After DLI, 50% of the patients developed higher-grade acute GVHD (grades > 2). Survival at 2 years for all patients was 55%, and progression-free survival was 42%. The 14 patients receiving DLI showed a better 2-year progression-free survival of 65% when compared with a historical cohort of MM patients. This study also highlights the importance of patient selection and management, since only 58% of the included patients could actually receive DLI.

A long-term follow-up and single-center study of prophylactic DLI [13] recently underlined these findings, but also highlighted the complexity of the alloSCT treatment platform [14]. This study had a long-term follow-up of >5 years. A total of 61 patients with MM, who did not relapse nor develop disease progression after alloSCT, were treated with prophylactic escalating DLI, including a total of 132 DLI procedures. The overall response rate was high (77%). Thirty-three patients (54%) upgraded their remission status, with a quarter of patients even achieving molecular remission. The cumulative incidence of acute GVHD was moderate (33%), and no treatment-related mortality was observed. After a median follow-up of 69 months from the first DLI, 8-year progression-free and overall survival were 43% and 67%, respectively, with rates of 62% and 83% for patients in molecular remission. In multivariable analysis, molecular remission was the only independent prognostic factor for progression-free survival, while for overall survival, only cytogenetics were significantly associated with survival (i.e., worse outcome for high-risk cytogenetics). In that study, no impact of novel agents was observed. However, the use of novel agents was associated with more DLI procedures [13,15,16]. Furthermore, patients who received unstimulated DLI had a higher risk of acute GVHD, which was not associated with higher response rates in comparison with those who received G-CSF-stimulated T cells that were obtained from the original alloSCT product. These findings are in line with a recent comparison of stimulated and unstimulated DLI, showing no significant differences regarding response, survival, and safety [17]. The main results of the studies in both the prophylactic and salvage setting are listed in Tables 1 and 2.

Table 1. Results of prophylactic donor lymphocyte infusion (DLI).

Study (Year)	N	Graft Type	Dose (Range), ×10⁶ Cells/kg	Response, %	Acute GVHD, n	Survival
Alyea [12] (2001)	14	MRD	10–30	86	7	PFS: 65% 2y
Badros [18] (2001)	14	MRD	120–220	86	10	OS: 69% 1y
Peggs [19] (2003)	20	MRD/MUD	1–100	50	3	PFS: 30% 2y OS: 71% 2y
Kröger [10] (2009)	32	MRD/MUD	0.5–200	78	13	PFS: 54% 5y
Gröger [13] (2018)	61	MRD/MUD	0.3–100	77	7	PFS: 43% 8y OS: 67% 8y

Abbreviations: MRD, matched related donor; MUD, matched unrelated donor; GVHD, graft-versus-host disease; y, years; m, months; N, number; DLI, donor lymphocyte infusion; PFS, progression-free survival; OS, overall survival.

Table 2. Results of salvage DLI.

Study (Year)	N	Graft Type	Dose (Range), ×10⁶ Cells/kg	Response, %	Acute GVHD, n	Survival
Lokhorst [9] (1997)	13	MRD	1–330	62	9	54% 1y
Salama [20] (2000)	25	MRD/MUD	2–224	36	13	48% 1y
Lokhorst [21] (2004)	54	MRD	1–500	52	31	PFS: 19m OS: 23m
El-Cheikh [22] (2012)	9	MRD/MUD	10–100	75	1	PFS: 50% 2y OS: 69% 2y
Montefusco [23] (2013)	19	MRD/MUD	0.5–100	68	2	PFS: 31% 3y OS: 73% 3y

Abbreviations: MRD, matched related donor; MUD, matched unrelated donor; GVHD, graft-versus-host disease; y, years; m, months; N, number; DLI, donor lymphocyte infusion; PFS, progression-free survival; OS, overall survival.

3. Salvage Setting

Donor lymphocyte infusions have long been an important strategy for patients with hematologic malignancies who have experienced relapse after alloSCT [24]. Early on, the most impressive results have been obtained in patients with post-alloSCT relapsed chronic myelogenous leukemia, especially when initiated in patients with cytogenetic relapse or in those who have relapsed into the chronic phase [25,26]. In the late 1990s, the first reports suggested antitumor effects in MM patients. In 1996, Tricot et al. [8] reported the achievement of complete remission with a single dose of CD3+ cells in an MM patient who had progressed after alloSCT, providing the first proof-of-concept for utilizing DLI to induce a GVM effect.

Soon after that, one retrospective study evaluated the impact of DLI in 13 patients with relapsed MM after alloSCT [9]. The patients received a total of 29 DLIs with T-cell doses ranging from 1×10^6/kg to 33×10^7/kg. Doses, sometimes with escalated levels, were repeated if no response or another relapse was observed after DLI. Eight patients responded, with 4 even achieving complete remission, while the others achieved partial remission. Median time from dli to response was 6 weeks. Major toxicities were secondary to GVHD, which was observed in >50% of patients and in >80% of the responders. Fatal aplasia was seen in 2 patients who responded. The only prognostic factors for response were single T-cell doses $>1 \times 10^8$/kg and the occurrence of acute GVHD. This first experience identified the importance of individual dosing schemes and acute GVHD, suggesting escalating doses until the maximum response has been achieved.

A follow-up and extension included 27 patients who received 52 DLI courses for a median of 30 months after alloSCT [21]. Fourteen patients (52%) responded to DLI, with

6 patients achieving complete remission (22%). Five patients remained in remission for more than 30 months after DLI. Acute GVHD was present in 55% of the patients. Two patients died due to aplasia. The median overall survival was 18 months. Comparing responders and DLI-resistant patients, the median survival was not reached compared with 11 months. In two patients, sustained molecular remission was observed. Again, one key factor that was associated with response was a cell dose $>1 \times 10^8$/kg.

Subsequently, a study from 4 Dutch transplant centers was reported [27], analyzing 54 patients (with a median age of 52 years), of whom 50 showed relapse following myeloablative partially T-cell-depleted alloSCT, and 4 following non-T-cell-depleted myeloablative alloSCT. Most patients received high-dose cyclophosphamide and total body irradiation (12 Gy) conditioning. A total of 95 DLI procedures (range, 1–7) for a median of 20 months were given. The T-cell doses of DLI varied between 1×10^6 and 5×10^8 cells/kg. Most patients received a starting dose of 1×10^7 cells/kg. Dose escalation was done in the absence of response and acute GVHD until 3 months after the first DLI. Forty patients received reinduction therapy before DLI with vincristine/adriamycin/dexamethasone, dexamethasone alone, or melphalan alone. Response rates were comparable with previous findings, and progression-free and overall survival were 19 and 23 months, respectively. Acute GVHD after DLI was the strongest predictor of response. In patients with deletion of chromosome 13, as determined by double-color fluorescence in situ hybridization (FISH), no difference in outcome was seen.

Another study on dose-escalating salvage DLI was undergone in patients receiving reduced-intensity conditioning [28]. Grade 3–4 acute GVHD was found in 14% of patients and 1 patient died because of grade 4 acute GVHD. Despite the lower median cell dose for unrelated DLI (1×10^6 compared with 4.7×10^6 CD3+ cells/kg for related DLI), only the unrelated DLI recipients showed acute GVHD. With respect to responses, 19% showed complete response and partial remission, respectively. Stable disease was seen in 29%, while 33% of patients showed progressive disease. Median time from dli and response was 2 months. One-third of patients showed response after the first DLI. The median follow-up from DLI was 7 months, and 71% of the patients were alive, with three patients still in complete remission at the last follow-up at 8–14 months.

To assess the impact of combination approaches, a prospective phase 2 study evaluated the efficacy and safety of the combination of bortezomib/dexamethasone followed by DLI [23]. Patients received 3 cycles of bortezomib/dexamethasone followed by escalated doses of DLIs in the cases of response or at least stable disease. Fourteen days after the third course, and in the absence of acute GVHD, DLI was administered every 6 weeks at escalating cell doses, for up to 4 infusions. For the transplants from HLA-identical siblings, the infusions were done at the following cell doses: 5×10^6 CD3+/kg, 1×10^7 CD3+/kg, 5×10^7 CD3+/kg, and 1×10^8 CD3+/kg. For transplants from HLA-mismatched siblings or matched unrelated donors, the infusion scheme consisted of 5×10^5 CD3+/kg, 1×10^6 CD3+/kg, 5×10^6 CD3+/kg, and 1×10^7 CD3+/kg. In the case of complete remission before the first DLI, the patients received only the first 2 DLI doses. The study included 19 patients with a median age of 57 years. Fourteen patients received HLA-identical sibling alloSCT and 5 received matched unrelated donor alloSCT. Before DLI, the response rate was 62%, including 1 complete remission. After DLI, the response rate was 68%, observing a significant deepening of responses, showing 3 stringent complete responses and 2 complete responses. At a median follow-up of 40 months, 3-year progression-free survival and overall survival rates were 31% and 73%, respectively. Notably, no severe GVHD was seen.

4. Prognostic Factors in Salvage Setting

Importantly, it needs to be stressed that most analyses included only a small number of patients and may not depict accurate relations because of the lack of control settings. In a retrospective study of 48 relapsed MM patients and 15 patients with persistent disease after non-myeloablative alloSCT, prognostic factors for efficacy of DLI were analyzed [29]. The conditioning consisted of TBI (Total body irradiation) only, TBI and fludarabine, melphalan only, or thiotepa and cyclophosphamide. The overall survival after DLI was 24 months (1–51 months). The median overall survival was not reached for responders while non-responders showed a median survival of 24 months. Progression-free survival was remarkably higher in patients with complete response (28 months), compared with those achieving only partial remission (7 months). The only significant prognostic factor for response to DLI was the occurrence of acute GVHD, and patients who received their DLI earlier after alloSCT appeared to benefit more than patients who received their DLI one year after alloSCT.

5. DLI and Patterns of Disease Progression

To date, the clinical kinetics of alloreactive T cells in controlling MM progression or even inducing regression are not fully understood. An efficient GVM response requires accurate targeting of malignant cells by antigen-specific T cells in all sites of MM infiltration. While homing of T cells to the bone marrow was found to happen constitutively, other tissues may need ligand specificity of T cells, or inflammatory environments [30,31]. As a result, the strength of the immune response may differ and result in differential progression patterns of MM after cellular therapy such as alloSCT and DLI [32].

One study hypothesized that alloSCT and DLI modulate patterns of MM progression. To test this, marrow and focal progression were assessed as separate events in a cohort of 43 patients who underwent alloSCT with planned DLI in comparison with outcomes of a cohort of 12 patients who did not receive alloSCT [33]. After DLI, complete disappearance of MM cells in the bone marrow occurred in 86% of evaluable patients. The probabilities of so-called bone marrow progression-free survival at 2 years after DLI was 62%. In contrast, the probability of focal progression-free survival was 28%. In sum, donor-derived T-cell responses effectively reduce bone marrow infiltration, while focal progression did not seem to be successfully influenced.

In contrast, one study from Minnema et al. [32] showed that the treatment of extramedullary relapse after alloSCT, using DLI in combination with bortezomib or thalidomide, showed complete responses and did not differ in comparison with those who did not have extramedullary relapse. Notably, patients with only skin involvement showed complete response after DLI, while patients with multiple involvements of the kidney, skin, and lymph nodes showed no response. Whether antitumor effects are not only site-specific when comparing marrow and extramedullary sites, but also organ-specific, needs to be addressed in future studies.

6. Improving DLI Effects

6.1. Enhance the Immune Response

Despite the impressive results of recent long-term outcome data of prophylactic DLI [13], and due to the consistent refinement of novel agent treatment schedules combining steroids, immunomodulation, and monoclonal antibodies, alloSCT is nowadays no longer considered part of the standard upfront or sometimes even second-line therapy for MM. Therefore, strategies to alter the balance between GVM and GVHD, and diminish toxicity, need to be explored.

Based on findings from animal models, the presence of host-dendritic cells (host-DC) in mixed chimeric recipients is considered crucial for the development of an adequate antitumor effect. Host-DCs are more able to prime donor T cells against the host antigens expressed on malignant cells [34–36]. However, after alloSCT, MM patients rapidly convert to complete donor chimerism in the DC compartment, often before the establishment of an effective anti-MM response [37]. Therefore, combining DLI with the infusion of host-DC was hypothesized to maximize GVM. However, the host-DCs may be infused as such to induce a GVM effect, as they already express the mismatched minor histocompatibility antigens. On the other hand and in addition, host-DCs may be loaded with the host hematopoietic minor histocompatibility antigens to guide the immune response towards MM cells [38]. One clinical phase 1/2 study tested this hypothesis [39]. Myeloma patients with persistent measurable disease after alloSCT and a first DLI were included. From 15 patients, 11 received a second equivalent dose of DLI combined with the repeated administration of a host-DC vaccine. The first 7 patients were treated with unloaded host-DCs, whereas the last four patients received a minor histocompatibility antigen-loaded host-DC vaccine. A portion of the vaccine included a control antigen. No new GVHD occurred and toxicity was mild. All evaluable patients developed objective T-cell responses against the control, 60% demonstrated anti-host T-cell responses, and 25% of patients with minor histocompatibility antigen-loaded host-DC vaccine induced an objective T-cell response against the relevant minor histocompatibility antigen peptide. However, only one patient showed stringent complete response. Despite its safety, this approach may need refinement, by developing more immunogenic products or by combining this vaccine with other immune boosting strategies [39,40].

6.2. Tumor-Specific T Cells

Another option could be the tumor-specific T cells. Previously, emerging tumor-specific T cells targeting the Wilms' tumor 1 (WT1) protein were associated with increased relapse-free survival in patients with hematologic malignancies after alloSCT [41,42]. In MM, one study examined responses after WT1-specific cytotoxic T lymphocytes (CTL) in relapsed MM and high-risk cytogenetics who were undergoing T-cell-depleted alloSCT followed by DLI [43]. Of 24 patients, all showed WT1-CTL responses before alloSCT, which were associated with pre-alloSCT tumor burden. All patients subsequently developed increased WT1-CTL frequencies, in the absence of graft-versus-host disease. Immunohistochemical analyses of WT1 and CD138 in bone marrow specimens demonstrated consistent coexpression within MM cells. Furthermore, WT1 expression in the bone marrow correlated with disease outcome. These first evaluations suggested an association of emerging WT1-CTL and GVM, supporting the idea of combined adoptive immunotherapies. However, translations into the clinical reality for MM patients are lacking.

Since GVM responses involve T-cell recognition of tumor-specific peptides presented by major histocompatibility complex molecules, it may be possible to identify and select donor T cells that provide beneficial antitumor responses but minimal GVHD risk. In this regard, immune transcriptome analyses of T-cell receptor (TCR) Vβ CDR3-size and -sequence is being used to characterize alloreactive versus tumor-specific T-cell responses. Previous studies showed that the Vβ families were involved in the GVM and GVH response in an MM alloSCT model, and found that the Vβ 2, 3 and 8.3 families of T cells were specifically involved in the GVM response [44]. The implication of these results would be that MM-specific T-cell subfamilies might be positively selected from the donor and could therefore be infused into MM patients after alloSCT [45]. As a result, no prior definition of target antigens would be needed. To test this rationale, one recent study used an allogeneic B10.D2→Balb/c alloSCT model with MOPC315.BM MM cells, first demonstrating that MM-bearing Balb/c mice initially respond to irradiation and auto-alloSCT but eventually relapse, similar to MM patients in the real world. After infusing mice with B10.D2 T cells from only the TCR Vβ 2, 3 and 8.3 repertoire, which was pre-activated in vitro, consistent GVM without GVHD or disease relapse was observed. These data highlight the possibility that tumor-specific allogeneic T-cell therapy may lead to long-term disease-free survival without GVHD in patients with MM.

6.3. Cancer/Testis Antigens

The specific expression of cancer/testis antigen patterns has been associated with disease stage and poor clinical prognostic indictors in MM [46]. Due to the immunosuppressive characteristics of MM, cancer/testis antigens have been studied in several treatment strategies. Responses specifically to New York esophageal squamous cell carcinoma 1 (NY-ESO-1) and melanoma-associated antigen (MAGE) have been the most reported, by simultaneously detecting serum antibodies as well as antigen-specific CD8+ T cells [47,48]. Importantly, strong antibody responses against cancer/testis antigens were preferentially found in patients undergoing alloSCT, which could therefore be targets for future post-alloSCT immunotherapy [49]. Moreover, primary autoantibodies against intracellular MM-specific tumor antigens such as NY-ESO-1 were rare but functional. Theoretically, they may have the ability to affect cellular anti-tumor immunity by developing monovalent and polyvalent immune complexes [50]. To further increase anti-MM responses, vaccines against these antigen targets may also provide treatment opportunities, using NY-ESO-1 pre-exposed dendritic cells or recombinant MAGE peptide plasmids [51]. However, no robust clinical trial data are currently existing, and more research is needed to find avenues identifying and realizing the full potential of cancer/testis antigens in MM and alloSCT.

6.4. Novel Agents

One study aimed to combine reduced-intensity alloSCT and escalating DLI with novel agents (thalidomide, bortezomib, and lenalidomide) to target complete remission [10]. Thirty-two patients achieving only partial remission after alloSCT were included. Complete remission was achieved >50%. After a median follow-up of 56 months, progression-free survival for patients who achieved complete remission was 58% in comparison with 35% for those who did not, while overall survival was 90% compared with 62%, respectively. Patients with molecular complete remission had significantly better progression-free and overall survival than patients without, showing 84% compared with 38% and 100% compared with 71%, respectively. Incidence of acute GVHD grades >2 was 33% and severe grade 3 GVHD was 7%. None of the patients developed grade 4 GVHD. These findings highlighted the utility of combination therapy post-alloSCT to deepen responses and, subsequently, improve outcomes with signals for cure in some patients.

7. Conclusions

Donor lymphocyte infusion, especially in the prophylactic setting, has the potential to significantly deepen the response after alloSCT, thereby offering the opportunity for long-term progression-free and, most importantly, overall survival for patients with MM. However, the dissection of the subgroup of patients who may benefit from alloSCT from those who may benefit from less toxic novel agent approaches remains crucial [52]. Limited evidence points to subgroups with high-risk MM patients, young and motivated patients [53–55]. Moreover, DLI application is a complex procedure, whereby many factors need to be considered (e.g., patient-oriented factors prior to application, disease-specific factors, as well as possible combinations with further therapies during and after DLI). The incorporation of novel agents showed similar responses and survival after DLI. To date, no specific information is available on the efficacy and safety of DLI after different transplant settings or maintenance approaches. Moreover, other cellular therapy approaches such as chimeric antigen receptor T-cell therapy, which was most recently approved for relapsed/refractory MM [56], and other immunotherapeutic approaches such as bispecific antibodies, will surely challenge alloSCT and DLI even further [57]. With promising responses across immunotherapeutic approaches, the myeloma community may be confident that immunotherapy will manifest itself for personalized myeloma therapy, although a cure does not seem achievable yet using these new treatment options.

Considering alloSCT, updated and larger evaluations are urgently needed to determine the specific role of multiple variables in such a complex treatment environment of alloSCT in an ever-evolving field of MM.

Author Contributions: N.G. and N.K. wrote the manuscript. All authors have read and agreed to the published version of the manuscript.

Funding: This research received no external funding.

Institutional Review Board Statement: Not applicable.

Informed Consent Statement: Not applicable.

Conflicts of Interest: The authors declare no conflict of interest.

References

1. Costa, L.J.; Iacobelli, S.; Pasquini, M.C.; Modi, R.; Giaccone, L.; Blade, J.; Schonland, S.; Evangelista, A.; Perez-Simon, J.A.; Hari, P.; et al. Long-term survival of 1338 MM patients treated with tandem autologous vs. autologous-allogeneic transplantation. *Bone Marrow Transplant.* **2020**, *55*, 1810–1816. [CrossRef]
2. Sobh, M.; Michallet, M.; Gahrton, G.; Iacobelli, S.; van Biezen, A.; Schönland, S.; Petersen, E.; Schaap, N.; Bonifazi, F.; Volin, L.; et al. Allogeneic hematopoietic cell transplantation for multiple myeloma in Europe: Trends and outcomes over 25 years. A study by the EBMT Chronic Malignancies Working Party. *Leukemia* **2016**, *30*, 2047–2054. [CrossRef] [PubMed]
3. Mina, R.; Lonial, S. Is there still a role for stem cell transplantation in multiple myeloma? *Cancer* **2019**, *125*, 2534–2543. [CrossRef] [PubMed]
4. Shah, U.A.; Mailankody, S. Emerging immunotherapies in multiple myeloma. *BMJ* **2020**, *370*, m3176. [CrossRef] [PubMed]
5. Gahrton, G.; Iacobelli, S.; Garderet, L.; Yakoub-Agha, I.; Schönland, S. Allogeneic Transplantation in Multiple Myeloma-Does It Still Have a Place? *J. Clin. Med.* **2020**, *9*, 2180. [CrossRef] [PubMed]
6. Malek, E.; El-Jurdi, N.; Kröger, N.; de Lima, M. Allograft for Myeloma: Examining Pieces of the Jigsaw Puzzle. *Front. Oncol.* **2017**, *7*, 287. [CrossRef]
7. Gahrton, G.; Iacobelli, S.; Björkstrand, B.; Hegenbart, U.; Gruber, A.; Greinix, H.; Volin, L.; Narni, F.; Carella, A.M.; Beksac, M.; et al. Autologous/reduced-intensity allogeneic stem cell transplantation vs. autologous transplantation in multiple myeloma: Long-term results of the EBMT-NMAM2000 study. *Blood* **2013**, *121*, 5055–5063. [CrossRef]
8. Tricot, G.; Vesole, D.H.; Jagannath, S.; Hilton, J.; Munshi, N.; Barlogie, B. Graft-versus-myeloma effect: Proof of principle. *Blood* **1996**, *87*, 1196–1198. [CrossRef]
9. Lokhorst, H.M.; Schattenberg, A.; Cornelissen, J.J.; Thomas, L.L.; Verdonck, L.F. Donor leukocyte infusions are effective in relapsed multiple myeloma after allogeneic bone marrow transplantation. *Blood* **1997**, *90*, 4206–4211. [CrossRef]
10. Kröger, N.; Badbaran, A.; Lioznov, M.; Schwarz, S.; Zeschke, S.; Hildebrand, Y.; Ayuk, F.; Atanackovic, D.; Schilling, G.; Zabelina, T.; et al. Post-transplant immunotherapy with donor-lymphocyte infusion and novel agents to upgrade partial into complete and molecular remission in allografted patients with multiple myeloma. *Exp. Hematol.* **2009**, *37*, 791–798. [CrossRef]
11. Donato, M.L.; Siegel, D.S.; Vesole, D.H.; McKiernan, P.; Nyirenda, T.; Pecora, A.L.; Baker, M.; Goldberg, S.L.; Mato, A.; Goy, A.; et al. The graft-versus-myeloma effect: Chronic graft-versus-host disease but not acute graft-versus-host disease prolongs survival in patients with multiple myeloma receiving allogeneic transplantation. *Biol. Blood Marrow Transplant.* **2014**, *20*, 1211–1216. [CrossRef] [PubMed]
12. Alyea, E.; Weller, E.; Schlossman, R.; Canning, C.; Webb, I.; Doss, D.; Mauch, P.; Marcus, K.; Fisher, D.; Freeman, A.; et al. T-cell–depleted allogeneic bone marrow transplantation followed by donor lymphocyte infusion in patients with multiple myeloma: Induction of graft-versus-myeloma effect. *Blood* **2001**, *98*, 934–939. [CrossRef]
13. Gröger, M.; Gagelmann, N.; Wolschke, C.; von Pein, U.-M.; Klyuchnikov, E.; Christopeit, M.; Zander, A.; Ayuk, F.; Kröger, N. Long-Term Results of Prophylactic Donor Lymphocyte Infusions for Patients with Multiple Myeloma after Allogeneic Stem Cell Transplantation. *Biol. Blood Marrow Transplant.* **2018**, *24*, 1399–1405. [CrossRef]
14. Kröger, N.; Perez-Simon, J.A.; Myint, H.; Klingemann, H.; Shimoni, A.; Nagler, A.; Martino, R.; Alegre, A.; Tomas, J.F.; Schwerdtfeger, R.; et al. Relapse to prior autograft and chronic graft-versus-host disease are the strongest prognostic factors for outcome of melphalan/fludarabine-based dose-reduced allogeneic stem cell transplantation in patients with multiple myeloma. *Biol. Blood Marrow Transplant.* **2004**, *10*, 698–708. [CrossRef]
15. Kröger, N.; Shimoni, A.; Zagrivnaja, M.; Ayuk, F.; Lioznov, M.; Schieder, H.; Renges, H.; Fehse, B.; Zabelina, T.; Nagler, A.; et al. Low-dose thalidomide and donor lymphocyte infusion as adoptive immunotherapy after allogeneic stem cell transplantation in patients with multiple myeloma. *Blood* **2004**, *104*, 3361–3363. [CrossRef]
16. Van de Donk, N.W.C.J.; Kröger, N.; Hegenbart, U.; Corradini, P.; San Miguel, J.F.; Goldschmidt, H.; Perez-Simon, J.A.; Zijlmans, M.; Raymakers, R.A.; Montefusco, V.; et al. Remarkable activity of novel agents bortezomib and thalidomide in patients not responding to donor lymphocyte infusions following nonmyeloablative allogeneic stem cell transplantation in multiple myeloma. *Blood* **2006**, *107*, 3415–3416. [CrossRef]
17. Lamure, S.; Paul, F.; Gagez, A.-L.; Delage, J.; Vincent, L.; Fegueux, N.; Sirvent, A.; Gehlkopf, E.; Veyrune, J.L.; Yang, L.Z.; et al. A Retrospective Comparison of DLI and gDLI for Post-Transplant Treatment. *J. Clin. Med.* **2020**, *9*. [CrossRef]
18. Badros, A.; Barlogie, B.; Morris, C.; Desikan, R.; Martin, S.R.; Munshi, N.; Zangari, M.; Mehta, J.; Toor, A.; Cottler-Fox, M.; et al. High response rate in refractory and poor-risk multiple myeloma after allotransplantation using a nonmyeloablative conditioning regimen and donor lymphocyte infusions. *Blood* **2001**, *97*, 2574–2579. [CrossRef]
19. Peggs, K.S.; Mackinnon, S.; Williams, C.D.; D'Sa, S.; Thuraisundaram, D.; Kyriakou, C.; Morris, E.C.; Hale, G.; Waldmann, H.; Linch, D.C.; et al. Reduced-intensity transplantation with in vivo T-cell depletion and adjuvant dose-escalating donor lymphocyte infusions for chemotherapy-sensitive myeloma: Limited efficacy of graft-versus-tumor activity. *Biol. Blood Marrow Transplant.* **2003**, *9*, 257–265. [CrossRef] [PubMed]
20. Salama, M.; Nevill, T.; Marcellus, D.; Parker, P.; Johnson, M.; Kirk, A.; Porter, D.; Giralt, S.; Levine, J.E.; Drobyski, W.; et al. Donor leukocyte infusions for multiple myeloma. *Bone Marrow Transplant.* **2000**, *26*, 1179–1184. [CrossRef] [PubMed]
21. Lokhorst, H.M.; Wu, K.; Verdonck, L.F.; Laterveer, L.L.; van de Donk, N.W.C.J.; van Oers, M.H.J.; Cornelissen, J.J.; Schattenberg, A.V. The occurrence of graft-versus-host disease is the major predictive factor for response to donor lymphocyte infusions in multiple myeloma. *Blood* **2004**, *103*, 4362–4364. [CrossRef]

22. El-Cheikh, J.; Crocchiolo, R.; Furst, S.; Ladaique, P.; Castagna, L.; Faucher, C.; Granata, A.; Oudin, C.; Lemarie, C.; Calmels, B.; et al. Lenalidomide plus donor-lymphocytes infusion after allogeneic stem-cell transplantation with reduced-intensity conditioning in patients with high-risk multiple myeloma. *Exp. Hematol.* **2012**, *40*, 521–527. [CrossRef] [PubMed]
23. Montefusco, V.; Spina, F.; Patriarca, F.; Offidani, M.; Bruno, B.; Montanari, M.; Mussetti, A.; Sperotto, A.; Scortechini, I.; Dodero, A.; et al. Bortezomib plus dexamethasone followed by escalating donor lymphocyte infusions for patients with multiple myeloma relapsing or progressing after allogeneic stem cell transplantation. *Biol. Blood Marrow Transplant.* **2013**, *19*, 424–428. [CrossRef] [PubMed]
24. Greiner, J.; Götz, M.; Bunjes, D.; Hofmann, S.; Wais, V. Immunological and Clinical Impact of Manipulated and Unmanipulated DLI after Allogeneic Stem Cell Transplantation of AML Patients. *J. Clin. Med.* **2019**, *9*, 39. [CrossRef] [PubMed]
25. Kolb, H.J.; Schattenberg, A.; Goldman, J.M.; Hertenstein, B.; Jacobsen, N.; Arcese, W.; Ljungman, P.; Ferrant, A.; Verdonck, L.; Niederwieser, D.; et al. Graft-versus-leukemia effect of donor lymphocyte transfusions in marrow grafted patients. *Blood* **1995**, *86*, 2041–2050. [CrossRef]
26. Collins, R.H.; Shpilberg, O.; Drobyski, W.R.; Porter, D.L.; Giralt, S.; Champlin, R.; Goodman, S.A.; Wolff, S.N.; Hu, W.; Verfaillie, C.; et al. Donor leukocyte infusions in 140 patients with relapsed malignancy after allogeneic bone marrow transplantation. *J. Clin. Oncol.* **1997**, *15*, 433–444. [CrossRef]
27. Lokhorst, H.M.; Schattenberg, A.; Cornelissen, J.J.; van Oers, M.H.; Fibbe, W.; Russell, I.; Donk, N.W.; Verdonck, L.F. Donor lymphocyte infusions for relapsed multiple myeloma after allogeneic stem-cell transplantation: Predictive factors for response and long-term outcome. *J. Clin. Oncol.* **2000**, *18*, 3031–3037. [CrossRef]
28. Ayuk, F.; Shimoni, A.; Nagler, A.; Schwerdtfeger, R.; Kiehl, M.; Sayer, H.G.; Zabelina, T.; Zander, A.R.; Kröger, N. Efficacy and toxicity of low-dose escalating donor lymphocyte infusion given after reduced intensity conditioning allograft for multiple myeloma. *Leukemia* **2004**, *18*, 659–662. [CrossRef]
29. Van de Donk, N.W.C.J.; Kröger, N.; Hegenbart, U.; Corradini, P.; San Miguel, J.F.; Goldschmidt, H.; Perez-Simon, J.A.; Zijlmans, M.; Raymakers, R.A.; Montefusco, V.; et al. Prognostic factors for donor lymphocyte infusions following non-myeloablative allogeneic stem cell transplantation in multiple myeloma. *Bone Marrow Transplant.* **2006**, *37*, 1135–1141. [CrossRef]
30. Brinkman, C.C.; Rouhani, S.J.; Srinivasan, N.; Engelhard, V.H. Peripheral tissue homing receptors enable T cell entry into lymph nodes and affect the anatomical distribution of memory cells. *J. Immunol.* **2013**, *191*, 2412–2425. [CrossRef]
31. Van der Voort, R.; Volman, T.J.H.; Verweij, V.; Linssen, P.C.M.; Maas, F.; Hebeda, K.M.; Dolstra, H. Homing characteristics of donor T cells after experimental allogeneic bone marrow transplantation and posttransplantation therapy for multiple myeloma. *Biol. Blood Marrow Transplant.* **2013**, *19*, 378–386. [CrossRef] [PubMed]
32. Minnema, M.C.; van de Donk, N.W.C.J.; Zweegman, S.; Hegenbart, U.; Schonland, S.; Raymakers, R.; Zijlmans, J.M.J.M.; Kersten, M.J.; Bos, G.M.J.; Lokhorst, H.M. Extramedullary relapses after allogeneic non-myeloablative stem cell transplantation in multiple myeloma patients do not negatively affect treatment outcome. *Bone Marrow Transplant.* **2008**, *41*, 779–784. [CrossRef]
33. Eefting, M.; de Wreede, L.C.; von dem Borne, P.A.; Halkes, C.J.M.; Kersting, S.; Marijt, E.W.A.; Putter, H.; Veelken, H.; Schetelig, J.; Falkenburg, J.H.F. Donor T-cell responses and disease progression patterns of multiple myeloma. *Bone Marrow Transplant.* **2017**, *52*, 1609–1615. [CrossRef]
34. Shlomchik, W.D.; Couzens, M.S.; Tang, C.B.; McNiff, J.; Robert, M.E.; Liu, J.; Shlomchik, M.J.; Emerson, S.G. Prevention of graft versus host disease by inactivation of host antigen-presenting cells. *Science* **1999**, *285*, 412–415. [CrossRef]
35. Duffner, U.A.; Maeda, Y.; Cooke, K.R.; Reddy, P.; Ordemann, R.; Liu, C.; Ferrara, J.L.M.; Teshima, T. Host dendritic cells alone are sufficient to initiate acute graft-versus-host disease. *J. Immunol.* **2004**, *172*, 7393–7398. [CrossRef]
36. Mapara, M.Y.; Kim, Y.-M.; Wang, S.-P.; Bronson, R.; Sachs, D.H.; Sykes, M. Donor lymphocyte infusions mediate superior graft-versus-leukemia effects in mixed compared to fully allogeneic chimeras: A critical role for host antigen-presenting cells. *Blood* **2002**, *100*, 1903–1909. [CrossRef]
37. Auffermann-Gretzinger, S.; Lossos, I.S.; Vayntrub, T.A.; Leong, W.; Grumet, F.C.; Blume, K.G.; Stockerl-Goldstein, K.E.; Levy, R.; Shizuru, J.A. Rapid establishment of dendritic cell chimerism in allogeneic hematopoietic cell transplant recipients. *Blood* **2002**, *99*, 1442–1448. [CrossRef] [PubMed]
38. Oostvogels, R.; Minnema, M.C.; van Elk, M.; Spaapen, R.M.; te Raa, G.D.; Giovannone, B.; Buijs, A.; van Baarle, D.; Kater, A.P.; Griffioen, M.; et al. Towards effective and safe immunotherapy after allogeneic stem cell transplantation: Identification of hematopoietic-specific minor histocompatibility antigen UTA2-1. *Leukemia* **2013**, *27*, 642–649. [CrossRef] [PubMed]
39. Oostvogels, R.; Kneppers, E.; Minnema, M.C.; Doorn, R.C.; Franssen, L.E.; Aarts, T.; Emmelot, M.E.; Spierings, E.; Slaper-Cortenbach, I.; Westinga, K.; et al. Efficacy of host-dendritic cell vaccinations with or without minor histocompatibility antigen loading, combined with donor lymphocyte infusion in multiple myeloma patients. *Bone Marrow Transplant.* **2017**, *52*, 228–237. [CrossRef] [PubMed]
40. Franssen, L.E.; Roeven, M.W.H.; Hobo, W.; Doorn, R.; Oostvogels, R.; Falkenburg, J.H.F.; van de Donk, N.W.; Kester, M.G.D.; Fredrix, H.; Westinga, K.; et al. A phase I/II minor histocompatibility antigen-loaded dendritic cell vaccination trial to safely improve the efficacy of donor lymphocyte infusions in myeloma. *Bone Marrow Transplant.* **2017**, *52*, 1378–1383. [CrossRef]
41. Rezvani, K.; Yong, A.S.M.; Savani, B.N.; Mielke, S.; Keyvanfar, K.; Gostick, E.; Price, D.A.; Douek, D.C.; Barrett, A.J. Graft-versus-leukemia effects associated with detectable Wilms tumor-1 specific T lymphocytes after allogeneic stem-cell transplantation for acute lymphoblastic leukemia. *Blood* **2007**, *110*, 1924–1932. [CrossRef] [PubMed]

42. Kapp, M.; Stevanović, S.; Fick, K.; Tan, S.M.; Loeffler, J.; Opitz, A.; Tonn, T.; Stuhler, G.; Einsele, H.; Grigoleit, G.U. CD8+ T-cell responses to tumor-associated antigens correlate with superior relapse-free survival after allo-SCT. *Bone Marrow Transplant.* **2009**, *43*, 399–410. [CrossRef] [PubMed]
43. Tyler, E.M.; Jungbluth, A.A.; O'Reilly, R.J.; Koehne, G. WT1-specific T-cell responses in high-risk multiple myeloma patients undergoing allogeneic T cell-depleted hematopoietic stem cell transplantation and donor lymphocyte infusions. *Blood* **2013**, *121*, 308–317. [CrossRef] [PubMed]
44. Binsfeld, M.; Beguin, Y.; Belle, L.; Otjacques, E.; Hannon, M.; Briquet, A.; Heusschen, R.; Drion, P.; Zilberberg, J.; Bogen, B.; et al. Establishment of a murine graft-versus-myeloma model using allogeneic stem cell transplantation. *PLoS ONE* **2014**, *9*, e113764. [CrossRef] [PubMed]
45. Yado, S.; Luboshits, G.; Hazan, O.; Or, R.; Firer, M.A. Long-term survival without graft-versus-host-disease following infusion of allogeneic myeloma-specific Vβ T cell families. *J. Immunother. Cancer* **2019**, *7*, 301. [CrossRef]
46. Atanackovic, D.; Hildebrandt, Y.; Jadczak, A.; Cao, Y.; Luetkens, T.; Meyer, S.; Kobold, S.; Bartels, K.; Pabst, C.; Lajmi, N.; et al. Cancer-testis antigens MAGE-C1/CT7 and MAGE-A3 promote the survival of multiple myeloma cells. *Haematologica* **2010**, *95*, 785–793. [CrossRef] [PubMed]
47. Rapoport, A.P.; Stadtmauer, E.A.; Binder-Scholl, G.K.; Goloubeva, O.; Vogl, D.T.; Lacey, S.F.; Badros, A.Z.; Garfall, A.; Weiss, B.; Finklestein, J.; et al. NY-ESO-1-specific TCR-engineered T cells mediate sustained antigen-specific antitumor effects in myeloma. *Nat. Med.* **2015**, *21*, 914–921. [CrossRef] [PubMed]
48. Lajmi, N.; Luetkens, T.; Yousef, S.; Templin, J.; Cao, Y.; Hildebrandt, Y.; Bartels, K.; Kröger, N.; Atanackovic, D. Cancer-testis antigen MAGEC2 promotes proliferation and resistance to apoptosis in Multiple Myeloma. *Br. J. Haematol.* **2015**, *171*, 752–762. [CrossRef]
49. Atanackovic, D.; Arfsten, J.; Cao, Y.; Gnjatic, S.; Schnieders, F.; Bartels, K.; Schilling, G.; Faltz, C.; Wolschke, C.; Dierlamm, J.; et al. Cancer-testis antigens are commonly expressed in multiple myeloma and induce systemic immunity following allogeneic stem cell transplantation. *Blood* **2007**, *109*, 1103–1112. [CrossRef]
50. Luetkens, T.; Kobold, S.; Cao, Y.; Ristic, M.; Schilling, G.; Tams, S.; Bartels, B.M.; Templin, J.; Bartels, K.; Hildebrandt, Y.; et al. Functional autoantibodies against SSX-2 and NY-ESO-1 in multiple myeloma patients after allogeneic stem cell transplantation. *Cancer Immunol. Immunother.* **2014**, *63*, 1151–1162. [CrossRef]
51. Rapoport, A.P.; Aqui, N.A.; Stadtmauer, E.A.; Vogl, D.T.; Xu, Y.Y.; Kalos, M.; Cai, L.; Fang, H.-B.; Weiss, B.M.; Badros, A.; et al. Combination immunotherapy after ASCT for multiple myeloma using MAGE-A3/Poly-ICLC immunizations followed by adoptive transfer of vaccine-primed and costimulated autologous T cells. *Clin. Cancer Res.* **2014**, *20*, 1355–1365. [CrossRef]
52. Sonneveld, P.; Avet-Loiseau, H.; Lonial, S.; Usmani, S.; Siegel, D.; Anderson, K.C.; Chng, W.-J.; Moreau, P.; Attal, M.; Kyle, R.A.; et al. Treatment of multiple myeloma with high-risk cytogenetics: A consensus of the International Myeloma Working Group. *Blood* **2016**, *127*, 2955–2962. [CrossRef]
53. Maffini, E.; Storer, B.E.; Sandmaier, B.M.; Bruno, B.; Sahebi, F.; Shizuru, J.A.; Chauncey, T.R.; Hari, P.; Lange, T.; Pulsipher, M.A.; et al. Long-term follow up of tandem autologous-allogeneic hematopoietic cell transplantation for multiple myeloma. *Haematologica* **2019**, *104*, 380–391. [CrossRef] [PubMed]
54. Jurgensen-Rauch, A.; Gibbs, S.; Farrell, M.; Aries, J.; Grantham, M.; Eccersley, L.; Gribben, J.; Hallam, S.; Oakervee, H.; Cavenagh, J.; et al. Reduced intensity allogeneic hematopoietic stem cell transplantation is a safe and effective treatment option in high-risk myeloma patients—A single centre experience. *Br. J. Haematol.* **2021**. [CrossRef] [PubMed]
55. Gagelmann, N.; Eikema, D.-J.; de Wreede, L.C.; Rambaldi, A.; Iacobelli, S.; Koster, L.; Caillot, D.; Blaise, D.; Remémyi, P.; Bulabois, C.-E.; et al. Upfront stem cell transplantation for newly diagnosed multiple myeloma with del(17p) and t(4;14): A study from the CMWP-EBMT. *Bone Marrow Transplant.* **2021**, *56*, 210–217. [CrossRef] [PubMed]
56. Bruno, B.; Wäsch, R.; Engelhardt, M.; Gay, F.; Giaccone, L.; D'Agostino, M.; Rodríguez-Lobato, L.-G.; Danhof, S.; Gagelmann, N.; Kröger, N.; et al. European Myeloma Network perspective on CAR T-Cell therapies for multiple myeloma. *Haematologica* **2021**. [CrossRef]
57. Rasche, L.; Hudecek, M.; Einsele, H. What is the future of immunotherapy in multiple myeloma? *Blood* **2020**, *136*, 2491–2497. [CrossRef] [PubMed]

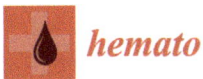

Review

Role and Modulation of NK Cells in Multiple Myeloma

Marie Thérèse Rubio [1],*, Adèle Dhuyser [2] and Stéphanie Nguyen [3]

1. Service d'Hématologie, Hopital Brabois, CHRU Nancy, CNRS UMR 7563 IMoPa, Biopole de l'Université de Lorraine, 54500 Vandoeuvre-les-Nancy, France
2. Laboratoire HLA, Hopital Brabois, CHRU Nancy, CNRS UMR 7563 IMoPa, Biopole de l'Université de Lorraine, 54500 Vandoeuvre-les-Nancy, France; adele.dhuyser@gmail.com
3. Service d'Hématologie Clinique, Groupe Hospitalier Pitié-Salpêtrière APHP.6, Pavillon Georges Heuyer and INSERM CNRS 1135, NK and T Cell Immunity, Virus and Cancer, Centre d'Immunologie et des Pathologies Infectieuses (CIMI), Sorbonne Université, 47–83 Bd de l'Hôpital, CEDEX 13, 75651 Paris, France; stephanie.nguyen-quoc@aphp.fr
* Correspondence: m.rubio@chru-nancy.fr; Tel.: +33-385-153-282; Fax: +33-385-153-558

Abstract: Myeloma tumor cells are particularly dependent on their microenvironment and sensitive to cellular antitumor immune response, including natural killer (NK) cells. These later are essential innate lymphocytes implicated in the control of viral infections and cancers. Their cytotoxic activity is regulated by a balance between activating and inhibitory signals resulting from the complex interaction of surface receptors and their respective ligands. Myeloma disease evolution is associated with a progressive alteration of NK cell number, phenotype and cytotoxic functions. We review here the different therapeutic approaches that could restore or enhance NK cell functions in multiple myeloma. First, conventional treatments (immunomodulatory drugs-IMids and proteasome inhibitors) can enhance NK killing of tumor cells by modulating the expression of NK receptors and their corresponding ligands on NK and myeloma cells, respectively. Because of their ability to kill by antibody-dependent cell cytotoxicity, NK cells are important effectors involved in the efficacy of anti-myeloma monoclonal antibodies targeting the tumor antigens CD38, CS1 or BCMA. These complementary mechanisms support the more recent therapeutic combination of IMids or proteasome inhibitors to monoclonal antibodies. We finally discuss the ongoing development of new NK cell-based immunotherapies, such as ex vivo expanded killer cell immunoglobulin-like receptors (KIR)-mismatched NK cells, chimeric antigen receptors (CAR)-NK cells, check point and KIR inhibitors.

Keywords: myeloma; NK cells; immunomodulation; cell therapy; immunotherapy

Citation: Rubio, M.T.; Dhuyser, A.; Nguyen, S. Role and Modulation of NK Cells in Multiple Myeloma. *Hemato* **2021**, *2*, 167–181. https://doi.org/10.3390/hemato2020010

Academic Editor: Nicolaus Kröger

Received: 5 March 2021
Accepted: 28 March 2021
Published: 2 April 2021

Publisher's Note: MDPI stays neutral with regard to jurisdictional claims in published maps and institutional affiliations.

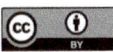

Copyright: © 2021 by the authors. Licensee MDPI, Basel, Switzerland. This article is an open access article distributed under the terms and conditions of the Creative Commons Attribution (CC BY) license (https://creativecommons.org/licenses/by/4.0/).

1. Introduction

Multiple myeloma (MM) is a mature B-cell hematologic neoplasia characterized by the clonal proliferation of plasma cells in the bone marrow [1]. It evolves in a multistep way from the pre-malignant monoclonal gammopathy of undetermined significance (MGUS) through a phase of asymptomatic smoldering myeloma until the symptomatic phase of MM, often presenting with bone lesions, hypercalcemia, renal failure and anemia [2]. Cytogenetic and epigenetic events both contribute to the progression towards a more active disease and the failure of immune surveillance with a progressive impairment of both innate and adaptive antitumor immune responses [3]. Natural killer (NK) cells are innate lymphoid cells that have been shown to play a major role in the anti-myeloma immune response [4]. Despite the development of multiple treatment strategies, including chemotherapy, proteasome inhibitors, immunomodulatory drugs, monoclonal antibodies and hematopoietic stem cell transplantation, MM remains incurable. Many patients evolve to a relapse and refractory (R/R) MM. One goal of the new treatment strategies in MM is to restore an effective immune response against myeloma cells. This review provides an overview of NK cells' role in the development and treatment of MM and discusses potentially new NK-based immunotherapies that may improve clinical outcomes.

2. Biology of NK Cells

NK cells are innate lymphoid cells representing the first effectors against malignant or virus-infected cells. By contrast with T cells, NK cells can kill without prior sensitization or recognition of presented antigens [5]. Human NK cells are defined as $CD3^{neg}$ $CD56^+$ and represent 5 to 15% of peripheral blood lymphocytes among which, two subtypes have been phenotypically and functionally described: the $CD56^{dim}$ and $CD56^{bright}$ cells. $CD56^{dim}$ cells are characterized by cytotoxic activities, while $CD56^{bright}$ cells mainly produce cytokines, such as IFN-γ and TNF-α and are implicated in immune regulation [6]. They also can express CD16 (FCγRIIIa), which binds human IgG through their Fc fragment, allowing antibody-dependent cellular cytotoxicity (ADCC) to occur [5]. While the majority of circulating NK cells in the peripheral blood are $CD16^{bright}/CD56^{dim}$ with high cytotoxic capacities and low proliferative response to IL-2, NK cells localized in secondary lymphoid tissues or inflammation sites is $CD16^{dim/neg}/CD56^{bright}$, highly express IL2-R$\alpha$ and have high proliferative capacities, but lower cytotoxicity [5]. NK cell kills their target cells by releasing the content of their lytic granules (perforin, granzyme), by expressing death molecules (Fas-L, TRAIL) at their surface and by secreting INF-γ and TNF-α; all of them induce apoptosis through caspase-dependent and independent pathways [7].

NK cell function depends on integrating signals from the interaction between activating and inhibiting surface receptors and their respective ligands. The initial description of the "missing-self" mechanism of cell death (i.e., lack of expression of HLA class I molecules on target cells spotted by NK inhibitory receptors) has been since revisited. Regulation of NK function is recognized to be more complex and dependent on the relative balance between inhibitory and activating signals induced by the engagement of inhibitory versus activating receptors according to the presence or absence of cognate ligands on target cells [5].

Inhibitory receptors include killer cell immunoglobulin-like receptors (KIR) and non-KIR inhibitory receptors. Among the inhibitory KIRs, three are critical for NK cell function: KIR2DL1, KIR2DL2/3 and KIR3DL1, specific for HLA class I molecules (HLA-Cw antigens belonging to the HLA C2 and HLA C1 families, and HLA-Bw4 antigens, respectively). Identified non-KIR inhibitory receptors so far are the C-type lectin-like receptors CD94/NKG2A heterodimer (CD159a), specific for HLA-E; ILT2 (LILRB1, CD85) recognizing various class I antigens; NKR-P1A (CD161) recognizing the lectin-like transcript 1 (LLT1); and the carcinoembryonic antigen-related cell adhesion molecule 1 (CEACAM-1, CD66a) specific for CD66 ligand [8]. In addition, NK cells can express the checkpoint inhibitors, such as programmed cell death protein-1 (PD-1), T-cell immunoglobulin and mucin containing protein-3 (TIM-3) and T cell immunoreceptor with Ig and ITIM domains (TIGIT). They can be inhibited by interaction with the corresponding ligands often expressed on tumor cells: PD-L1 or PD-L2 for PD-1; HMGB1 (high mobility group B1 protein), CEACAM-1, phosphatidylserine or Galectin-9 for TIM-3; PVR (poliovirus receptor, CD155) and nectin-2 (CD112) for TIGIT [9] (Figure 1).

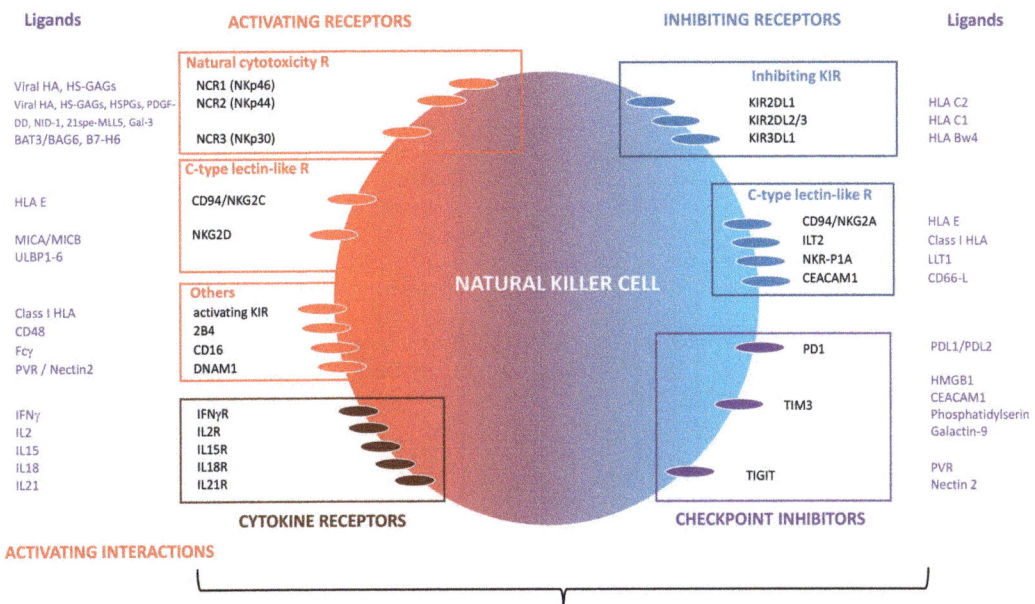

Figure 1. Natural killer (NK) cell inhibitory and activating receptors and ligands.

NK cells also express activating receptors. In addition to CD16 (FcγRIIIa), they can express natural cytotoxicity receptors NCRs: NKP46 (NCR1, CD335); NKp44 (NCR2, CD336) and NKp30 (NCR3, CD337), which ligands are partially characterized. The main ligands are derived from infectious agents (mainly viral hemagglutinins), cell-membrane, or extracellular matrix-derived proteins, such as heparan sulfate (HS) glycosaminoglycans (GAGs) or molecules expressed on tumor cells [10]. In the context of cancers, NKp46 can bind HS-GAGs, NKp44 can be activated by HS-proteoglycans (HSPGs), platelet-derived growth factor-DD (PDGF-DD), nidogen-1 (NID-1), an isoform of mixed-lineage leukemia protein-5 (21spe-MLL5) and Galectin 3 (Gla-3), while NKp30 recognizes HLA-B associated transcript 3/Bcl-2 associated pathogens 6 (BAT3/BAG6) and B7-H6 [10]. Other activating receptors include C-type lectin-like receptors, such as NKG2D (CD314) and the heterodimer CD94/NKG2C (CD159c) recognizing stress-induced cell surface ligands, such as the MHC-related ligands A and B (MICA, MICB) and the UL16-binding proteins 1–6 (ULBP1–6) for the first one and HLA-E for the later. Activating receptors include SLAM-related 2B4 (CD244), which engages CD48 and the DNAX accessory molecule-1 (DNAM1, CD226). recognizing PVR (polio virus receptor or CD155) and nectin-2 (CD112). Some KIRs recognizing classical and non-classical class I HLA molecules can be activating [8] (Figure 1).

NK cells express receptors for several cytokines (IFN-γ, IL-2, IL-15, IL-18, IL-21) involved in their survival, differentiation, activation and proliferation (Figure 1). IL-2 induces NK proliferation and increases NKG2D and NKp44 expression, while IL-15 drives NK cell differentiation and proliferation. The combination of IL-2 and IL-15 improves NK cell viability in vitro. IL-18 stimulates IFN-γ production and provides costimulatory activation, while IL-21 enhances NK cells' maturation [11]. Upon activation and Fc binding, NK cells express CD137 (4-1BB), and anti-CD157 mAbs enhance their cytotoxic properties [12].

3. NK Cells as Immunotherapeutic Effectors: Lessons from Allogeneic HSCT

In an autologous setting and the absence of stress, NK cells fail to kill autologous tumor cells as they are inhibited by the interaction between NK-inhibitory surface receptors (mainly KIR and CD94/NKG2A) and self HLA-class I ligands.

The proof of concept that NK cells may have an immunotherapeutic action against malignant cells first came from allogeneic hematopoietic stem cell (HSC) transplantation performed with haplo-HLA-mismatched donors (haplo-HSCT). The Perugia's group developed a platform of haplo-HSCT combining the use of a myeloablative conditioning regimen and the administration of a T-cell depleted megadose of CD34$^+$ selected HSCs allowing the engraftment of haplo-mismatched HSC with the absence of acute or chronic graft-versus-host disease (GVHD) [13]. This ex vivo T cell-depleted haplo-HSCT platform represented an ideal in vivo model to investigate the role of NK cells in the absence of confounding factors, such as alloreactive T cells or immunosuppressive drugs. In such an environment, donor KIR-mismatched NK cell clones expand after transplantation and have the capacity to kill recipient HSC, antigen-presenting cells (APC) and leukemic cells, thus facilitating engraftment and the graft-versus-leukemia effect without GVHD [14,15]. Other studies from the same group demonstrated that NK alloreactivity could be predicted by the "KIR–ligand mismatch" model based on the principle that when the donor carry at least one KIR ligand (i.e., HLA CLASS I Bw4, C1 or C2) absent in the transplant recipient, donor NK cells, supposed to express the corresponding inhibitory KIRs, will kill recipient cells missing the HLA Class I allele [16]. The role of alloreactive KIR-mismatched NK cells in the anti-leukemic effect has been confirmed by other models of in vitro T-cell depleted haplo-HSCT [17–19].

Because KIR and HLA genes are localized in distinct chromosomes (chromosome 19q13.4 and 6p21, respectively) and thus segregate independently, an HLA matched donor-recipient pair can be KIR-mismatched. More recent studies exploring NK alloreactivity on transplant outcomes have then been performed in T-cell repleted haploidentical, mismatched unrelated, cord-blood, but also in matched unrelated HSCT (MUD). In allo-HSCT performed with MUD and mismatched MUD, the group of Kroger showed a reduction of relapse in MM patients transplanted with a KIR–ligand-mismatched donor [20]. However, in these settings, the role of the KIR–ligand mismatches has been a matter of debate, with some studies showing no advantage or even a negative impact [21–25].

The development of KIR genotyping, considering both inhibitory and activating KIRs, has provided better predictive tools. Cooley et al. demonstrated that the assigned presence of a donor KIR genotype enriched in activating KIRs (Bx haplotype) was associated with better disease-free survival in AML transplanted with unrelated donors [26,27]. The combination of both donor KIR genotyping and donor/recipient HLA typing seems to represent the best approach to predict the potential impact of NK cells on post-transplant outcomes [28]. Impaired immune NK cell reconstitution after haplo-HSCT may also contribute to the contradictory clinical impact of NK cell alloreactivity reported so far [24,29].

Despite some controversial reports due to the use of distinct predictive models and to an imperfect understanding of NK cell interactions and regulation, it is acknowledged that NK cells play a role in the control of hematological malignancies.

4. NK Cells in MM

Several studies have pointed to the crucial role of NK cells in the control of MM. First, human plasma cells have been shown to be sensitive to NK cell killing from healthy donors [30]. Indeed, in MGUS and early-stage MM, plasma cells can be recognized and killed by NK cells through their expression of ligands for NK-activating receptors, such as the NKG2D ligands MICA and MICB, NKp30 ligand B7-H6, and DNAM-1 ligands nectin-2 and PVR, in combination with the reduced engagement of inhibitory KIR due to low HLA class I expression on myeloma cells [31,32].

However, both quantitative and qualitative alterations of NK cells have been reported in the progression from MGUS to MM. Compared to healthy individuals, a number of peripheral blood (PB) NK cells seem to decrease from the higher or normal value at the stage of MGUS or early-stage untreated MM to reduced numbers in advanced-stage untreated patients [33]. Functional studies have shown that NK remains cytotoxic in MGUS patients, while they may lose their cytotoxic capacities in advanced MM [34,35]. Decreased cytotoxicity is associated with reduced expression of activating receptors like CD16, NKG2D, NCRs, 2B4 and DNAM-1 in PB and/or BM NK cells of MM patients [32,36,37] and increase expression of the inhibitory receptors KIR2DL1 and PD1 [38,39]. After autologous HSCT, a higher expression of the activating receptor KIR2DS4 and decreased expression of the inhibitory CD94/NKG2A has been observed in patients with detectable minimal residual disease (MRD), analyzed by flow cytometry, compared with those with negative MRD [40].

Alterations of NK cell phenotype and functions are explained by the transformation of myeloma tumor cells and their microenvironment during disease evolution [41]. Many cellular and soluble factors have been involved in the alteration of NK cell phenotype and functions during the progression of the disease. Among those, TGF-β produced in MM by plasma cells [42], regulatory T cells (Tregs) [43] or potentially by myeloid-derived suppressive cells (MDSCs) [44] has been described to downregulate NK-activating receptors and to impair NK functions [45,46]. Increased levels of IL-6 and IL-10 are also observed in MM [47,48]. These cytokines act as growth factors for plasma cells and promote the development of NK-resistant tumor phenotype by inhibiting NK cell activity [49,50]. Prostaglandin E2 (PGE2), produced in cultures of BM from MM patients [51], may inhibit activating signals transduced by NCRs, NKG2D and CD16 [52]. Indoleamine 2,3-deoxygenase (IDO) produced by stromal dendritic cells when they interact with CD28 expressed on plasma cells can impair NK-mediated lysis by inhibiting the expression of NKp46 and NKG2D [53,54].

In parallel, myeloma plasma cells progressively develop different strategies to escape NK cell killing. High levels of expression of HLA class I and of HLA-E (ligands for inhibitory KIRs and CD94/NKG2A, respectively) are observed in tumor cells from advanced MM patients, which was associated with reduced degranulation of NK cells in vitro [55]. Another way for MM to escape NK cell lysis is to cleave the surface expression of the NKG2D–ligands MICA and MICB [56]. Indeed, soluble MIC ligands induce the internalization of NKG2D and NCRs and promote the accumulation of MDSCs and immunosuppressive macrophages [57,58]. Plasma cells can escape immune lymphocytes by expressing PDL-1 [38]. Finally, myeloma cells can alter the chemokine microenvironment to promote the migration of NK cells (expressing CXCR3 or CXCR4) outside the BM, consequently to the upregulation of serum levels of the CXCR3–ligand CXCL10 and the downregulated expression of the CXCR4–ligand CXCL12 in the BM [59].

5. Therapeutic Modulation of NK Cells in MM

Most of the therapeutic agents used in the treatment of MM either modulate or require NK cell functions (Figure 2).

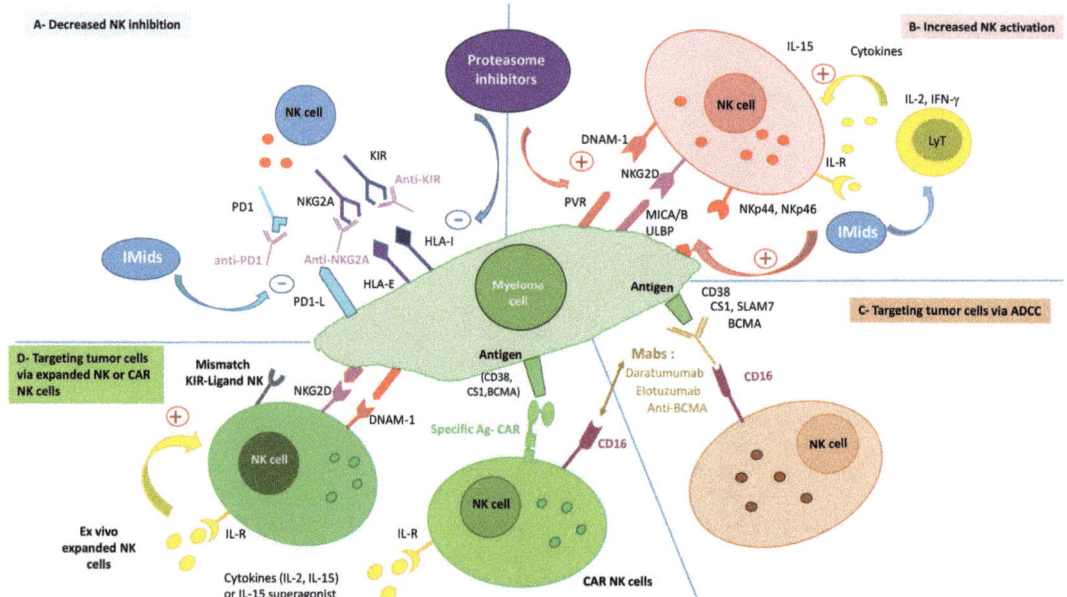

Figure 2. Restauration and enhancement of NK cell functions in multiple myeloma (MM). (**A**). Decreased inhibition of NK cells: the inhibitory signaling can be overrided by several ways: infusion of haploidentical NK cells (haplo) with a killer cell immunoglobulin-like receptors (KIR)–ligand mismatch, the use of anti-KIR, anti-NKG2A or anti-PD1 monoclonal antibodies (mAbs), or by reducing tumor cell surface expression of HLA-I by proteasome inhibitors (PI) or that of PDL-1 by immunomodulatory drugs (IMIDs) (**B**). Increased activation of NK cells: PIs and IMIDs can increase the tumor expression of ligands of activating receptors (polio virus receptor-PVR, MHC-related ligands (MICA), UL16-binding protein (ULBP)) and the corresponding receptors DNAX accessory molecule (DNAM-1) and NKG2D on NK cells. IMIDs or IL-15 can favor the activation and proliferation of NK cells (**C**). Targeting tumor cells via antibody-dependent cellular cytotoxicity (ADCC). CD16 (Fc-receptor) expressed on NK cells can bind to anti-CD38 (daratumumab), anti-CS1/SLAM7 (elotuzumab) or anti-BCMA mAbs and induce tumor killing by ADCC. (**D**). Targeting tumor cells via ex vivo expanded or chimeric antigen receptors (CAR) NK cells: Ex vivo expanded and activated NK cells expressing NK-activating receptors can kill tumor cells. CAR-NK cells can be engineered against various myeloma targets (see 2C). CD16 expressed on CAR NK cells can also mediate a synergistic effect in combination with antigen-specific mAbs.

5.1. Modulation of NK Cells by Immunomodulatory Drugs and Monoclonal Abs

Immunomodulatory drugs thalidomide, lenalidomide and pomalidomide stimulate the production of IL-2 and IFN-γ by T cells, which, in turn, increases the proliferation of NK cells and their cytotoxicity against myeloma cells [60–62]. They increase the expression of NK-cell-activating ligands MICA, ULBP1 and PVR on myeloma cells and that of NK-activating receptors (NKG2D, NKp30, NKp46) on NK cells [62,63]. In addition, lenalidomide has been shown to enhance the expression of Fas-L and TRAIL on NK cells [61] while reducing PDL1 [38] on myeloma cells (Figure 2A,B). Importantly, the effects of IMids on NK cells are maintained when they are combined with a low dose of dexamethasone [64,65].

Proteasome inhibitors bortezomib and carfilzomib also enhance NK-cell-mediated myeloma cell killing. Both downregulate the expression of HLA class I molecules on myeloma cells [66,67], thus sensitizing them to NK cytotoxicity. In addition, bortezomib upregulates the expression of the ligands for NKG2D (MICA/MICB) and for DNAM-1 (PVR and nectin-2) on tumor cells [68,69], and carfilzomib increases the expression of the CD107a thus the degranulation of NK cells [67] (Figure 2A,B).

Through their expression of CD16 (FCγRIIIa), NK cells are recruited by monoclonal antibodies (mAbs) targeting tumor antigens and participate in tumor killing by antibody-dependent cellular cytotoxicity (ADCC) [70] (Figure 2C). Daratumumab, a fully human IgG1, targets CD38, a transmembrane glycoprotein highly expressed on myeloma cells, but also on other hematopoietic cells, including NK cells [71]. Despite the associated killing of $CD38^{+/\ bright}$ NK cells, daratumumab mediates its anti-MM effect via ADCC through remaining $CD38^{neg/low}$ NK cells, which have higher expansion and cytotoxicity capacities [71]. Elotuzumab is a humanized IgG1 directed against CS1/SLAM-7, a transmembrane glycoprotein highly expressed on myeloma cells and at lower levels on NK and CD8 T, NKT cells and activated monocytes [72]. Elotuzumab enhances NK-mediated myeloma cell killing by ADCC, but also by direct recognition of CS1 on NK cells. This latter induces the activation of NK cells through the signaling intermediate EAT2, which is not expressed on myeloma cells, inducing tumor cell lysis in complement to ADCC [73].

The combination of IMids or proteasome inhibitors to mAbs have shown synergistic effects on NK cell activation and ADCC induction in preclinical models as well as in clinical trials (lenalidomide or pomalidomide + elotuzumab, bortezomib or lenalidomide + daratumumab) [74–79].

5.2. Expanded NK Cells for Cellular Immunotherapy in MM

The anti-leukemic effects of NK cells in haplo-HSCT led to the development of NK cell therapies in several hematologic malignancies. Miller et al. reported that administration of activated HLA-haploidentical NK cells combined with in vivo subcutaneous injections of IL-2 after a lymphodepleting conditioning regimen (high-dose cyclophosphamide and fludarabine) resulted in an in vivo expansion of donor NK cells and the induction of anti-leukemic responses without GVHD in 5 out of 19 patients with poor-prognosis acute myeloid leukemia (AML), with higher responses in case of a KIR ligand-mismatched donor [80]. The same group demonstrated enhanced NK cell activity by concomitant depletion of Tregs by administration of IL-2-diphtheria fusion protein (IL-2DT) [81]. The potential curative or preventive effect of KIR ligand mismatched NK cell therapies in AML has been since reported by others [82,83].

Because of the role of NK cells in the development of MM, the administration of activated NK cells represents an attractive therapeutic approach in this disease. Expansion of NK cells from PBMC of MM patients can be achieved in co-culture with feeder K562 cells transfected with CD137-L and IL-15, which activate and enhance the proliferation of highly cytotoxic NK cells expressing NKG2D and DNAM-1 [84] (Figure 2D). Such ex vivo expanded NK cells from myeloma patients have been infused in heavily pretreated patients with no serious adverse events, and responses lasting at least six months were observed in two out of seven patients [85]. In vitro expansion of PBMC-derived NK cells can also be performed in co-culture with polyvalent immunoglobulins, platelet lysate and lenalidomide, allowing an 80-fold expansion rated and the generation of highly cytotoxic and polyfunctional NK cells [86].

Administration of allogeneic KIR ligand-mismatched NK cells from haploidentical family donors was performed after conditioning regimen with melphalan and fludarabine in patients with advanced MM followed by delayed rescue with autologous stem cells. This approach led to short survival and in vivo expansion of donor NK cells but uncourageous response rates with 50% of near-complete remission [87]. A phase I study evaluated the safety and efficacy of sequential infusions of autologous ex vivo expanded NK cells in combination with lenalidomide or bortezomib-based treatments in 5 relapsed or refractory MM patients to 2 to 7 lines of treatment. After four cycles of treatment with 2 NK cell infusions per cycle, four patients had stable disease, 2 showed a reduction in bone marrow plasma cell infiltration of 50%, and one had a response lasting for more than a year [88]. Umbilical cord blood-derived NK cells have also been used in combination with autologous HSCT in 12 heavily pretreated and high cytogenetic risk MM [89]. An in vivo expansion of activated NKG2D$^+$/NKP30$^+$ NK cells was observed in 6 patients, and most patients achieved prolonged near CR (n = 8) or very good partial response (n = 2).

IL-15 has the advantage over IL-2 to not support the maintenance of Tregs and to protect effector memory T cells as well. In a MM mouse model, the administration of the IL-15 superagonist ALT-803 increased T and NK-mediated-cell lysis of myeloma cells compared to conventional IL-15 [90,91]. In vitro-primed CD56^{bright} NK cells by IL-15 have become more cytotoxic against myeloma cell lines, and a phase I study of administration of ALT-803 in MM patients showed a transient expansion of CD56^{bright} NK cells in vivo with cytotoxic activity against U266 myeloma cell line [92]. A phase I study combining ALT-803 and expanded non-HLA matched allogeneic NK cells in hematologic malignancies, including MM, is ongoing (NCT02890758).

Overall, these studies suggest the therapeutic activity of NK cells for the treatment of MM when those are activated ex vivo and express activating KIRs or NCR to be able to overcome the high expression of HLA class I molecules on myeloma cells.

5.3. CAR-NK in MM

Genetic modifications of T cells with chimeric antigen receptors (CAR), first developed against CD19 for the treatment of lymphoid malignancies, have been explored in MM with different antigen targets (BCMA, CD38, CD138, SLMAF7, NKG2D, CD56) (reviewed in [93,94]). Among those, the most advanced are CAR-T cells recently targeting BCMA approved for the treatment of R/R MM patients [95]. With a median progression-free survival of 9 months, results of CAR-T cells in MM could be improved.

Compared to CAR-T cells, CAR-NK cells have several potential advantages [96] (i) they do not induce GVHD and can be safely used in an allogeneic setting, (ii) their shorter in vivo persistence in the allogeneic context and their mixed cytokine profile (both anti- and proinflammatory and proapoptotic) may reduce cytokine release syndrome and other side effects, (iii) their expression of activating receptors may enhance their efficacy by nonCAR-dependent tumor lysis and (iv) their expression of CD16 could allow a synergistic effect in combination with monoclonal therapeutic antibodies. In addition, several sources of CAR-NK cells can be considered: primary NK cells, NK cell lines (NK-92), umbilical cord blood or induced pluripotent stem cells (iPSCs) [97]. CAR-NK cells are, therefore, under investigation in several hematologic malignancies. The most impressive results have been reported with cord blood-derived NK cells transduced with an anti-CD19 and IL-15-containing CAR construct tested in 11 patients with refractory lymphoid malignancies in a phase I study [98]. Despite HLA mismatches between CAR-NK cells and patients, none of them developed CRS, neurotoxicity or GVHD. Eight patients (73%) responded within the first month, including 7 CR (64%), and NK-CAR cells were detectable for up to one year after administration independently of the administered dose, possibly because of the persistent production of IL-15 included in the CAR construct [98,99]. The clinical efficacy of CAR-NK is difficult to assess as most patients received a consolidation therapy (lenalidomide, allogeneic HSCT, etc.), but those preliminary results are very encouraging.

In MM, CAR-NK cells targeting CD138, BCMA, NKG2D or CS1/SLAMF7 have been explored in preclinical studies [100–102] (Figure 2D). Jiang et al. demonstrated that NK-92 cells transduced with an anti-CD138 CAR kill myeloma cell lines and primary tumor plasma cells in vitro and that administration of irradiated CAR-NK-92 cells has strong antitumor activity towards CD138-positive MM cells in the xenograft NOD-SCID mouse model [100]. Chu et al. reported similar results with NK-92 cells expressing an anti-CS1/SLAMF7 CAR [101]. Another group observed similar efficacy between anti-NKG2D and anti-BCMA NK cells in eradicating myeloma cells [102]. A phase I trial with anti-BCMA CAR NK-92 cells for R/R myeloma patients is ongoing in China (NCT03940833). A combination of anti-CD38 monoclonal antibody daratumumab and anti-CS1 CAR CD38^{neg} NK cells has been described to treat relapsed MM with the hypothesis of a synergistic effect of Daratumumab and CAR-CD38^{neg} NK cells [103] (Figure 2D).

5.4. KIR and Check Point Inhibitors in MM

Blocking NK cell inhibitory molecules by monoclonal antibodies represents another way to increase the efficacy of NK cells against tumor cells (Figure 2A).

The interest of targeting the PD1/PDL1 axis in MM was first described by Benson et al., who showed that the anti-PD1 antibody CT-011 could enhance NK cell function against primary myeloma cells expressing PDL-1, with a synergistic effect when combined with lenalidomide, which reduces PDL1 expression on myeloma cells [38]. In a preclinical model, the combination of anti-PD1 mAb and lenalidomide enhanced the effect of DC-based immunotherapy by inhibition of suppressive cells (MDSCs, Tregs and M2 macrophages) and activation of T and NK cytotoxic effector cells [104]. In humans, inhibition of the PD1/PDL1 axis with mAbs in monotherapy failed to demonstrate efficacy [105]. In combination with IMids, despite a good safety profile and some interesting responses observed in the first phase I-II studies evaluating the combination of pembrolizumab (anti-PD-1) to lenalidomide or pomalidomide and dexamethasone [106–108], the unpredictable occurrence of immune-related adverse events reported in R/R MM receiving a combination of anti-PD1 and IMids, conducted the FDA to discontinue all the trials exploring such combination of drugs [9]. Inhibition of the PD1/PDL1 axis is currently explored in R/R MM patients receiving anti-BCMA CAR T cells with a CAR also expressing a PD1-Fc fusion protein capable of inhibiting PD1/PDL1 (NCT04162119).

The KIR inhibitor mAb 1-7F9 was developed to inhibit different inhibitory KIRs (KIR2DL-1, -2 and -3) and enhance NK antitumor effect. This anti-KIR inhibitor mAb increases NK-cell-mediated killing of HLA-C expressing tumor cells in vitro and in vivo [109]. The combination of lenalidomide and IPH2101 (formerly 1-7F9) was shown to enhance NK cell-mediated anti-myeloma responses in a preclinical model [110]. IPH2101 was, therefore, tested in phase I and II trials in MM. The first phase I included 32 patients with R/R MM, who received up to four cycles of 28-day intravenous administration of IPH2101 at different doses demonstrated that the drug was well-tolerated, and the treatment was associated with the full saturation of inhibitory KIRs and anti-myeloma cell NK-mediated killing [111]. Another phase I study explored the combination of lenalidomide and IPH2101 in 15 MM patients and showed a response in 5 patients, but severe adverse events were observed in 5 patients [112]. However, in smoldering MM patients, IPH2101 failed to reach a 50% decline of the M-protein [113]. Lirilumab, a recombinant version of IPH2101 that also recognizes the activating KIRs KIR2DS1 and -2, has been tested in combination with the anti-PD1 nivolumab in a phase I study in R/R lymphoid malignancies, but no objective response was observed in MM patients [114]. Actually, because of its inhibition of both inhibitory and activating KIRs, the effect of lirilumab will depend on MHC class I expression and KIR receptor repertoire. In addition, it has been reported that KIR2D molecules are removed from NK cells by monocyte trogocytosis under the pressure of IPH2101, a phenomenon associated with a reduction of NK cell cytotoxicity in vivo [115]. Altogether, these results suggest using anti-inhibitory KIRs in association with other immunomodulatory drugs rather than as a single-agent. Results of a phase analyzing the combination of elotuzumab with lirilumab or urelumab (anti-4-1BB mAb) in MM are pending (NCT02252263).

Monalizumab, a humanized mAb, was developed to block the heterodimer CD94/NKG2A and reverse the inhibitory signaling induced by NKG2A on NK cells and HLA-E on tumor cells [116]. An ongoing phase I trial is investigating the safety of monalizumab in hematologic malignancies, including MM relapsing after allo-HSTC (NCT02921685).

6. Conclusions

Multiple myeloma is a multiple-step evoluting disease. During disease evolution, tumor cells escape to immune surveillance, particularly to NK cell control. Restoring NK cell cytotoxicity against myeloma tumor plasma cells is a major goal of MM treatment strategies. Conventional treatments (IMids, proteasome inhibitors and monoclonal antibodies) can modulate and enhance NK cell recognition and killing of myeloma plasma cells. NK cell-based therapies, such as expanded and activated KIR mismatched and particularly CAR NK cells, are promising, as well as blocking NK cell inhibitory checkpoint and receptors. The actions of all these treatment approaches are complementary and synergistic. Future studies will help to define the best combination strategies and the respective place of conventional versus cellular and/or inhibitor blockers in the therapeutic care of multiple myeloma.

Author Contributions: M.T.R. wrote and reviewed the manuscript, A.D. and S.N.-Q. made figures and reviewed the manuscript. All authors have read and agreed to the published version of the manuscript.

Funding: This research received no external funding.

Institutional Review Board Statement: Not applicable.

Informed Consent Statement: Not applicable.

Data Availability Statement: Not applicable.

Conflicts of Interest: The authors declare no conflict of interest.

References

1. Raab, M.S.; Podar, K.; Breitkreutz, I.; Richardson, P.G.; Anderson, K.C. Multiple myeloma. *Lancet* **2009**, *374*, 324–339. [CrossRef]
2. Blade, J.; Rosinol, L.; Cibeira, M.T.; de Larrea, C.F. Pathogenesis and progression of monoclonal gammapathy of undetermined significance. *Leukemia* **2008**, *22*, 1651–1657. [CrossRef]
3. Kawano, Y.; Roccaro, A.M.; Ghobrial, I.M.; Azzi, J. Multiple Myeloma and the Immune Microenvironment. *Curr. Cancer Drug Targets* **2017**, *17*, 806–818. [CrossRef] [PubMed]
4. Dosani, T.; Carlsten, M.; Maric, I.; Landgren, O. The cellular immune system in myelomagenesis: NK cells and T cells in the development of myeloma [corrected] and their uses in immunotherapies. *Blood Cancer J.* **2015**, *5*, e306. [CrossRef] [PubMed]
5. Vivier, E.; Tomasello, E.; Baratin, M.; Walzer, T.; Ugolini, S. Functions of natural killer cells. *Nat. Immunol.* **2008**, *9*, 503–510. [CrossRef]
6. Campbell, K.S.; Hasegawa, J. Natural killer cell biology: An update and future directions. *J. Allergy Clin. Immunol.* **2013**, *132*, 536–544. [CrossRef]
7. Kumar, S. Natural killer cell cytotoxicity and its regulation by inhibitory receptors. *Immunology* **2018**, *154*, 383–393. [CrossRef]
8. Pegram, H.J.; Andrews, D.M.; Smyth, M.J.; Darcy, P.K.; Kershaw, M.H. Activating and inhibitory receptors of natural killer cells. *Immunol. Cell Biol.* **2011**, *89*, 216–224. [CrossRef]
9. Alfarra, H.; Weir, J.; Grieve, S.; Reiman, T. Targeting NK Cell Inhibitory Receptors for Precision Multiple Myeloma Immunotherapy. *Front. Immunol.* **2020**, *11*, 575609. [CrossRef] [PubMed]
10. Barrow, A.D.; Martin, C.J.; Colonna, M. The Natural Cytotoxicity Receptors in Health and Disease. *Front. Immunol.* **2019**, *10*, 909. [CrossRef]
11. Lupo, K.B.; Matosevic, S. Natural Killer Cells as Allogeneic Effectors in Adoptive Cancer Immunotherapy. *Cancers* **2019**, *11*, 769. [CrossRef]
12. Lin, W.; Voskens, C.J.; Zhang, X.; Schindler, D.G.; Wood, A.; Burch, E.; Wei, Y.; Chen, L.; Tian, G.; Tamada, K.; et al. Fc-dependent expression of CD137 on human NK cells: Insights into "agonistic" effects of anti-CD137 monoclonal antibodies. *Blood* **2008**, *112*, 699–707. [CrossRef] [PubMed]
13. Aversa, F.; Tabilio, A.; Velardi, A.; Cunningham, I.; Terenzi, A.; Falzetti, F.; Ruggeri, L.; Barbabietola, G.; Aristei, C.; Latini, P.; et al. Treatment of high-risk acute leukemia with T-cell-depleted stem cells from related donors with one fully mismatched HLA haplotype. *N. Engl. J. Med.* **1998**, *339*, 1186–1193. [CrossRef] [PubMed]
14. Ruggeri, L.; Capanni, M.; Casucci, M.; Volpi, I.; Tosti, A.; Perruccio, K.; Urbani, E.; Negrin, R.S.; Martelli, M.F.; Velardi, A. Role of natural killer cell alloreactivity in HLA-mismatched hematopoietic stem cell transplantation. *Blood* **1999**, *94*, 333–339. [CrossRef] [PubMed]
15. Ruggeri, L.; Capanni, M.; Urbani, E.; Perruccio, K.; Shlomchik, W.D.; Tosti, A.; Posati, S.; Rogaia, D.; Frassoni, F.; Aversa, F.; et al. Effectiveness of donor natural killer cell alloreactivity in mismatched hematopoietic transplants. *Science* **2002**, *295*, 2097–2100. [CrossRef]
16. Velardi, A.; Ruggeri, L.; Alessandro Moretta Moretta, L. NK cells: A lesson from mismatched hematopoietic transplantation. *Trends Immunol.* **2002**, *23*, 438–444. [CrossRef]
17. Aversa, F.; Terenzi, A.; Tabilio, A.; Falzetti, F.; Carotti, A.; Ballanti, S.; Felicini, R.; Falcinelli, F.; Velardi, A.; Ruggeri, L.; et al. Full haplotype-mismatched hematopoietic stem-cell transplantation: A phase II study in patients with acute leukemia at high risk of relapse. *J. Clin. Oncol.* **2005**, *23*, 3447–3454. [CrossRef]

18. Pende, D.; Marcenaro, S.; Falco, M.; Martini, S.; Bernardo, M.E.; Montagna, D.; Romeo, E.; Cognet, C.; Martinetti, M.; Maccario, R.; et al. Anti-leukemia activity of alloreactive NK cells in KIR ligand-mismatched haploidentical HSCT for pediatric patients: Evaluation of the functional role of activating KIR and redefinition of inhibitory KIR specificity. *Blood* **2009**, *113*, 3119–3129. [CrossRef]
19. Locatelli, F.; Bauquet, A.; Palumbo, G.; Moretta, F.; Bertaina, A. Negative depletion of alpha/beta+ T cells and of CD19+ B lymphocytes: A novel frontier to optimize the effect of innate immunity in HLA-mismatched hematopoietic stem cell transplantation. *Immunol. Lett.* **2013**, *155*, 21–23. [CrossRef] [PubMed]
20. Kroger, N.; Shaw, B.; Iacobelli, S.; Zabelina, T.; Peggs, K.; Shimoni, A.; Nagler, A.; Binder, T.; Eiermann, T.; Madrigal, A.; et al. Comparison between antithymocyte globulin and alemtuzumab and the possible impact of KIR-ligand mismatch after dose-reduced conditioning and unrelated stem cell transplantation in patients with multiple myeloma. *Br. J. Haematol.* **2005**, *129*, 631–643. [CrossRef] [PubMed]
21. Davies, S.M.; Ruggieri, L.; DeFor, T.; Wagner, J.E.; Weisdorf, D.J.; Miller, J.S.; Velardi, A.; Blazar, B.R. Evaluation of KIR ligand incompatibility in mismatched unrelated donor hematopoietic transplants. Killer immunoglobulin-like receptor. *Blood* **2002**, *100*, 3825–3827. [CrossRef]
22. Farag, S.S.; Bacigalupo, A.; Eapen, M.; Hurley, C.; Dupont, B.; Caligiuri, M.A.; Boudreau, C.; Nelson, G.; Oudshoorn, M.; van Rood, J.; et al. The effect of KIR ligand incompatibility on the outcome of unrelated donor transplantation: A report from the center for international blood and marrow transplant research, the European blood and marrow transplant registry, and the Dutch registry. *Biol. Blood Marrow Transplant.* **2006**, *12*, 876–884. [CrossRef]
23. Brunstein, C.G.; Wagner, J.E.; Weisdorf, D.J.; Cooley, S.; Noreen, H.; Barker, J.N.; DeFor, T.; Verneris, M.R.; Blazar, B.R.; Miller, J.S. Negative effect of KIR alloreactivity in recipients of umbilical cord blood transplant depends on transplantation conditioning intensity. *Blood* **2009**, *113*, 5628–5634. [CrossRef]
24. Russo, A.; Oliveira, G.; Berglund, S.; Greco, R.; Gambacorta, V.; Cieri, N.; Toffalori, C.; Zito, L.; Lorentino, F.; Piemontese, S.; et al. NK cell recovery after haploidentical HSCT with posttransplant cyclophosphamide: Dynamics and clinical implications. *Blood* **2018**, *131*, 247–262. [CrossRef] [PubMed]
25. Nguyen, S.; Beziat, V.; Roos-Weil, D.; Vieillard, V. Role of natural killer cells in hematopoietic stem cell transplantation: Myth or reality? *J. Innate. Immun.* **2011**, *3*, 383–394. [CrossRef] [PubMed]
26. Cooley, S.; Trachtenberg, E.; Bergemann, T.L.; Saeteurn, K.; Klein, J.; Le, C.T.; Marsh, S.G.; Guethlein, L.A.; Parham, P.; Miller, J.S.; et al. Donors with group B KIR haplotypes improve relapse-free survival after unrelated hematopoietic cell transplantation for acute myelogenous leukemia. *Blood* **2009**, *113*, 726–732. [CrossRef] [PubMed]
27. Cooley, S.; Weisdorf, D.J.; Guethlein, L.A.; Klein, J.P.; Wang, T.; Le, C.T.; Marsh, S.G.; Geraghty, D.; Spellman, S.; Haagenson, M.D.; et al. Donor selection for natural killer cell receptor genes leads to superior survival after unrelated transplantation for acute myelogenous leukemia. *Blood* **2010**, *116*, 2411–2419. [CrossRef] [PubMed]
28. Venstrom, J.M.; Pittari, G.; Gooley, T.A.; Chewning, J.H.; Spellman, S.; Haagenson, M.; Gallagher, M.M.; Malkki, M.; Petersdorf, E.; Dupont, B.; et al. HLA-C-dependent prevention of leukemia relapse by donor activating KIR2DS1. *N. Engl. J. Med.* **2012**, *367*, 805–816. [CrossRef] [PubMed]
29. Nguyen, S.; Dhedin, N.; Vernant, J.P.; Kuentz, M.; Al Jijakli, A.; Rouas-Freiss, N.; Carosella, E.D.; Boudifa, A.; Debre, P.; Vieillard, V. NK-cell reconstitution after haploidentical hematopoietic stem-cell transplantations: Immaturity of NK cells and inhibitory effect of NKG2A override GvL effect. *Blood* **2005**, *105*, 4135–4142. [CrossRef] [PubMed]
30. Frohn, C.; Hoppner, M.; Schlenke, P.; Kirchner, H.; Koritke, P.; Luhm, J. Anti-myeloma activity of natural killer lymphocytes. *Br. J. Haematol.* **2002**, *119*, 660–664. [CrossRef] [PubMed]
31. Carbone, E.; Neri, P.; Mesuraca, M.; Fulciniti, M.T.; Otsuki, T.; Pende, D.; Groh, V.; Spies, T.; Pollio, G.; Cosman, D.; et al. HLA class I, NKG2D, and natural cytotoxicity receptors regulate multiple myeloma cell recognition by natural killer cells. *Blood* **2005**, *105*, 251–258. [CrossRef] [PubMed]
32. El-Sherbiny, Y.M.; Meade, J.L.; Holmes, T.D.; McGonagle, D.; Mackie, S.L.; Morgan, A.W.; Cook, G.; Feyler, S.; Richards, S.J.; Davies, F.E.; et al. The requirement for DNAM-1, NKG2D, and NKp46 in the natural killer cell-mediated killing of myeloma cells. *Cancer Res.* **2007**, *67*, 8444–8449. [CrossRef] [PubMed]
33. Tienhaara, A.; Pelliniemi, T.T. Peripheral blood lymphocyte subsets in multiple myeloma and monoclonal gammopathy of undetermined significance. *Clin. Lab. Haematol.* **1994**, *16*, 213–223. [CrossRef] [PubMed]
34. Famularo, G.; D'Ambrosio, A.; Quintieri, F.; Di Giovanni, S.; Parzanese, I.; Pizzuto, F.; Giacomelli, R.; Pugliese, O.; Tonietti, G. Natural killer cell frequency and function in patients with monoclonal gammopathies. *J. Clin. Lab. Immunol.* **1992**, *37*, 99–109. [PubMed]
35. Jurisic, V.; Srdic, T.; Konjevic, G.; Markovic, O.; Colovic, M. Clinical stage-depending decrease of NK cell activity in multiple myeloma patients. *Med. Oncol.* **2007**, *24*, 312–317. [CrossRef]
36. Fauriat, C.; Mallet, F.; Olive, D.; Costello, R.T. Impaired activating receptor expression pattern in natural killer cells from patients with multiple myeloma. *Leukemia* **2006**, *20*, 732–733. [CrossRef]
37. Costello, R.T.; Boehrer, A.; Sanchez, C.; Mercier, D.; Baier, C.; Le Treut, T.; Sebahoun, G. Differential expression of natural killer cell activating receptors in blood versus bone marrow in patients with monoclonal gammopathy. *Immunology* **2013**, *139*, 338–341. [CrossRef]

38. Benson, D.M., Jr.; Bakan, C.E.; Mishra, A.; Hofmeister, C.C.; Efebera, Y.; Becknell, B.; Baiocchi, R.A.; Zhang, J.; Yu, J.; Smith, M.K.; et al. The PD-1/PD-L1 axis modulates the natural killer cell versus multiple myeloma effect: A therapeutic target for CT-011, a novel monoclonal anti-PD-1 antibody. *Blood* **2010**, *116*, 2286–2294. [CrossRef]
39. Konjevic, G.; Vuletic, A.; Mirjacic Martinovic, K.; Colovic, N.; Colovic, M.; Jurisic, V. Decreased CD161 activating and increased CD158a inhibitory receptor expression on NK cells underlies impaired NK cell cytotoxicity in patients with multiple myeloma. *J. Clin. Pathol.* **2016**, *69*, 1009–1016. [CrossRef]
40. Bhutani, M.; Foureau, D.; Zhang, Q.; Robinson, M.; Wynn, A.S.; Steuerwald, N.M.; Druhan, L.J.; Guo, F.; Rigby, K.; Turner, M.; et al. Peripheral Immunotype Correlates with Minimal Residual Disease Status and Is Modulated by Immunomodulatory Drugs in Multiple Myeloma. *Biol. Blood Marrow Transplant.* **2019**, *25*, 459–465. [CrossRef]
41. Bianchi, G.; Munshi, N.C. Pathogenesis beyond the cancer clone(s) in multiple myeloma. *Blood* **2015**, *125*, 3049–3058. [CrossRef] [PubMed]
42. Urashima, M.; Ogata, A.; Chauhan, D.; Hatziyanni, M.; Vidriales, M.B.; Dedera, D.A.; Schlossman, R.L.; Anderson, K.C. Transforming growth factor-beta1: Differential effects on multiple myeloma versus normal B cells. *Blood* **1996**, *87*, 1928–1938. [CrossRef]
43. Beyer, M.; Kochanek, M.; Giese, T.; Endl, E.; Weihrauch, M.R.; Knolle, P.A.; Classen, S.; Schultze, J.L. In vivo peripheral expansion of naive CD4+CD25high FoxP3+ regulatory T cells in patients with multiple myeloma. *Blood* **2006**, *107*, 3940–3949. [CrossRef]
44. Van Valckenborgh, E.; Schouppe, E.; Movahedi, K.; De Bruyne, E.; Menu, E.; De Baetselier, P.; Vanderkerken, K.; Van Ginderachter, J.A. Multiple myeloma induces the immunosuppressive capacity of distinct myeloid-derived suppressor cell subpopulations in the bone marrow. *Leukemia* **2012**, *26*, 2424–2428. [CrossRef] [PubMed]
45. Li, H.; Han, Y.; Guo, Q.; Zhang, M.; Cao, X. Cancer-expanded myeloid-derived suppressor cells induce anergy of NK cells through membrane-bound TGF-beta 1. *J. Immunol.* **2009**, *182*, 240–249. [CrossRef] [PubMed]
46. Castriconi, R.; Cantoni, C.; Della Chiesa, M.; Vitale, M.; Marcenaro, E.; Conte, R.; Biassoni, R.; Bottino, C.; Moretta, L.; Moretta, A. Transforming growth factor beta 1 inhibits expression of NKp30 and NKG2D receptors: Consequences for the NK-mediated killing of dendritic cells. *Proc. Natl. Acad. Sci. USA* **2003**, *100*, 4120–4125. [CrossRef]
47. Sharma, A.; Khan, R.; Joshi, S.; Kumar, L.; Sharma, M. Dysregulation in T helper 1/T helper 2 cytokine ratios in patients with multiple myeloma. *Leuk. Lymphoma* **2010**, *51*, 920–927. [CrossRef] [PubMed]
48. Bataille, R.; Jourdan, M.; Zhang, X.G.; Klein, B. Serum levels of interleukin 6, a potent myeloma cell growth factor, as a reflect of disease severity in plasma cell dyscrasias. *J. Clin. Investig.* **1989**, *84*, 2008–2011. [CrossRef]
49. Tsuruma, T.; Yagihashi, A.; Hirata, K.; Torigoe, T.; Araya, J.; Watanabe, N.; Sato, N. Interleukin-10 reduces natural killer (NK) sensitivity of tumor cells by downregulating NK target structure expression. *Cell. Immunol.* **1999**, *198*, 103–110. [CrossRef]
50. Cifaldi, L.; Prencipe, G.; Caiello, I.; Bracaglia, C.; Locatelli, F.; De Benedetti, F.; Strippoli, R. Inhibition of natural killer cell cytotoxicity by interleukin-6: Implications for the pathogenesis of macrophage activation syndrome. *Arthritis Rheumatol.* **2015**, *67*, 3037–3046. [CrossRef]
51. Lu, Z.Y.; Bataille, R.; Poubelle, P.; Rapp, M.J.; Harousseau, J.L.; Klein, B. An interleukin 1 receptor antagonist blocks the IL-1-induced IL-6 paracrine production through a prostaglandin E2-related mechanism in multiple myeloma. *Stem Cells* **1995**, *13* (Suppl. S2), 28–34.
52. Martinet, L.; Jean, C.; Dietrich, G.; Fournie, J.J.; Poupot, R. PGE2 inhibits natural killer and gamma delta T cell cytotoxicity triggered by NKR and TCR through a cAMP-mediated PKA type I-dependent signaling. *Biochem. Pharmacol.* **2010**, *80*, 838–845. [CrossRef]
53. Nair, J.R.; Carlson, L.M.; Koorella, C.; Rozanski, C.H.; Byrne, G.E.; Bergsagel, P.L.; Shaughnessy, J.P., Jr.; Boise, L.H.; Chanan-Khan, A.; Lee, K.P. CD28 expressed on malignant plasma cells induces a prosurvival and immunosuppressive microenvironment. *J. Immunol.* **2011**, *187*, 1243–1253. [CrossRef]
54. Della Chiesa, M.; Carlomagno, S.; Frumento, G.; Balsamo, M.; Cantoni, C.; Conte, R.; Moretta, L.; Moretta, A.; Vitale, M. The tryptophan catabolite L-kynurenine inhibits the surface expression of NKp46- and NKG2D-activating receptors and regulates NK-cell function. *Blood* **2006**, *108*, 4118–4125. [CrossRef]
55. Sarkar, S.; van Gelder, M.; Noort, W.; Xu, Y.; Rouschop, K.M.; Groen, R.; Schouten, H.C.; Tilanus, M.G.; Germeraad, W.T.; Martens, A.C.; et al. Optimal selection of natural killer cells to kill myeloma: The role of HLA-E and NKG2A. *Cancer Immunol. Immunother.* **2015**, *64*, 951–963. [CrossRef] [PubMed]
56. Jinushi, M.; Vanneman, M.; Munshi, N.C.; Tai, Y.T.; Prabhala, R.H.; Ritz, J.; Neuberg, D.; Anderson, K.C.; Carrasco, D.R.; Dranoff, G. MHC class I chain-related protein A antibodies and shedding are associated with the progression of multiple myeloma. *Proc. Natl. Acad. Sci. USA* **2008**, *105*, 1285–1290. [CrossRef]
57. Groh, V.; Wu, J.; Yee, C.; Spies, T. Tumour-derived soluble MIC ligands impair expression of NKG2D and T-cell activation. *Nature* **2002**, *419*, 734–738. [CrossRef] [PubMed]
58. Xiao, G.; Wang, X.; Sheng, J.; Lu, S.; Yu, X.; Wu, J.D. Soluble NKG2D ligand promotes MDSC expansion and skews macrophage to the alternatively activated phenotype. *J. Hematol. Oncol.* **2015**, *8*, 13. [CrossRef] [PubMed]
59. Ponzetta, A.; Benigni, G.; Antonangeli, F.; Sciume, G.; Sanseviero, E.; Zingoni, A.; Ricciardi, M.R.; Petrucci, M.T.; Santoni, A.; Bernardini, G. Multiple Myeloma Impairs Bone Marrow Localization of Effector Natural Killer Cells by Altering the Chemokine Microenvironment. *Cancer Res.* **2015**, *75*, 4766–4777. [CrossRef]

60. Davies, F.E.; Raje, N.; Hideshima, T.; Lentzsch, S.; Young, G.; Tai, Y.T.; Lin, B.; Podar, K.; Gupta, D.; Chauhan, D.; et al. Thalidomide and immunomodulatory derivatives augment natural killer cell cytotoxicity in multiple myeloma. *Blood* **2001**, *98*, 210–216. [CrossRef] [PubMed]
61. Quach, H.; Ritchie, D.; Stewart, A.K.; Neeson, P.; Harrison, S.; Smyth, M.J.; Prince, H.M. Mechanism of action of immunomodulatory drugs (IMiDS) in multiple myeloma. *Leukemia* **2010**, *24*, 22–32. [CrossRef]
62. Hayashi, T.; Hideshima, T.; Akiyama, M.; Podar, K.; Yasui, H.; Raje, N.; Kumar, S.; Chauhan, D.; Treon, S.P.; Richardson, P.; et al. Molecular mechanisms whereby immunomodulatory drugs activate natural killer cells: Clinical application. *Br. J. Haematol.* **2005**, *128*, 192–203. [CrossRef]
63. Lagrue, K.; Carisey, A.; Morgan, D.J.; Chopra, R.; Davis, D.M. Lenalidomide augments actin remodeling and lowers NK-cell activation thresholds. *Blood* **2015**, *126*, 50–60. [CrossRef]
64. Sehgal, K.; Das, R.; Zhang, L.; Verma, R.; Deng, Y.; Kocoglu, M.; Vasquez, J.; Koduru, S.; Ren, Y.; Wang, M.; et al. Clinical and pharmacodynamic analysis of pomalidomide dosing strategies in myeloma: Impact of immune activation and cereblon targets. *Blood* **2015**, *125*, 4042–4051. [CrossRef]
65. Paiva, B.; Mateos, M.V.; Sanchez-Abarca, L.I.; Puig, N.; Vidriales, M.B.; Lopez-Corral, L.; Corchete, L.A.; Hernandez, M.T.; Bargay, J.; de Arriba, F.; et al. Immune status of high-risk smoldering multiple myeloma patients and its therapeutic modulation under LenDex: A longitudinal analysis. *Blood* **2016**, *127*, 1151–1162. [CrossRef] [PubMed]
66. Shi, J.; Tricot, G.J.; Garg, T.K.; Malaviarachchi, P.A.; Szmania, S.M.; Kellum, R.E.; Storrie, B.; Mulder, A.; Shaughnessy, J.D., Jr.; Barlogie, B.; et al. Bortezomib down-regulates the cell-surface expression of HLA class I and enhances natural killer cell-mediated lysis of myeloma. *Blood* **2008**, *111*, 1309–1317. [CrossRef]
67. Yang, G.; Gao, M.; Zhang, Y.; Kong, Y.; Gao, L.; Tao, Y.; Han, Y.; Wu, H.; Meng, X.; Xu, H.; et al. Carfilzomib enhances natural killer cell-mediated lysis of myeloma linked with decreasing expression of HLA class I. *Oncotarget* **2015**, *6*, 26982–26994. [CrossRef] [PubMed]
68. Niu, C.; Jin, H.; Li, M.; Zhu, S.; Zhou, L.; Jin, F.; Zhou, Y.; Xu, D.; Xu, J.; Zhao, L.; et al. Low-dose bortezomib increases the expression of NKG2D and DNAM-1 ligands and enhances induced NK and gammadelta T cell-mediated lysis in multiple myeloma. *Oncotarget* **2017**, *8*, 5954–5964. [CrossRef] [PubMed]
69. Soriani, A.; Zingoni, A.; Cerboni, C.; Iannitto, M.L.; Ricciardi, M.R.; Di Gialleonardo, V.; Cippitelli, M.; Fionda, C.; Petrucci, M.T.; Guarini, A.; et al. ATM-ATR-dependent up-regulation of DNAM-1 and NKG2D ligands on multiple myeloma cells by therapeutic agents results in enhanced NK-cell susceptibility and is associated with a senescent phenotype. *Blood* **2009**, *113*, 3503–3511. [CrossRef]
70. Wang, W.; Erbe, A.K.; Hank, J.A.; Morris, Z.S.; Sondel, P.M. NK Cell-Mediated Antibody-Dependent Cellular Cytotoxicity in Cancer Immunotherapy. *Front. Immunol.* **2015**, *6*, 368. [CrossRef] [PubMed]
71. Wang, Y.; Zhang, Y.; Hughes, T.; Zhang, J.; Caligiuri, M.A.; Benson, D.M.; Yu, J. Fratricide of NK Cells in Daratumumab Therapy for Multiple Myeloma Overcome by Ex Vivo-Expanded Autologous NK Cells. *Clin. Cancer Res.* **2018**, *24*, 4006–4017. [CrossRef]
72. Ritchie, D.; Colonna, M. Mechanisms of Action and Clinical Development of Elotuzumab. *Clin. Transl. Sci.* **2018**, *11*, 261–266. [CrossRef]
73. Collins, S.M.; Bakan, C.E.; Swartzel, G.D.; Hofmeister, C.C.; Efebera, Y.A.; Kwon, H.; Starling, G.C.; Ciarlariello, D.; Bhaskar, S.; Briercheck, E.L.; et al. Elotuzumab directly enhances NK cell cytotoxicity against myeloma via CS1 ligation: Evidence for augmented NK cell function complementing ADCC. *Cancer Immunol. Immunother.* **2013**, *62*, 1841–1849. [CrossRef] [PubMed]
74. Nijhof, I.S.; Groen, R.W.; Noort, W.A.; van Kessel, B.; de Jong-Korlaar, R.; Bakker, J.; van Bueren, J.J.; Parren, P.W.; Lokhorst, H.M.; van de Donk, N.W.; et al. Preclinical Evidence for the Therapeutic Potential of CD38-Targeted Immuno-Chemotherapy in Multiple Myeloma Patients Refractory to Lenalidomide and Bortezomib. *Clin. Cancer Res.* **2015**, *21*, 2802–2810. [CrossRef] [PubMed]
75. Van der Veer, M.S.; de Weers, M.; van Kessel, B.; Bakker, J.M.; Wittebol, S.; Parren, P.W.; Lokhorst, H.M.; Mutis, T. Towards effective immunotherapy of myeloma: Enhanced elimination of myeloma cells by combination of lenalidomide with the human CD38 monoclonal antibody daratumumab. *Haematologica* **2011**, *96*, 284–290. [CrossRef] [PubMed]
76. Dimopoulos, M.A.; Lonial, S.; Betts, K.A.; Chen, C.; Zichlin, M.L.; Brun, A.; Signorovitch, J.E.; Makenbaeva, D.; Mekan, S.; Sy, O.; et al. Elotuzumab plus lenalidomide and dexamethasone in relapsed/refractory multiple myeloma: Extended 4-year follow-up and analysis of relative progression-free survival from the randomized ELOQUENT-2 trial. *Cancer* **2018**, *124*, 4032–4043. [CrossRef]
77. Dimopoulos, M.A.; Dytfeld, D.; Grosicki, S.; Moreau, P.; Takezako, N.; Hori, M.; Leleu, X.; LeBlanc, R.; Suzuki, K.; Raab, M.S.; et al. Elotuzumab plus Pomalidomide and Dexamethasone for Multiple Myeloma. *N. Engl. J. Med.* **2018**, *379*, 1811–1822. [CrossRef]
78. Dimopoulos, M.A.; Oriol, A.; Nahi, H.; San-Miguel, J.; Bahlis, N.J.; Usmani, S.Z.; Rabin, N.; Orlowski, R.Z.; Komarnicki, M.; Suzuki, K.; et al. Daratumumab, Lenalidomide, and Dexamethasone for Multiple Myeloma. *N. Engl. J. Med.* **2016**, *375*, 1319–1331. [CrossRef]
79. Palumbo, A.; Chanan-Khan, A.; Weisel, K.; Nooka, A.K.; Masszi, T.; Beksac, M.; Spicka, I.; Hungria, V.; Munder, M.; Mateos, M.V.; et al. Daratumumab, Bortezomib, and Dexamethasone for Multiple Myeloma. *N. Engl. J. Med.* **2016**, *375*, 754–766. [CrossRef] [PubMed]

80. Miller, J.S.; Soignier, Y.; Panoskaltsis-Mortari, A.; McNearney, S.A.; Yun, G.H.; Fautsch, S.K.; McKenna, D.; Le, C.; Defor, T.E.; Burns, L.J.; et al. Successful adoptive transfer and in vivo expansion of human haploidentical NK cells in patients with cancer. *Blood* **2005**, *105*, 3051–3057. [CrossRef]
81. Bachanova, V.; Cooley, S.; Defor, T.E.; Verneris, M.R.; Zhang, B.; McKenna, D.H.; Curtsinger, J.; Panoskaltsis-Mortari, A.; Lewis, D.; Hippen, K.; et al. Clearance of acute myeloid leukemia by haploidentical natural killer cells is improved using IL-2 diphtheria toxin fusion protein. *Blood* **2014**, *123*, 3855–3863. [CrossRef] [PubMed]
82. Rubnitz, J.E.; Inaba, H.; Ribeiro, R.C.; Pounds, S.; Rooney, B.; Bell, T.; Pui, C.H.; Leung, W. NKAML: A pilot study to determine the safety and feasibility of haploidentical natural killer cell transplantation in childhood acute myeloid leukemia. *J. Clin. Oncol.* **2010**, *28*, 955–959. [CrossRef] [PubMed]
83. Curti, A.; Ruggeri, L.; D'Addio, A.; Bontadini, A.; Dan, E.; Motta, M.R.; Trabanelli, S.; Giudice, V.; Urbani, E.; Martinelli, G.; et al. Successful transfer of alloreactive haploidentical KIR ligand-mismatched natural killer cells after infusion in elderly high risk acute myeloid leukemia patients. *Blood* **2011**, *118*, 3273–3279. [CrossRef] [PubMed]
84. Garg, T.K.; Szmania, S.M.; Khan, J.A.; Hoering, A.; Malbrough, P.A.; Moreno-Bost, A.; Greenway, A.D.; Lingo, J.D.; Li, X.; Yaccoby, S.; et al. Highly activated and expanded natural killer cells for multiple myeloma immunotherapy. *Haematologica* **2012**, *97*, 1348–1356. [CrossRef]
85. Szmania, S.; Lapteva, N.; Garg, T.; Greenway, A.; Lingo, J.; Nair, B.; Stone, K.; Woods, E.; Khan, J.; Stivers, J.; et al. Ex vivo-expanded natural killer cells demonstrate robust proliferation in vivo in high-risk relapsed multiple myeloma patients. *J. Immunother.* **2015**, *38*, 24–36. [CrossRef]
86. Trebeden-Negre, H.; Vieillard, V.; Rosenzwajg, M.; Garderet, L.; Cherai, M.; Nguyen-Quoc, S.; Tanguy, M.L.; Norol, F. Polyvalent immunoglobulins, platelet lysate and lenalidomide: Cocktail for polyfunctional NK cells expansion for multiple myeloma. *Bone Marrow Transplant.* **2017**, *52*, 480–483. [CrossRef]
87. Shi, J.; Tricot, G.; Szmania, S.; Rosen, N.; Garg, T.K.; Malaviarachchi, P.A.; Moreno, A.; Dupont, B.; Hsu, K.C.; Baxter-Lowe, L.A.; et al. Infusion of haplo-identical killer immunoglobulin-like receptor ligand mismatched NK cells for relapsed myeloma in the setting of autologous stem cell transplantation. *Br. J. Haematol.* **2008**, *143*, 641–653. [CrossRef]
88. Leivas, A.; Perez-Martinez, A.; Blanchard, M.J.; Martin-Clavero, E.; Fernandez, L.; Lahuerta, J.J.; Martinez-Lopez, J. Novel treatment strategy with autologous activated and expanded natural killer cells plus anti-myeloma drugs for multiple myeloma. *Oncoimmunology* **2016**, *5*, e1250051. [CrossRef]
89. Shah, N.; Li, L.; McCarty, J.; Kaur, I.; Yvon, E.; Shaim, H.; Muftuoglu, M.; Liu, E.; Orlowski, R.Z.; Cooper, L.; et al. Phase I study of cord blood-derived natural killer cells combined with autologous stem cell transplantation in multiple myeloma. *Br. J. Haematol.* **2017**, *177*, 457–466. [CrossRef]
90. Xu, W.; Jones, M.; Liu, B.; Zhu, X.; Johnson, C.B.; Edwards, A.C.; Kong, L.; Jeng, E.K.; Han, K.; Marcus, W.D.; et al. Efficacy and mechanism-of-action of a novel superagonist interleukin-15: Interleukin-15 receptor alphaSu/Fc fusion complex in syngeneic murine models of multiple myeloma. *Cancer Res.* **2013**, *73*, 3075–3086. [CrossRef]
91. Wong, H.C.; Jeng, E.K.; Rhode, P.R. The IL-15-based superagonist ALT-803 promotes the antigen-independent conversion of memory CD8(+) T cells into innate-like effector cells with antitumor activity. *Oncoimmunology* **2013**, *2*, e26442. [CrossRef] [PubMed]
92. Wagner, J.A.; Rosario, M.; Romee, R.; Berrien-Elliott, M.M.; Schneider, S.E.; Leong, J.W.; Sullivan, R.P.; Jewell, B.A.; Becker-Hapak, M.; Schappe, T.; et al. CD56bright NK cells exhibit potent antitumor responses following IL-15 priming. *J. Clin. Investig.* **2017**, *127*, 4042–4058. [CrossRef] [PubMed]
93. Kriegsmann, K.; Kriegsmann, M.; Cremer, M.; Schmitt, M.; Dreger, P.; Goldschmidt, H.; Muller-Tidow, C.; Hundemer, M. Cell-based immunotherapy approaches for multiple myeloma. *Br. J. Cancer* **2019**, *120*, 38–44. [CrossRef] [PubMed]
94. Shah, U.A.; Mailankody, S. CAR T and CAR NK cells in multiple myeloma: Expanding the targets. *Best Pract. Res. Clin. Haematol.* **2020**, *33*, 101141. [CrossRef] [PubMed]
95. Raje, N.; Berdeja, J.; Lin, Y.; Siegel, D.; Jagannath, S.; Madduri, D.; Liedtke, M.; Rosenblatt, J.; Maus, M.V.; Turka, A.; et al. Anti-BCMA CAR T-Cell Therapy bb2121 in Relapsed or Refractory Multiple Myeloma. *N. Engl. J. Med.* **2019**, *380*, 1726–1737. [CrossRef] [PubMed]
96. Kloess, S.; Oberschmidt, O.; Dahlke, J.; Vu, X.K.; Neudoerfl, C.; Kloos, A.; Gardlowski, T.; Matthies, N.; Heuser, M.; Meyer, J.; et al. Preclinical Assessment of Suitable Natural Killer Cell Sources for Chimeric Antigen Receptor Natural Killer-Based "Off-the-Shelf" Acute Myeloid Leukemia Immunotherapies. *Hum. Gene Ther.* **2019**, *30*, 381–401. [CrossRef]
97. Rezvani, K. Adoptive cell therapy using engineered natural killer cells. *Bone Marrow Transplant.* **2019**, *54* (Suppl. S2), 785–788. [CrossRef]
98. Liu, E.; Marin, D.; Banerjee, P.; Macapinlac, H.A.; Thompson, P.; Basar, R.; Nassif Kerbauy, L.; Overman, B.; Thall, P.; Kaplan, M.; et al. Use of CAR-Transduced Natural Killer Cells in CD19-Positive Lymphoid Tumors. *N. Engl. J. Med.* **2020**, *382*, 545–553. [CrossRef]
99. Liu, E.; Tong, Y.; Dotti, G.; Shaim, H.; Savoldo, B.; Mukherjee, M.; Orange, J.; Wan, X.; Lu, X.; Reynolds, A.; et al. Cord blood NK cells engineered to express IL-15 and a CD19-targeted CAR show long-term persistence and potent antitumor activity. *Leukemia* **2018**, *32*, 520–531. [CrossRef]

100. Jiang, H.; Zhang, W.; Shang, P.; Zhang, H.; Fu, W.; Ye, F.; Zeng, T.; Huang, H.; Zhang, X.; Sun, W.; et al. Transfection of chimeric anti-CD138 gene enhances natural killer cell activation and killing of multiple myeloma cells. *Mol. Oncol.* **2014**, *8*, 297–310. [CrossRef]
101. Chu, J.; Deng, Y.; Benson, D.M.; He, S.; Hughes, T.; Zhang, J.; Peng, Y.; Mao, H.; Yi, L.; Ghoshal, K.; et al. CS1-specific chimeric antigen receptor (CAR)-engineered natural killer cells enhance in vitro and in vivo antitumor activity against human multiple myeloma. *Leukemia* **2014**, *28*, 917–927. [CrossRef] [PubMed]
102. Maroto-Martin, E.E.J.; Garcia-Ortiz, A.; Alonso, R.; Leivas, A.; Paciello, M.L. NKG2D and BCMA-CAR NK cells efficiently eliminate multiple myeloma cells. A comprehensive comparison between two clinically relevant CARs. *HemaSphere* **2019**, *3*, 550–551. [CrossRef]
103. Wang, Y.; Zhang, Y.; Bnson, D.; Caligiuri, M.; Yu, J. Daratumumab combined with CD38(-) natural killer cells armed with a CS1 chimeric antigen receptor for the treatment of relapsed multiple myeloma. [abstract 4617]. In Proceedings of the American Association for Cancer Research, Washington, DC, USA, 1–5 April 2017; Volume 77.
104. Vo, M.C.; Jung, S.H.; Chu, T.H.; Lee, H.J.; Lakshmi, T.J.; Park, H.S.; Kim, H.J.; Rhee, J.H.; Lee, J.J. Lenalidomide and Programmed Death-1 Blockade Synergistically Enhances the Effects of Dendritic Cell Vaccination in a Model of Murine Myeloma. *Front. Immunol.* **2018**, *9*, 1370. [CrossRef] [PubMed]
105. Jelinek, T.; Paiva, B.; Hajek, R. Update on PD-1/PD-L1 Inhibitors in Multiple Myeloma. *Front. Immunol.* **2018**, *9*, 2431. [CrossRef] [PubMed]
106. Badros, A.Z.; Ma, N.; Rapoport, A.P.; Lederer, E.; Lesokhin, A.M. Long-term remissions after stopping pembrolizumab for relapsed or refractory multiple myeloma. *Blood Adv.* **2019**, *3*, 1658–1660. [CrossRef]
107. Mateos, M.V.; Orlowski, R.Z.; Ocio, E.M.; Rodriguez-Otero, P.; Reece, D.; Moreau, P.; Munshi, N.; Avigan, D.E.; Siegel, D.S.; Ghori, R.; et al. Pembrolizumab combined with lenalidomide and low-dose dexamethasone for relapsed or refractory multiple myeloma: Phase I KEYNOTE-023 study. *Br. J. Haematol.* **2019**, *186*, e117–e121. [CrossRef]
108. D'Souza, A.; Hari, P.; Pasquini, M.; Braun, T.; Johnson, B.; Lundy, S.; Couriel, D.; Hamadani, M.; Magenau, J.; Dhakal, B.; et al. A Phase 2 Study of Pembrolizumab during Lymphodepletion after Autologous Hematopoietic Cell Transplantation for Multiple Myeloma. *Biol. Blood Marrow Transplant.* **2019**, *25*, 1492–1497. [CrossRef]
109. Romagne, F.; Andre, P.; Spee, P.; Zahn, S.; Anfossi, N.; Gauthier, L.; Capanni, M.; Ruggeri, L.; Benson, D.M., Jr.; Blaser, B.W.; et al. Preclinical characterization of 1-7F9, a novel human anti-KIR receptor therapeutic antibody that augments natural killer-mediated killing of tumor cells. *Blood* **2009**, *114*, 2667–2677. [CrossRef]
110. Benson, D.M., Jr.; Bakan, C.E.; Zhang, S.; Collins, S.M.; Liang, J.; Srivastava, S.; Hofmeister, C.C.; Efebera, Y.; Andre, P.; Romagne, F.; et al. IPH2101, a novel anti-inhibitory KIR antibody, and lenalidomide combine to enhance the natural killer cell versus multiple myeloma effect. *Blood* **2011**, *118*, 6387–6391. [CrossRef]
111. Benson, D.M., Jr.; Hofmeister, C.C.; Padmanabhan, S.; Suvannasankha, A.; Jagannath, S.; Abonour, R.; Bakan, C.; Andre, P.; Efebera, Y.; Tiollier, J.; et al. A phase 1 trial of the anti-KIR antibody IPH2101 in patients with relapsed/refractory multiple myeloma. *Blood* **2012**, *120*, 4324–4333. [CrossRef]
112. Benson, D.M., Jr.; Cohen, A.D.; Jagannath, S.; Munshi, N.C.; Spitzer, G.; Hofmeister, C.C.; Efebera, Y.A.; Andre, P.; Zerbib, R.; Caligiuri, M.A. A Phase I Trial of the Anti-KIR Antibody IPH2101 and Lenalidomide in Patients with Relapsed/Refractory Multiple Myeloma. *Clin. Cancer Res.* **2015**, *21*, 4055–4061. [CrossRef] [PubMed]
113. Korde, N.; Carlsten, M.; Lee, M.J.; Minter, A.; Tan, E.; Kwok, M.; Manasanch, E.; Bhutani, M.; Tageja, N.; Roschewski, M.; et al. A phase II trial of pan-KIR2D blockade with IPH2101 in smoldering multiple myeloma. *Haematologica* **2014**, *99*, e81–e83. [CrossRef] [PubMed]
114. Armand, P.; Lesokhin, A.; Borrello, I.; Timmerman, J.; Gutierrez, M.; Zhu, L.; Popa McKiver, M.; Ansell, S.M. A phase 1b study of dual PD-1 and CTLA-4 or KIR blockade in patients with relapsed/refractory lymphoid malignancies. *Leukemia* **2020**, *35*, 777–786. [CrossRef] [PubMed]
115. Carlsten, M.; Korde, N.; Kotecha, R.; Reger, R.; Bor, S.; Kazandjian, D.; Landgren, O.; Childs, R.W. Checkpoint Inhibition of KIR2D with the Monoclonal Antibody IPH2101 Induces Contraction and Hyporesponsiveness of NK Cells in Patients with Myeloma. *Clin. Cancer Res.* **2016**, *22*, 5211–5222. [CrossRef]
116. Andre, P.; Denis, C.; Soulas, C.; Bourbon-Caillet, C.; Lopez, J.; Arnoux, T.; Blery, M.; Bonnafous, C.; Gauthier, L.; Morel, A.; et al. Anti-NKG2A mAb Is a Checkpoint Inhibitor that Promotes Anti-tumor Immunity by Unleashing Both T and NK Cells. *Cell* **2018**, *175*, 1731–1743. [CrossRef]

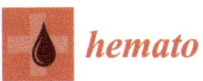

Review

Immunotherapy with Antibodies in Multiple Myeloma: Monoclonals, Bispecifics, and Immunoconjugates

Christie P. M. Verkleij, Wassilis S. C. Bruins, Sonja Zweegman and Niels W. C. J. van de Donk *

Department of Hematology, Cancer Center Amsterdam, Amsterdam UMC, Vrije Universiteit Amsterdam, 1081HV Amsterdam, The Netherlands; c.verkleij@amsterdamumc.nl (C.P.M.V.); w.s.bruins@amsterdamumc.nl (W.S.C.B.); s.zweegman@vumc.nl (S.Z.)
* Correspondence: n.vandedonk@amsterdamumc.nl; Tel.: +31-(0)-20-4442604

Abstract: In the 2010s, immunotherapy revolutionized the treatment landscape of multiple myeloma. CD38-targeting antibodies were initially applied as monotherapy in end-stage patients, but are now also approved by EMA/FDA in combination with standards-of-care in newly diagnosed disease or in patients with early relapse. The approved SLAMF7-targeting antibody can also be successfully combined with lenalidomide or pomalidomide in relapsed/refractory myeloma. Although this has resulted in improved clinical outcomes, there remains a high unmet need in patients who become refractory to immunomodulatory drugs, proteasome inhibitors and CD38-targeting antibodies. Several new antibody formats, such as antibody–drug conjugates (e.g., belantamab mafodotin, which was approved in 2020 and targets BCMA) and T cell redirecting bispecific antibodies (e.g., teclistamab, talquetamab, cevostamab, AMG-420, and CC-93269) are active in these triple-class refractory patients. Based on their promising efficacy, it is expected that these new antibody formats will also be combined with other agents in earlier disease settings.

Keywords: multiple myeloma; immunotherapy; antibodies; monoclonal; bispecific; immunoconjugates; antibody-drug conjugates

Citation: Verkleij, C.P.M.; Bruins, W.S.C.; Zweegman, S.; van de Donk, N.W.C.J. Immunotherapy with Antibodies in Multiple Myeloma: Monoclonals, Bispecifics, and Immunoconjugates. *Hemato* **2021**, *2*, 116–130. https://doi.org/10.3390/hemato2010007

Received: 6 February 2021
Accepted: 24 February 2021
Published: 1 March 2021

Publisher's Note: MDPI stays neutral with regard to jurisdictional claims in published maps and institutional affiliations.

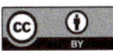

Copyright: © 2021 by the authors. Licensee MDPI, Basel, Switzerland. This article is an open access article distributed under the terms and conditions of the Creative Commons Attribution (CC BY) license (https://creativecommons.org/licenses/by/4.0/).

1. Introduction

The survival of multiple myeloma (MM) patients has substantially improved over the last three decades because of the introduction of autologous stem cell transplantation and novel agents, such as immunomodulatory drugs (IMiDs; e.g., thalidomide, lenalidomide, and pomalidomide) and proteasome inhibitors (PIs; e.g., bortezomib, ixazomib, and carfilzomib). More recently, the incorporation of CD38- and SLAMF7-specific antibodies in treatment regimens for patients with newly diagnosed or relapsed/refractory disease, has further improved the clinical outcomes of MM patients. Based on the activity and favorable toxicity profile of these naked antibodies, several new antibody formats are now evaluated in clinical trials in extensively pretreated patients. In this review, we will discuss the efficacy and safety profile of naked antibodies as well as novel antibody formats such as bispecific antibodies and immunoconjugates.

2. Naked Antibodies

2.1. CD38-Targeting Antibodies

Naked CD38-targeting antibodies (approved: daratumumab and isatuximab; in clinical development: MOR202, SAR442085, and TAK-079) induce MM cell death via direct on-tumor effects such as the direct induction of apoptosis, complement-mediated cytotoxicity (CDC), antibody-dependent cellular cytotoxicity (ADCC), and antibody-dependent cellular phagocytosis (ADCP) (Figure 1) [1–3]. Although there is overlap in the mode of action of these antibodies, there are also some differences [3]. Daratumumab is most potent in terms of the induction of CDC, while isatuximab is more effective in the direct induction of cell death [3]. In addition, CD38-targeting antibodies have T cell stimulatory properties by eliminating CD38-positive regulatory T cells, regulatory B cells, and myeloid-derived suppressor cells [4–7].

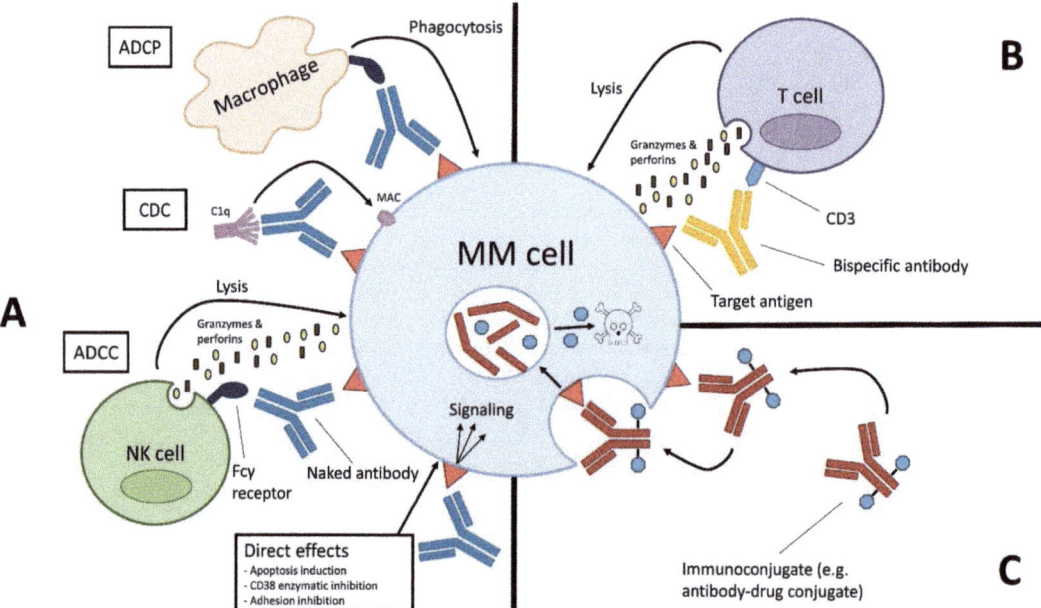

Figure 1. Immunotherapy with antibodies in multiple myeloma. Mode of action of naked antibodies (**A**), bispecific antibodies (**B**), and immunoconjugates (**C**). Abbreviations: MM, multiple myeloma; CDC, complement-mediated cytotoxicity; ADCC, antibody-dependent cellular cytotoxicity; ADCP, antibody-dependent cellular phagocytosis; MAC, membrane attack complex.

CD38-targeting antibodies were first explored as monotherapy in patients with disease exposed to IMiDs and PIs. At that time, these double-refractory patients had a very poor outcome with a median overall survival of only nine months [8]. The overall response rate with CD38-targeting antibodies as a single agent was approximately 30% [9–12]. Importantly, long-term follow-up of the GEN501 and Sirius studies, which evaluated daratumumab monotherapy in patients with advanced MM, showed a remarkably long overall survival (median overall survival: 20.5 months, with a three-year overall survival rate of 36.5%) [13]. This survival is much longer than what was observed in a similar patient population, who did not receive CD38-targeted therapy [8]. Equally important is the favorable toxicity profile of CD38-targeting antibodies. The most frequent side effect observed with CD38-targeting antibodies as monotherapy is the development of infusion-related reactions, most often observed during the first infusion. Premedication with acetaminophen, antihistamine and a steroid is important to prevent infusion reactions, which are characterized by fever, chills, coughing, and sometimes dyspnea. The leukotriene receptor antagonist montelukast is also helpful to prevent infusion-related reactions. Another issue of CD38-targeting antibodies is that these therapeutic antibodies can be detected in laboratory assays such as serum protein electrophoresis (SPEP) and immune fixation electrophoresis (IFE) assays. When the therapeutic antibodies co-migrate with the M-protein of the patient, and are of the same isotype, laboratory personnel may be unable to differentiate between a very good partial response and a complete response. The daratumumab interference reflex assay (DIRA) is able to shift the migration pattern of daratumumab, which enables the correct quantification of the patient's M-protein [14–17]. Blood banks also need to be informed when a patient is treated with a CD38-targeting antibody. Red blood cells express low levels of CD38; thus, CD38-targeting antibodies interfere with the indirect Coombs test, which is used by blood transfusion laboratories to assess the presence of anti-red blood cell antibodies [18]. Several mitigation strategies are now available to solve this issue, including the phenotyping (before start of CD38-targeting antibody treatment) or genotyping of clinically relevant red blood cell antigens [16]. Furthermore, the use of dithiothreitol (DTT) to remove CD38 on the surface of red blood cells can be used to safely provide blood to CD38-targeting antibody-treated patients. Because DTT denatures Kell antigens, K-negative units are provided to these patients [18].

2.2. Combination Therapy with CD38-Targeting Antibodies

Based on the excellent balance between safety and activity, CD38-targeting antibodies are attractive partners for combination strategies in both newly diagnosed and relapsed/refractory patients.

2.2.1. IMiD-Based Combinations

The MAIA study [19], which enrolled newly diagnosed, transplant ineligible MM patients, and the POLLUX [20] study, which included patients with at least one prior line of therapy, showed that adding daratumumab to the standard-of-care regimen lenalidomide–dexamethasone (Rd) improved response rates, including the proportion of patients with minimal-residual disease negative complete remissions (Table 1). The superior response rate translated into a longer progression-free survival of the daratumumab-based triplet, compared to Rd alone. Although cross-trial comparisons should be performed with caution, given the heterogeneity in patient populations, in the relapse setting daratumumab plus Rd has the longest progression-free survival (median 44.5 vs. 17.5 months) with the best hazard ratio (HR: 0.44), compared to other lenalidomide-based triplets such as Rd plus elotuzumab (median progression-free survival, 19.4 versus 14.9 months, HR 0.71), ixazomib (median progression-free survival, 20.6 months versus 14.7 months, HR: 0.74) or carfilzomib (median progression-free survival, 26.1 versus 16.6 months, HR: 0.66) [21–26]. Daratumumab and isatuximab can also effectively be combined with pomalidomide–dexamethasone in patients with prior lenalidomide exposure [27–29]. In the phase 3 APOLLO (median of two prior lines of therapy) and IKARIA (median of three prior lines of therapy) studies, there was roughly a doubling in response rate ($\geq$PR: 46 versus 69% in APOLLO, and 35 versus 60% in IKARIA) and doubling in progression-free survival (APOLLO: median progression-free survival 6.9 versus 12.4 months, HR 0.63; IKARIA: median progression-free survival 6.5 versus 11.5 months, HR 0.60) when either daratumumab or isatuximab was added to the standard-of-care regimen pomalidomide–dexamethasone [28,29].

Table 1. Selected phase 3 studies evaluating IMiD-based antibody combinations.

Study	Regimens	Patient Population
MAIA	Lenalidomide–dexamethasone +/− DARA	Newly diagnosed myeloma patients not eligible for immediate autologous stem cell transplant
POLLUX	Lenalidomide–dexamethasone +/− DARA	At least one prior line of therapy
APOLLO	Pomalidomide–dexamethasone +/− DARA	$\geq$1 prior line of therapy including lenalidomide and a proteasome inhibitor; patients with only 1 prior line of therapy were required to be refractory to lenalidomide.
ICARIA	Pomalidomide–dexamethasone +/− ISA	$\geq$2 previous lines of treatment, including lenalidomide and a proteasome inhibitor
ELOQUENT-2	Lenalidomide–dexamethasone +/− ELO	1–3 prior lines of therapy
ELOQUENT-3	Pomalidomide–dexamethasone +/− ELO	$\geq$2 prior lines of therapy, including at least two consecutive cycles of lenalidomide and a proteasome inhibitor alone or in combination.

Abbreviations: DARA, daratumumab; ISA, isatuximab; ELO, elotuzumab.

2.2.2. PI-Based Combinations

The proteasome inhibitors bortezomib and carfilzomib are effective partner drugs with CD38-targeting antibodies in patients with relapsed/refractory MM (Table 2). The

CASTOR study randomized patients with at least one prior line of therapy between bortezomib–dexamethasone and daratumumab plus bortezomib–dexamethasone [30]. The triplet regimen resulted in a higher response rate and superior progression-free survival across most subgroups [30]. The combination of carfilzomib–dexamethasone plus a CD38-targeting antibody was evaluated in two phase 3 trials in patients with 1–3 prior lines of therapy: isatuximab in the IKEMA and daratumumab in the CANDOR study [31,32]. In both studies, the triplet with a CD38-targeting antibody significantly improved response and progression-free survival with a favorable benefit-risk profile. In the IKEMA study, the overall response was 86% versus 83% with a median progression-free survival of not reached versus 19.2 months (HR: 0.53) in the treatment arm with isatuximab and without isatuximab, respectively. In the CANDOR study, the overall response rate was 84% versus 75%, and median progression-free survival was not reached versus 15.8 months (HR: 0.63) in the daratumumab arm and control arm, respectively. Adding a CD38 antibody to the carfilzomib–dexamethasone backbone also improved the proportion of patients who achieved minimal residual disease-negativity. Both triplets are excellent treatment options for patients with a first lenalidomide-refractory relapse [33].

Table 2. Selected phase 3 studies evaluating proteasome inhibitor-based antibody combinations.

Study	Regimens	Patient Population
ALCYONE	Bortezomib–melphalan–prednisone (VMP) +/− DARA	Newly diagnosed myeloma patients not eligible for immediate autologous stem cell transplantation
CASTOR	Bortezomib–dexamethasone +/− DARA	At least one prior line of therapy
CANDOR	Carfilzomib–dexamethasone +/− DARA	1–3 prior lines of therapy
IKEMA	Carfilzomib–dexamethasone +/− ISA	1–3 prior lines of therapy

Abbreviations: DARA, daratumumab; ISA, isatuximab.

2.2.3. CD38-Targeting Antibody Based Quadruplets

Younger transplant-eligible patients with newly diagnosed disease are frequently treated with high-dose melphalan and autologous stem cell transplantation. Prior to high-dose therapy, these patients receive induction therapy, typically a bortezomib-based triplet such as bortezomib–lenalidomide–dexamethasone (VRD), bortezomib–thalidomide–dexamethasone (VTD), or bortezomib–cyclophosphamide–dexamethasone (VCD) [34]. Because of the favorable activity and safety profile of CD38-targeting antibodies, several studies have evaluated or are currently evaluating the value of adding a CD38-targeting antibody to these triplets (Table 3). The CASSIOPEIA study showed the superiority of daratumumab plus VTD versus VTD alone before and as consolidation after transplantation [35]. The complete response (CR) rate was 39% in the daratumumab group and 26% in the control group, and 64% versus 44% a achieved minimal residual disease-negativity (10^{-5} sensitivity threshold, assessed by multiparametric flow cytometry. The improved response rate resulted in a significantly improved progression-free survival (hazard ratio 0.47) [35]. The randomized phase 2 GRIFFIN study also showed a higher quality of response when daratumumab was added to VRD, compared to VRD alone [36]. In this study, there is not yet a progression-free survival advantage observed in the daratumumab-treated patients. The phase 3 PERSEUS study, which is ongoing, also compares VRD plus or minus daratumumab in a larger number of transplant-eligible patients. The combination of carfilzomib–lenalidomide–dexamethasone (KRd) plus a CD38-targeting antibody is also evaluated in transplant-eligible patients with newly diagnosed disease (e.g., in the ISKIA study). In addition, phase 3 trials (e.g., PERSEUS, CASSIOPEIA, and AURIGA) are also investigating CD38-targeting antibodies alone or in combination with lenalidomide as maintenance treatment post-transplant [35,36].

Table 3. Selected phase 3 studies evaluating IMiD + proteasome inhibitor-based antibody combinations.

Study	Regimens	Patient Population
CASSIOPEIA	Bortezomib–thalidomide–dexamethasone +/− DARA	Newly diagnosed myeloma patients eligible for autologous stem cell transplant and aged ≤65
PERSEUS	Bortezomib–lenalidomide–dexamethasone +/− DARA	Newly diagnosed myeloma patients eligible for autologous stem cell transplant and aged ≤70
CEPHEUS	Bortezomib–lenalidomide–dexamethasone +/− DARA	Newly diagnosed myeloma patients for whom transplant is not intended as initial therapy
IMROZ	Bortezomib–lenalidomide–dexamethasone +/− ISA	Newly diagnosed myeloma patients not eligible for autologous stem cell transplantation

Abbreviations: DARA, daratumumab; ISA, isatuximab.

Elderly, non-transplant eligible patients can be treated with several approved regimens such as the doublet lenalidomide–dexamethasone and the triplets daratumumab–lenalidomide–dexamethasone or bortezomib–melphalan–prednisone (VMP). In addition, based on results from the ALCYONE study, there is now one quadruplet regimen approved for these patients. In the ALCYONE study, non-transplant eligible MM patients received either nine cycles of bortezomib–melphalan–prednisone (VMP) alone or with daratumumab until progression [37,38]. The daratumumab group experienced superior clinical outcomes including an improved overall survival. Part of the improved outcomes with daratumumab–VMP may be related to the design of the study, with patients treated with VMP alone not receiving any maintenance after nine cycles of VMP, while daratumumab was continued until progression in the experimental arm. In addition, only a small proportion of patients who developed disease progression in the VMP only arm were treated with a CD38-targeting antibody at the time of relapse, which may explain part of the overall survival benefit in the daratumumab arm [37]. The combination of CD38-targeting antibody plus VRD is also evaluated in two phase 3 randomized trials with transplant-ineligible patients: CEPHEUS with daratumumab, and IMROZ with isatuximab. Importantly, a meta-analysis in newly diagnosed patients showed that daratumumab also improved progression-free survival in patients with high-risk cytogenetics such as del(17p), t(4;14), and t(14;16) [39].

2.2.4. Toxicity in Combination Regimens

When CD38-targeting antibodies are added to standard-of-care regimens, this is typically accompanied by a higher rate of infections. Particularly, the frequency of respiratory infections is increased. This may be caused by the reduction in already-suppressed polyclonal immunoglobulins [40] or NK cell depletion [41]. Furthermore, the higher rate of neutropenia, especially when a CD38-targeting antibody is combined with an IMiD, may contribute to the development of infections. Patients at high risk for infections (such as elderly patients, or those with elevated lactate dehydrogenase (LDH) low albumin, or elevated alanine aminotransferase (ALAT) may benefit from antibacterial prophylaxis [42].

2.2.5. Subcutaneous Administration

Daratumumab can also be administered via a 5 min subcutaneous injection [43]. The COLUMNA study demonstrated the non-inferiority of subcutaneous daratumumab versus intravenous daratumumab in terms of efficacy and pharmacokinetics [44]. Subcutaneous daratumumab also had an improved safety profile in patients with relapsed or refractory MM with a lower rate of infusion reactions [44]. Subcutaneous administration of daratumumab reduces the time spent in the outpatient infusion center, and thereby quality of life.

2.3. SLAMF7-Targeting Antibodies

Elotuzumab is the first-in-class naked SLAMF7-targeting antibody, which induces MM cell death via ADCC and ADCP [45]. Binding of elotuzumab to SLAMF7 present on the cell surface of NK cells results in NK cell activation and improved immune-mediated attack of MM cells [46,47]. Elotuzumab has no single agent activity in heavily pretreated MM patients, but it significantly enhances the anti-MM effects of IMiDs and PIs in patients with relapsed/refractory MM [21,48–50].

There are currently two elotuzumab-based triplets approved for the treatment of relapsed/refractory MM patients: elotuzumab–lenalidomide–dexamethasone [21] and elotuzumab–pomalidomide–dexamethasone [48]. The ELOQUENT-2 study demonstrated a superior response rate, as well as longer progression-free and overall survival with elotuzumab added to lenalidomide–dexamethasone compared to lenalidomide–dexamethasone alone in patients with 1–3 prior lines of therapy [21,25,42,51]. Similarly, a higher response rate (53 versus 26%) and longer progression-free survival (median progression-free survival: 10.3 versus 4.7 months) was reported in the ELOQUENT-3 study for elotuzumab plus pomalidomide–dexamethasone, compared to pomalidomide–dexamethasone alone in patients with at least two prior lines of therapy including an IMiD and PI [48]. The toxicity profile of elotuzumab is mild, with a low rate of infusion reactions.

Surprisingly, until now, the incorporation of elotuzumab has not been successful in the setting of newly diagnosed disease. Adding elotuzumab to VRD in high-risk, newly diagnosed MM patients did not improve clinical outcomes [52]. In addition, the phase 3 ELOQUENT-1 study showed that elotuzumab plus lenalidomide–dexamethasone was not superior to lenalidomide–dexamethasone alone in newly diagnosed transplant ineligible patients. Finally, elotuzumab plus VRD as induction therapy prior to transplantation did not improve response rate or response quality in the large German GMMG-HD6 study [53].

3. Triple-Class Refractory Myeloma

Although the survival of MM patients significantly improved through the introduction of IMiDs, PIs, and CD38-targeting antibodies, virtually all patients eventually develop resistance towards these agents. MM patients with disease which is resistant to IMiDs, PIs, and CD38-targeting antibodies (triple-class refractory disease) have a very poor outcome at this moment. One analysis showed that triple-class refractory patients have a median overall survival of less than 12 months [54]. Penta-refractory patients (disease refractory to lenalidomide, pomalidomide, bortezomib, carfilzomib, and a CD38-targeting antibody) have the worst prognosis, with a median overall survival of only 5.6 months [54].

These triple-class refractory patients benefit from newly approved drugs with novel mechanism of action such as selinexor, which inhibits XPO-1-mediated nuclear export [55], or the immunoconjugate belantamab mafodotin (see next section) [56]. One study with 34 patients (median of three prior lines of therapy) showed that selinexor can also be effectively combined with daratumumab and dexamethasone [57]. Common adverse events with this IMiD- and PI-free regimen included thrombocytopenia, nausea, and fatigue. The overall response rate was 73% with a median progression-free survival of 12.5 months in daratumumab-naïve patients. In addition, retreatment with drugs that were used in prior lines of therapy can also be considered [33]. However, these triple-class refractory patients should also be considered for clinical trial participation. In such trials, several promising new immunotherapies are evaluated, including chimeric antigen receptor (CAR) T cells and cereblon E3 ligase modulators (CelMods), but also with new antibody formats such as immunoconjugates and bispecific antibodies. The most common target for immunoconjugates and bispecific antibodies is B cell maturation antigen (BCMA). This cell surface protein is highly and uniformly expressed on normal plasma cells, MM cells, and a small subset of mature B cells. BCMA promotes MM cell survival and proliferation [58]. The first naked BCMA antibody evaluated in preclinical studies was SG1 [59]. Although it effectively eliminated MM cells, it was not further developed. A phase 1 study evaluating a humanized, non-fucosylated IgG1 anti-BCMA naked antibody is ongoing [60]. However, maybe more important is that the rather selective expression of BCMA on MM cells makes it possible to improve the cytotoxic capacity of the antibody. Indeed, at this moment powerful immunotherapeutic drugs targeting BCMA show promising results in heavily pretreated patients.

4. Immunoconjugates

Antibodies can also be used to specifically deliver a small molecule (antibody–drug conjugate (ADC)), toxin (immunotoxin), cytokine (immunocytokine) or radionuclide (radioimmunoconjugate) to the tumor cells (Figure 1) [61]. Several immunoconjugates are being investigated in preclinical or phase 1 clinical studies [61], but most advanced in its development is the ADC belantamab mafodotin.

Belantamab mafodotin is a BCMA-directed antibody conjugated by a protease-resistant maleimidocaproyl linker to the microtubule-disrupting agent, monomethyl auristatin F (MMAF). BCMA is specifically expressed on normal plasma cells, MM cells, and a small subset of mature B-cells; therefore, MMAF will be selectively targeted to the tumor cells. Belantamab mafodotin also has other modes of action, such as ADCC and the inhibition of BCMA receptor signaling. In the DREAMM-2 study, belantamab mafodotin was administered every three weeks to triple-class refractory patients. In the 2.5 mg/kg cohort the overall response rate was 31% with a median progression-free survival of 2.9 months, while in the 3.4 mg/kg cohort this was 34% and 4.9 months [56]. The approved dose for use in patients with at least four prior lines of therapy, including a CD38-targeting antibody, PI and IMiD, is 2.5 mg/kg, based on the lower rate of adverse events leading to dose delay or dose reductions in the 2.5 mg/kg cohort, compared to the 3.4 mg/kg cohort [56]. Toxicity of belantamab mafodotin consists of thrombocytopenia and corneal toxicity (keratopathy). Because of the corneal adverse events, close collaboration with an ophthalmologist is important, with ocular assessments at baseline and every cycle thereafter. Based on the activity observed in advanced MM, several combination studies with belantamab mafodotin are ongoing, also in earlier stages of the disease. This includes the DREAMM-6 study, which evaluates the combination of belantamab mafodotin with lenalidomide–dexamethasone or bortezomib–dexamethasone in patients with at least one prior line of therapy [62]. Preliminary data show an acceptable safety profile of belantamab mafodotin (2.5 mg/kg) plus bortezomib–dexamethasone, with keratopathy and thrombocytopenia as the most common adverse events. The three-drug combination induced an overall response rate of 78% in these patients with a median of three prior lines of therapy. Based on these results, the phase 3 DREAMM-7 study is now enrolling patients to evaluate bortezomib–dexamethasone with or without belantamab mafodotin in patients with at least one prior therapy. DREAMM-8 is another phase 3 study, which randomizes patients with at least one prior line of therapy (including lenalidomide) to pomalidomide–dexamethasone or pomalidomide–dexamethasone with belantamab mafodotin. Newly diagnosed transplant-ineligible MM patients can be enrolled in the DREAMM-9 study, which compares VRD with or without belantamab mafodotin.

Several other BCMA-targeting ADCs are in development, including AMG-224 and MEDI2228 [63,64]. AMG-224 is a BCMA antibody conjugated to the tubulin inhibitor mertansine (DM1). In a phase 1 study with 42 patients with a median of 7 prior lines of therapy, the overall response rate was 23% and the recommended phase 2 dose was determined as 3 mg/kg [63]. Ocular adverse events were reported in 21% in the escalation cohort and 36% in the expansion cohort, but no dose reduction or delays were reported due to ocular events [63]. MEDI2228 is another BCMA-specific ADC with a DNA cross-linking pyrrolobenzodiazepine (PBD) dimer as a warhead, which is currently under clinical evaluation [64]. The overall response rate in 41 patients (56% triple-class refractory) treated at the maximum tolerated dose (0.14 mg/kg, every three weeks) was 66% with a median duration of response of 5.9 months. Although keratopathy was not reported in the 0.14 mg/kg cohort, photophobia was commonly observed (all grade: 59%; grade $\geq$ 3: 17%). ADCs targeting other MM-associated antigens are also in (pre)clinical development, such as ADCs targeting CD38, CD138, CD46, and FcRL5 [61].

Importantly, several immunotoxins and immunocytokines are also in early phases of clinical development. This includes TAK-169, which comprises an anti-CD38 single-chain variable fragment fused to the Shiga-like toxin A-subunit [65], and TAK-573, a CD38-specific IgG4 antibody fused to an attenuated form of human IFNα2b [66]. TAK-573 not only has direct anti-tumor activity, but also has the ability to enhance immune cell function [67].

5. Bispecific Antibodies

Durable remissions in a subset of MM patients, who received an allogeneic stem cell transplantation (allo-SCT) or a donor lymphocyte infusion (DLI), provided evidence of the existence of a graft-versus-myeloma effect mediated by donor T cells [68–71]. However, because allo-SCT and DLI are also associated with the development of sometimes life-threatening, infections and graft-versus-host disease, several new strategies that use T cells to eliminate MM cells have been developed with high potency and a better safety profile, compared to allo-SCT. This includes T cells genetically modified to express a chimeric antigen receptor (CAR) that targets a surface antigen expressed on the MM cell. BCMA-specific CAR T cells are very promising, with high response rates and durable responses observed in heavily, often triple-class refractory, MM patients [72–76]. An alternative, off-the-shelf approach to redirect T cells to MM cells is the application of bispecific antibodies (Figure 1) [77,78].

The first-in-class T cell redirecting antibody used in MM is AMG-420 (Table 4) [79]. AMG-420 is a bispecific T cell engager, comprising two single-chain fragment variables and a peptide linker, and lacking an Fc domain. AMG-420 binds with one arm to the CD3 antigen present on the T cell surface, and with the other arm to BCMA, present on the MM cell. This coupling of T cells and MM cells results in T cell activation and degranulation, and subsequently, MM cell death. AMG-420 has a short half-life and needs to be administered via continuous intravenous infusion over four weeks of each six-week cycle [79]. The overall response rate of AMG-420 in patients (median of 3.5 prior lines of therapy), treated at the maximum tolerated dose was 70%, with cytokine release syndrome observed in 38%. Other side effects included infections, cytopenias, and polyneuropathy [79]. Clinical development of AMG-420 stopped because of the need for continuous infusion, which can be challenging for patients. A half-life extended variant, AMG-701, which can be administered once weekly, is now being evaluated in clinical trials with promising results from the phase 1 trial. The overall response rate was 83% in the most recent evaluable cohort, with four out of five responders being triple-class refractory [80].

Teclistamab is another IgG-like bispecific antibody with high activity in advanced MM [81]. In an ongoing phase 1 study, it is administered via intravenous (I.V.) infusion or subcutaneous (S.C.) injection [82]. Most active doses were 270–720 µg/kg I.V. and 720–3000 µg/kg S.C., with an overall response rate at these doses of 69% (overall response rate: 67% (18/27) in I.V. cohorts and 71% (29/41) in S.C. cohorts). The overall response rate at the recommended phase 2 dose of 1500 µg/kg (S.C. administration) was 73%, including at least a very good partial response (VGPR) in 55% of the patients (n = 22, 85% triple-class refractory) [82]. These responses were durable and improved over time. Teclistamab was well-tolerated at the dose of 1500 µg/kg S.C., with only grade 1 or 2 cytokine release syndrome (CRS) events, mainly occurring following the step-up dosing or first full dose. A phase 2 expansion study has started based on these promising results.

Preliminary results from other studies also show promising activity of IgG-like BCMA-targeting bispecific antibodies such as CC-93269, which is characterized by bivalent binding to BCMA [83]. Response to CC-93269 was dose-dependent, with an overall response rate of 43% in all patients (n = 30; 67% triple-class refractory) and 89% in the nine patients treated with 10 mg CC-93269, including CR in 44%. CRS occurred in 77% of patients, including one grade $\geq$ 3 event [83]. This study is ongoing to define the recommended phase 2 dose. Other BCMA/CD3-bispecific antibodies in clinical development are PF-06863135, REGN5458, and TNB-383B (see Table 4) [84–86].

Table 4. Selected studies with bispecific T cell engagers.

Drug Name	Company	Target	Format	Phase of Study	Administration Route	Number of Patients	Median Age (years)	Triple Class Refractory (%)	CRS (All Grade) (%)	CRS (Grade ≥ 3) (%)	≥PR	≥VGPR
AMG-420 [79]	AMGEN	BCMA	BiTE	1	Continuous I.V. infusion	42	65	≤21	38	2	70% at the MTD of 400 ug/day (n = 10)	60% at the MTD of 400 ug/day (n = 10)
AMG-701 [80]	AMGEN	BCMA	Half-life extended BiTE	1	I.V.	85	64	62	65	9	83% in most recent evaluable cohort (n = 6)	50% in most recent evaluable cohort (n = 6)
Teclistamab [82]	Janssen Pharmaceuticals	BCMA	Bispecific antibody	1	I.V. or S.C.	149	63	81	55	0	73% at the RP2D (1500 µg/kg SC) (n = 22)	55% at the RP2D (1500 µg/kg SC) (n = 22)
CC-93269 [83]	BMS/Celgene	BCMA	Bispecific antibody	1	I.V.	30	64	67	77	3	89% among patients with 10 mg (n = 9)	78% among patients with 10 mg (n = 9)
REGN5458 [85]	Regeneron	BCMA	Bispecific antibody	1	I.V.	49	64	100	39	0	63% at dose level 6 (n = 8)	63% at dose level 6 (n = 8)
PF-06863135 [84]	Pfizer	BCMA	Bispecific antibody	1	I.V. and S.C.	30	63	NR	73	0	80% at the 215–1000 µg/kg SC dose (n = 20)	NR
TNB-383B [86]	Tenebio	BCMA	Bispecific antibody	1	I.V.	58	66	64	45	0	80% at dose of 40–60 mg (n = 15)	73% at dose of 40–60 mg (n = 15)
Talquetamab [87]	Janssen Pharmaceuticals	GPRC5D	Bispecific antibody	1	I.V. or S.C.	157	64	82	54	3	69% at the RP2D (405 µg/kg SC) (n = 13)	39% at the RP2D (405 µg/kg SC) (n = 13)
Cevostamab [88]	Roche/Genentech	FcRH5	Bispecific antibody	1	I.V.	53	62	72	78	2	53% in ≥3.6/20 mg cohorts (n = 34)	32% in ≥3.6/20 mg cohorts (n = 34)

Abbreviations: PR, partial response; VGPR, very good partial response; S.C., subcutaneous; I.V., intravenous; RP2D, recommended phase 2 dose; MTD maximum-tolerated dose; NR, not reported.

Several studies are also evaluating bispecific antibodies targeting other MM-associated antigens such as GPRC5D and FcRH5. Talquetamab is the first-in-class GPRC5D-targeting bispecific antibody with high activity in triple-class refractory MM [87]. In an ongoing phase 1 study, talquetamab is administered once weekly via intravenous infusion or subcutaneous injection. Talquetamab has a tolerable safety profile at the recommended phase 2 dose of 405 µg/kg S.C. Frequent adverse events include CRS (no grade 3 events reported with S.C. dosing) and skin toxicity including nail disorders. The overall response rate in the 19 patients (68% triple-class refractory) treated with 405 µg/kg S.C. was 69%, including at least VGPR in 39% [87]. Finally, cevostamab is the first-in-class FcRH5-targeting bispecific antibody which is administered intravenously every three weeks [88]. Preliminary results of the first 53 patients (72% triple-class refractory) have been reported [88]. The overall response rate was 53% in 34 patients who received active doses. CRS was observed in 76% of patients (grade $\geq$ 3 in 2%).

6. Conclusions

The last decade has demonstrated substantial progress in immunotherapy of MM patients. Firstly, the incorporation of CD38-targeting antibodies into standard-of-care relapse and frontline regimens has markedly improved the outcomes of MM patients. In addition, more recently, several clinical studies have shown that new antibody formats such as immunoconjugates and bispecific antibodies have high activity in extensively pretreated, often triple-class refractory, patients. Given the high activity of these new immunotherapies, several ongoing studies are evaluating the value of these novel therapies in earlier phases of the disease (early relapse as well as newly diagnosed disease), frequently combined with other anti-MM agents, such as CD38 antibodies or IMiDs. Given the high single agent activity of bispecific antibodies, these agents may also be applied in patients, who remain minimal residual disease-positive after optimal induction therapy with or without transplant. Efforts are also ongoing to mitigate eye toxicity associated with the BCMA-targeting ADCs. Another open research question is which patients will benefit most from BCMA-targeting CAR T cells, bispecific antibodies, or ADCs. In this respect, not only are differences in efficacy of importance, but safety aspects also play a role. Pre-existing ocular toxicity may limit the applicability of belantamab mafodotin, while compromised cardio-pulmonary function may limit the use of bispecific antibodies or CAR T cells, which often induce CRS. Another important aspect is the direct "off-the-shelf" availability of bispecific antibodies and ADCs, while CAR T cell therapy needs more time for manufacturing. Patients with rapidly progressing disease may benefit most from such "off-the-shelf" approaches. However, in the future, allogeneic CAR T cells or NK cells may be able to overcome such logistical issues. The role of immune fitness also deserves further investigation, because the use of T cell redirection therapy with bispecific antibodies or CAR T cells early in the disease course may be more effective than in end-stage MM, where the cumulative exposure to immunosuppressive anti-MM agents has resulted in substantial impairment of T cell function. In the near future, we will learn whether earlier application of these novel immunotherapies, in combination with other agents, will lead to further improvements in the survival of MM patients.

Author Contributions: C.P.M.V., W.S.C.B., S.Z. and N.W.C.J.v.d.D. equally contributed to writing the manuscript and approved the final version. All authors have read and agreed to the published version of the manuscript.

Funding: This research received no external funding.

Institutional Review Board Statement: Not applicable.

Informed Consent Statement: Not applicable.

Conflicts of Interest: N.W.C.J.v.d.D.: Research support from Janssen Pharmaceuticals, Amgen, Celgene, Novartis, Cellectis, and Bristol-Myers Squibb; Advisory boards for Janssen Pharmaceuticals, Amgen, Celgene, Bristol-Myers Squibb, Novartis, Roche, Takeda, GSK, Sanofi, Bayer and Servier.

References

1. Nijhof, I.S.; Casneuf, T.; Van Velzen, J.; van Kessel, B.; Axel, A.E.; Syed, K.; Groen, R.W.; van Duin, M.; Sonneveld, P.; Minnema, M.C.; et al. CD38 expression and complement inhibitors affect response and resistance to daratumumab therapy in myeloma. *Blood* **2016**, *128*, 959–970. [CrossRef]
2. Nijhof, I.S.; Groen, R.W.; Noort, W.A.; van Kessel, B.; de Jong-Korlaar, R.; Bakker, J.; van Bueren, J.J.; Parren, P.W.; Lokhorst, H.M.; van de Donk, N.W.; et al. Preclinical Evidence for the Therapeutic Potential of CD38-Targeted Immuno-Chemotherapy in Multiple Myeloma Patients Refractory to Lenalidomide and Bortezomib. *Clin. Cancer Res.* **2015**, *21*, 2802–2810. [CrossRef]
3. Kinder, M.; Bahlis, N.J.; Malavasi, F.; De Goeij, B.; Babich, A.; Sendecki, J.; Rusbuldt, J.; Bellew, K.; Kane, C.; Van de Donk, N. Comparison of CD38 antibodies in vitro and ex vivo mechanisms of action in multiple myeloma. *Haematologica* **2021**. [CrossRef] [PubMed]
4. Krejcik, J.; Casneuf, T.; Nijhof, I.S.; Verbist, B.; Bald, J.; Plesner, T.; Syed, K.; Liu, K.; van de Donk, N.W.; Weiss, B.M.; et al. Daratumumab depletes CD38+ immune regulatory cells, promotes T-cell expansion, and skews T-cell repertoire in multiple myeloma. *Blood* **2016**, *128*, 384–394. [CrossRef]
5. van de Donk, N. Immunomodulatory effects of CD38-targeting antibodies. *Immunol. Lett.* **2018**, *199*, 16–22. [CrossRef]
6. Adams, H.C., 3rd; Stevenaert, F.; Krejcik, J.; Van der Borght, K.; Smets, T.; Bald, J.; Abraham, Y.; Ceulemans, H.; Chiu, C.; Vanhoof, G.; et al. High-Parameter Mass Cytometry Evaluation of Relapsed/Refractory Multiple Myeloma Patients Treated with Daratumumab Demonstrates Immune Modulation as a Novel Mechanism of Action. *Cytom. Part A* **2019**, *95*, 279–289. [CrossRef]
7. Atanackovic, D.; Yousef, S.; Shorter, C.; Tantravahi, S.K.; Steinbach, M.; Iglesias, F.; Sborov, D.; Radhakrishnan, S.V.; Chiron, M.; Miles, R.; et al. In vivo vaccination effect in multiple myeloma patients treated with the monoclonal antibody isatuximab. *Leukemia* **2020**, *34*, 317–321. [CrossRef]
8. Kumar, S.K.; Lee, J.H.; Lahuerta, J.J.; Morgan, G.; Richardson, P.G.; Crowley, J.; Haessler, J.; Feather, J.; Hoering, A.; Moreau, P.; et al. Risk of progression and survival in multiple myeloma relapsing after therapy with IMiDs and bortezomib: A multicenter international myeloma working group study. *Leukemia* **2012**, *26*, 149–157. [CrossRef]
9. Lokhorst, H.M.; Plesner, T.; Laubach, J.P.; Nahi, H.; Gimsing, P.; Hansson, M.; Minnema, M.C.; Lassen, U.; Krejcik, J.; Palumbo, A.; et al. Targeting CD38 with Daratumumab Monotherapy in Multiple Myeloma. *N. Engl. J. Med.* **2015**, *373*, 1207–1219. [CrossRef] [PubMed]
10. Lonial, S.; Weiss, B.M.; Usmani, S.Z.; Singhal, S.; Chari, A.; Bahlis, N.J.; Belch, A.; Krishnan, A.; Vescio, R.A.; Mateos, M.V.; et al. Daratumumab monotherapy in patients with treatment-refractory multiple myeloma (SIRIUS): An open-label, randomised, phase 2 trial. *Lancet* **2016**, *387*, 1551–1560. [CrossRef]
11. Martin, T.; Strickland, S.; Glenn, M.; Charpentier, E.; Guillemin, H.; Hsu, K.; Mikhael, J. Phase I trial of isatuximab monotherapy in the treatment of refractory multiple myeloma. *Blood Cancer J.* **2019**, *9*, 41. [CrossRef]
12. Krishnan, A.Y.; Patel, K.; Parameswaran, H.; Jagannath, S.; Niesvizky, R.; Silbermann, R. Preliminary Results from a Phase 1b Study of TAK-079, an Investigational Anti-CD38 Monoclonal Antibody (mAb) in Patients with Relapsed/Refractory Multiple Myeloma (RRMM). *Blood* **2019**, *134*, 140. [CrossRef]
13. Usmani, S.Z.; Nahi, H.; Plesner, T.; Weiss, B.M.; Bahlis, N.J.; Belch, A.; Voorhees, P.M.; Laubach, J.P.; van de Donk, N.; Ahmadi, T.; et al. Daratumumab monotherapy in patients with heavily pretreated relapsed or refractory multiple myeloma: Final results from the phase 2 GEN501 and SIRIUS trials. *Lancet Haematol.* **2020**, *7*, e447–e455. [CrossRef]
14. McCudden, C.R.; Axel, A.; Slaets, D.; Frans, S.; Bald, J.; Schecter, J. Assessing clinical response in multiple myeloma (MM) patients treated with monoclonal antibodies (mAbs): Validation of a daratumumab IFE reflex assay (DIRA) to distinguish malignant M-protein from therapeutic antibody. *J. Clin. Oncol.* **2015**, *33*, 8590. [CrossRef]
15. van de Donk, N.W.; Otten, H.G.; El Haddad, O.; Axel, A.; Sasser, A.K.; Croockewit, S.; Jacobs, J.F. Interference of daratumumab in monitoring multiple myeloma patients using serum immunofixation electrophoresis can be abrogated using the daratumumab IFE reflex assay (DIRA). *Clin. Chem. Lab. Med.* **2016**, *54*, 1105–1109. [CrossRef] [PubMed]
16. van de Donk, N.; Richardson, P.G.; Malavasi, F. CD38 antibodies in multiple myeloma: Back to the future. *Blood* **2018**, *131*, 13–29. [CrossRef]
17. van de Donk, N.W.; Moreau, P.; Plesner, T.; Palumbo, A.; Gay, F.; Laubach, J.P.; Malavasi, F.; Avet-Loiseau, H.; Mateos, M.V.; Sonneveld, P.; et al. Clinical efficacy and management of monoclonal antibodies targeting CD38 and SLAMF7 in multiple myeloma. *Blood* **2016**, *127*, 681–695. [CrossRef]
18. Chapuy, C.I.; Nicholson, R.T.; Aguad, M.D.; Chapuy, B.; Laubach, J.P.; Richardson, P.G.; Doshi, P.; Kaufman, R.M. Resolving the daratumumab interference with blood compatibility testing. *Transfusion* **2015**, *55*, 1545–1554. [CrossRef]
19. Facon, T.; Kumar, S.; Plesner, T.; Orlowski, R.Z.; Moreau, P.; Bahlis, N.; Basu, S.; Nahi, H.; Hulin, C.; Quach, H.; et al. Daratumumab plus Lenalidomide and Dexamethasone for Untreated Myeloma. *N. Engl. J. Med.* **2019**, *380*, 2104–2115. [CrossRef]
20. Dimopoulos, M.A.; Oriol, A.; Nahi, H.; San-Miguel, J.; Bahlis, N.J.; Usmani, S.Z.; Rabin, N.; Orlowski, R.Z.; Komarnicki, M.; Suzuki, K.; et al. Daratumumab, Lenalidomide, and Dexamethasone for Multiple Myeloma. *N. Engl. J. Med.* **2016**, *375*, 1319–1331. [CrossRef] [PubMed]
21. Lonial, S.; Dimopoulos, M.; Palumbo, A.; White, D.; Grosicki, S.; Spicka, I.; Walter-Croneck, A.; Moreau, P.; Mateos, M.V.; Magen, H.; et al. Elotuzumab Therapy for Relapsed or Refractory Multiple Myeloma. *N. Engl. J. Med.* **2015**, *373*, 621–631. [CrossRef]
22. Moreau, P.; Masszi, T.; Grzasko, N.; Bahlis, N.J.; Hansson, M.; Pour, L.; Sandhu, I.; Ganly, P.; Baker, B.W.; Jackson, S.R.; et al. Oral Ixazomib, Lenalidomide, and Dexamethasone for Multiple Myeloma. *N. Engl. J. Med.* **2016**, *374*, 1621–1634. [CrossRef] [PubMed]

23. Stewart, A.K.; Rajkumar, S.V.; Dimopoulos, M.A.; Masszi, T.; Spicka, I.; Oriol, A.; Hajek, R.; Rosinol, L.; Siegel, D.S.; Mihaylov, G.G.; et al. Carfilzomib, lenalidomide, and dexamethasone for relapsed multiple myeloma. *N. Engl. J. Med.* **2015**, *372*, 142–152. [CrossRef]
24. Bahlis, N.J.; Dimopoulos, M.A.; White, D.J.; Benboubker, L.; Cook, G.; Leiba, M.; Ho, P.J.; Kim, K.; Takezako, N.; Moreau, P.; et al. Daratumumab plus lenalidomide and dexamethasone in relapsed/refractory multiple myeloma: Extended follow-up of POLLUX, a randomized, open-label, phase 3 study. *Leukemia* **2020**, *34*, 1875–1884. [CrossRef]
25. Dimopoulos, M.A.; Lonial, S.; Betts, K.A.; Chen, C.; Zichlin, M.L.; Brun, A.; Signorovitch, J.E.; Makenbaeva, D.; Mekan, S.; Sy, O.; et al. Elotuzumab plus lenalidomide and dexamethasone in relapsed/refractory multiple myeloma: Extended 4-year follow-up and analysis of relative progression-free survival from the randomized ELOQUENT-2 trial. *Cancer* **2018**, *124*, 4032–4043. [CrossRef]
26. Siegel, D.S.; Dimopoulos, M.A.; Ludwig, H.; Facon, T.; Goldschmidt, H.; Jakubowiak, A.; San-Miguel, J.; Obreja, M.; Blaedel, J.; Stewart, A.K. Improvement in Overall Survival with Carfilzomib, Lenalidomide, and Dexamethasone in Patients with Relapsed or Refractory Multiple Myeloma. *J. Clin. Oncol.* **2018**, *36*, 728–734. [CrossRef]
27. Siegel, D.S.; Schiller, G.J.; Samaras, C.; Sebag, M.; Berdeja, J.; Ganguly, S.; Matous, J.; Song, K.; Seet, C.S.; Talamo, G.; et al. Pomalidomide, dexamethasone, and daratumumab in relapsed refractory multiple myeloma after lenalidomide treatment. *Leukemia* **2020**. [CrossRef]
28. Attal, M.; Richardson, P.G.; Rajkumar, S.V.; San-Miguel, J.; Beksac, M.; Spicka, I.; Leleu, X.; Schjesvold, F.; Moreau, P.; Dimopoulos, M.A.; et al. Isatuximab plus pomalidomide and low-dose dexamethasone versus pomalidomide and low-dose dexamethasone in patients with relapsed and refractory multiple myeloma (ICARIA-MM): A randomised, multicentre, open-label, phase 3 study. *Lancet* **2019**, *394*, 2096–2107. [CrossRef]
29. Dimopoulos, M.; Terpos, E.; Boccadoro, M.; Delimpasi, S.; Beksac, M.; Katodritou, E.; Moreau, P.; Baldini, L. Apollo: Phase 3 Randomized Study of Subcutaneous Daratumumab Plus Pomalidomide and Dexamethasone (D-Pd) Versus Pomalidomide and Dexamethasone (Pd) Alone in Patients (Pts) with Relapsed/Refractory Multiple Myeloma (RRMM). *Blood* **2020**, *130*, 412.
30. Palumbo, A.; Chanan-Khan, A.; Weisel, K.; Nooka, A.K.; Masszi, T.; Beksac, M.; Spicka, I.; Hungria, V.; Munder, M.; Mateos, M.V.; et al. Daratumumab, Bortezomib, and Dexamethasone for Multiple Myeloma. *N. Engl. J. Med.* **2016**, *375*, 754–766. [CrossRef] [PubMed]
31. Dimopoulos, M.; Quach, H.; Mateos, M.V.; Landgren, O.; Leleu, X.; Siegel, D.; Weisel, K.; Yang, H.; Klippel, Z.; Zahlten-Kumeli, A.; et al. Carfilzomib, dexamethasone, and daratumumab versus carfilzomib and dexamethasone for patients with relapsed or refractory multiple myeloma (CANDOR): Results from a randomised, multicentre, open-label, phase 3 study. *Lancet* **2020**, *396*, 186–197. [CrossRef]
32. Moreau, P.; Dimopoulos, M.; Mikhael, J.; Yong, K.; Capra, M.; Facon, T.; Hajek, R. Isatuximab plus carfilzomib and dexamethasone vs carfilzomib and dexamethasone in relapsed/refractory multiple myeloma (IKEMA): Interim analysis of a phase 3 randomized, open-label study. *EHA* **2020**, *16*, 4347–4358.
33. van de Donk, N. Sequencing multiple myeloma therapies with and after antibody therapies. *Hematol. Am. Soc. Hematol. Educ. Program* **2020**, *2020*, 248–258. [CrossRef]
34. van de Donk, N.; Pawlyn, C.; Yong, K.L. Multiple myeloma. *Lancet* **2021**, *397*, 410–427. [CrossRef]
35. Moreau, P.; Attal, M.; Hulin, C.; Arnulf, B.; Belhadj, K.; Benboubker, L.; Bene, M.C.; Broijl, A.; Caillon, H.; Caillot, D.; et al. Bortezomib, thalidomide, and dexamethasone with or without daratumumab before and after autologous stem-cell transplantation for newly diagnosed multiple myeloma (CASSIOPEIA): A randomised, open-label, phase 3 study. *Lancet* **2019**, *394*, 29–38. [CrossRef]
36. Voorhees, P.M.; Kaufman, J.L.; Laubach, J.; Sborov, D.W.; Reeves, B.; Rodriguez, C.; Chari, A.; Silbermann, R.; Costa, L.J.; Anderson, L.D., Jr.; et al. Daratumumab, lenalidomide, bortezomib, and dexamethasone for transplant-eligible newly diagnosed multiple myeloma: The GRIFFIN trial. *Blood* **2020**, *136*, 936–945. [CrossRef] [PubMed]
37. Mateos, M.V.; Cavo, M.; Blade, J.; Dimopoulos, M.A.; Suzuki, K.; Jakubowiak, A.; Knop, S.; Doyen, C.; Lucio, P.; Nagy, Z.; et al. Overall survival with daratumumab, bortezomib, melphalan, and prednisone in newly diagnosed multiple myeloma (ALCYONE): A randomised, open-label, phase 3 trial. *Lancet* **2020**, *395*, 132–141. [CrossRef]
38. Mateos, M.V.; Dimopoulos, M.A.; Cavo, M.; Suzuki, K.; Jakubowiak, A.; Knop, S.; Doyen, C.; Lucio, P.; Nagy, Z.; Kaplan, P.; et al. Daratumumab plus Bortezomib, Melphalan, and Prednisone for Untreated Myeloma. *N. Engl. J. Med.* **2018**, *378*, 518–528. [CrossRef]
39. Giri, S.; Grimshaw, A.; Bal, S.; Godby, K.; Kharel, P.; Djulbegovic, B.; Dimopoulos, M.A.; Facon, T.; Usmani, S.Z.; Mateos, M.V.; et al. Evaluation of Daratumumab for the Treatment of Multiple Myeloma in Patients with High-Risk Cytogenetic Factors: A Systematic Review and Meta-Analysis. *JAMA Oncol.* **2020**, *6*, 1–8. [CrossRef]
40. Frerichs, K.A.; Bosman, P.W.C.; van Velzen, J.F.; Fraaij, P.L.A.; Koopmans, M.P.G.; Rimmelzwaan, G.F.; Nijhof, I.S.; Bloem, A.C.; Mutis, T.; Zweegman, S.; et al. Effect of daratumumab on normal plasma cells, polyclonal immunoglobulin levels, and vaccination responses in extensively pre-treated multiple myeloma patients. *Haematologica* **2020**, *105*, e302–e306. [CrossRef]
41. Casneuf, T.; Xu, X.S.; Adams, H.C., 3rd; Axel, A.E.; Chiu, C.; Khan, I.; Ahmadi, T.; Yan, X.; Lonial, S.; Plesner, T.; et al. Effects of daratumumab on natural killer cells and impact on clinical outcomes in relapsed or refractory multiple myeloma. *Blood Adv.* **2017**, *1*, 2105–2114. [CrossRef] [PubMed]

42. Van de Donk, N.; Zweegman, S.; San Miguel, J.; Dimopoulos, M.; Cavo, M.; Suzuki, K.; Touzeau, C.; Usmani, S. Predictive Markers of High-Grade or Serious Treatment-Emergent Infections with Daratumumab-Based Regimens in Newly Diagnosed Multiple Myeloma (NDMM). *Blood* **2020**, *130*, 3209.
43. San-Miguel, J.; Usmani, S.Z.; Mateos, M.V.; van de Donk, N.; Kaufman, J.L.; Moreau, P.; Oriol, A.; Plesner, T.; Benboubker, L.; Liu, K.; et al. Subcutaneous daratumumab in patients with relapsed or refractory multiple myeloma: Part 2 of the open-label, multicenter, dose-escalation phase 1b study (PAVO). *Haematologica* **2020**. [CrossRef] [PubMed]
44. Mateos, M.V.; Nahi, H.; Legiec, W.; Grosicki, S.; Vorobyev, V.; Spicka, I.; Hungria, V.; Korenkova, S.; Bahlis, N.; Flogegard, M.; et al. Subcutaneous versus intravenous daratumumab in patients with relapsed or refractory multiple myeloma (COLUMBA): A multicentre, open-label, non-inferiority, randomised, phase 3 trial. *Lancet Haematol.* **2020**, *7*, e370–e380. [CrossRef]
45. Kurdi, A.T.; Glavey, S.V.; Bezman, N.A.; Jhatakia, A.; Guerriero, J.L.; Manier, S.; Moschetta, M.; Mishima, Y.; Roccaro, A.; Detappe, A.; et al. Antibody-Dependent Cellular Phagocytosis by Macrophages is a Novel Mechanism of Action of Elotuzumab. *Mol. Cancer Ther.* **2018**, *17*, 1454–1463. [CrossRef] [PubMed]
46. Hsi, E.D.; Steinle, R.; Balasa, B.; Szmania, S.; Draksharapu, A.; Shum, B.P.; Huseni, M.; Powers, D.; Nanisetti, A.; Zhang, Y.; et al. CS1, a potential new therapeutic antibody target for the treatment of multiple myeloma. *Clin. Cancer Res.* **2008**, *14*, 2775–2784. [CrossRef] [PubMed]
47. Collins, S.M.; Bakan, C.E.; Swartzel, G.D.; Hofmeister, C.C.; Efebera, Y.A.; Kwon, H.; Starling, G.C.; Ciarlariello, D.; Bhaskar, S.; Briercheck, E.L.; et al. Elotuzumab directly enhances NK cell cytotoxicity against myeloma via CS1 ligation: Evidence for augmented NK cell function complementing ADCC. *Cancer Immunol. Immunother.* **2013**, *62*, 1841–1849. [CrossRef]
48. Dimopoulos, M.A.; Dytfeld, D.; Grosicki, S.; Moreau, P.; Takezako, N.; Hori, M.; Leleu, X.; LeBlanc, R.; Suzuki, K.; Raab, M.S.; et al. Elotuzumab plus Pomalidomide and Dexamethasone for Multiple Myeloma. *N. Engl. J. Med.* **2018**, *379*, 1811–1822. [CrossRef]
49. Jakubowiak, A.; Offidani, M.; Pegourie, B.; De La Rubia, J.; Garderet, L.; Laribi, K.; Bosi, A.; Marasca, R.; Laubach, J.; Mohrbacher, A.; et al. Randomized phase 2 study: Elotuzumab plus bortezomib/dexamethasone vs bortezomib/dexamethasone for relapsed/refractory MM. *Blood* **2016**, *127*, 2833–2840. [CrossRef]
50. Jakubowiak, A.J.; Benson, D.M.; Bensinger, W.; Siegel, D.S.; Zimmerman, T.M.; Mohrbacher, A.; Richardson, P.G.; Afar, D.E.; Singhal, A.K.; Anderson, K.C. Phase I trial of anti-CS1 monoclonal antibody elotuzumab in combination with bortezomib in the treatment of relapsed/refractory multiple myeloma. *J. Clin. Oncol.* **2012**, *30*, 1960–1965. [CrossRef]
51. Dimopoulos, M.A.; Lonial, S.; White, D.; Moreau, P.; Palumbo, A.; San-Miguel, J.; Shpilberg, O.; Anderson, K.; Grosicki, S.; Spicka, I.; et al. Elotuzumab plus lenalidomide/dexamethasone for relapsed or refractory multiple myeloma: ELOQUENT-2 follow-up and post-hoc analyses on progression-free survival and tumour growth. *Br. J. Haematol.* **2017**, *178*, 896–905. [CrossRef] [PubMed]
52. Usmani, S.Z.; Hoering, A.; Ailawadhi, S.; Sexton, R.; Lipe, B.; Hita, S.F.; Valent, J.; Rosenzweig, M.; Zonder, J.A.; Dhodapkar, M.; et al. Bortezomib, lenalidomide, and dexamethasone with or without elotuzumab in patients with untreated, high-risk multiple myeloma (SWOG-1211): Primary analysis of a randomised, phase 2 trial. *Lancet Haematol.* **2021**, *8*, e45–e54. [CrossRef]
53. Goldschmidt, H.; Mai, E.; Salwender, H.; Bertsch, U.; Miah, K.; Kunz, C.; Fenk, R.; Blau, I. Bortezomib, lenalidomide and dexamethasone with or without elotuzumab as induction therapy for newly-diagnosed, transplant-eligible multiple myeloma. *EHA* **2020**, S203. Available online: https://library.ehaweb.org/eha/2020/eha25th/295023/hartmut.goldschmidt.bortezomib.lenalidomide.and.dexamethasone.with.or.without (accessed on 22 February 2021).
54. Gandhi, U.H.; Cornell, R.F.; Lakshman, A.; Gahvari, Z.J.; McGehee, E.; Jagosky, M.H.; Gupta, R.; Varnado, W.; Fiala, M.A.; Chhabra, S.; et al. Outcomes of patients with multiple myeloma refractory to CD38-targeted monoclonal antibody therapy. *Leukemia* **2019**, *33*, 2266–2275. [CrossRef]
55. Chari, A.; Vogl, D.T.; Gavriatopoulou, M.; Nooka, A.K.; Yee, A.J.; Huff, C.A.; Moreau, P.; Dingli, D.; Cole, C.; Lonial, S.; et al. Oral Selinexor-Dexamethasone for Triple-Class Refractory Multiple Myeloma. *N. Engl. J. Med.* **2019**, *381*, 727–738. [CrossRef]
56. Lonial, S.; Lee, H.C.; Badros, A.; Trudel, S.; Nooka, A.K.; Chari, A.; Abdallah, A.O.; Callander, N.; Lendvai, N.; Sborov, D.; et al. Belantamab mafodotin for relapsed or refractory multiple myeloma (DREAMM-2): A two-arm, randomised, open-label, phase 2 study. *Lancet Oncol.* **2020**, *21*, 207–221. [CrossRef]
57. Gasparetto, C.; Lentzsch, S.; Schiller, G.; Callander, N.; Tuchman, S.; Chen, C.; White, D.; Kotb, R.; Sutherland, H.; Sebag, M.; et al. Selinexor, daratumumab, and dexamethasone in patients with relapsed or refractory multiple myeloma. *eJHaem* **2021**, *2*, 56–65. [CrossRef]
58. Tai, Y.T.; Acharya, C.; An, G.; Moschetta, M.; Zhong, M.Y.; Feng, X.; Cea, M.; Cagnetta, A.; Wen, K.; van Eenennaam, H.; et al. APRIL and BCMA promote human multiple myeloma growth and immunosuppression in the bone marrow microenvironment. *Blood* **2016**, *127*, 3225–3236. [CrossRef] [PubMed]
59. Ryan, M.C.; Hering, M.; Peckham, D.; McDonagh, C.F.; Brown, L.; Kim, K.M.; Meyer, D.L.; Zabinski, R.F.; Grewal, I.S.; Carter, P.J. Antibody targeting of B-cell maturation antigen on malignant plasma cells. *Mol. Cancer Ther.* **2007**, *6*, 3009–3018. [CrossRef]
60. Abdallah, A.-O.A.; Hoffman, J.E.; Schroeder, M.A.; Jacquemont, C.; Li, H.; Wang, Y.; Epps, H.V.; Campbell, M.S. SGNBCMA-001: A phase 1 study of SEA-BCMA, a non-fucosylated monoclonal antibody, in subjects with relapsed or refractory multiple myeloma. *J. Clin. Oncol.* **2019**, *37*, TPS8054. [CrossRef]
61. Bruins, W.S.C.; Zweegman, S.; Mutis, T.; van de Donk, N. Targeted Therapy with Immunoconjugates for Multiple Myeloma. *Front. Immunol.* **2020**, *11*, 1155. [CrossRef] [PubMed]

62. Popat, R.; Nooka, A.; Stockerl-Goldstein, K.; Abonour, R.; Ramaekers, R.; Khot, A.; Forbes, A.; Lee, C.; Augustson, B.; Spencer, A.; et al. DREAMM-6: Safety, Tolerability and Clinical Activity of Belantamab Mafodotin (Belamaf) in Combination with Bortezomib/Dexamethasone (BorDex) in Relapsed/Refractory Multiple Myeloma (RRMM). *Blood* **2020**, *136*, 19–20. [CrossRef]
63. Lee, H.C.; Raje, N.S.; Landgren, O.; Upreti, V.V.; Wang, J.; Avilion, A.A.; Hu, X.; Rasmussen, E.; Ngarmchamnanrith, G.; Fujii, H.; et al. Phase 1 study of the anti-BCMA antibody-drug conjugate AMG 224 in patients with relapsed/refractory multiple myeloma. *Leukemia* **2021**, *35*, 255–258. [CrossRef] [PubMed]
64. Kumar, S.; Migkou, M.; Bhutani, M.; Spencer, A.; Ailawadhi, S.; Kalff, A.; Walcott, F.; Pore, N. Phase 1 First-in-Human Study of MEDI2228, a BCMA-Targeted ADC in Patients with Relapsed/Refractory Multiple Myeloma. *Blood* **2020**, *136*, 26. [CrossRef]
65. Willert, E.K.; Robinson, G.L.; Higgins, J.P.; Liu, J.; Lee, J.; Syed, S.; Zhang, Y.; Tavares, D.; Lublinsky, A.; Chattopadhyay, N.; et al. Abstract 2384: TAK-169, an exceptionally potent CD38 targeted engineered toxin body, as a novel direct cell kill approach for the treatment of multiple myeloma. *Cancer Res.* **2019**, *79*, 2384. [CrossRef]
66. Pogue, S.L.; Taura, T.; Bi, M.; Yun, Y.; Sho, A.; Mikesell, G.; Behrens, C.; Sokolovsky, M.; Hallak, H.; Rosenstock, M.; et al. Targeting Attenuated Interferon-Alpha to Myeloma Cells with a CD38 Antibody Induces Potent Tumor Regression with Reduced Off-Target Activity. *PLoS ONE* **2016**, *11*, e0162472. [CrossRef]
67. Pogue, S.; Bi, M.; Armanini, M.; Fatholahi, M.; Taura, T.; Valencia, M.; Yun, Y.; Sho, A.; Jamin, A.; Nock, S.; et al. Attenuated Interferon-α Targeted to CD38 Expressing Multiple Myeloma Tumor Cells Induces Robust and Durable Anti-Tumor Responses through Direct Anti-Proliferative Activity in Addition to Indirect Recruitment and Activation of M1 Macrophages. *Blood* **2017**, *130*, 3112. [CrossRef]
68. Lokhorst, H.M.; Schattenberg, A.; Cornelissen, J.J.; van Oers, M.H.; Fibbe, W.; Russell, I.; Donk, N.W.; Verdonck, L.F. Donor lymphocyte infusions for relapsed multiple myeloma after allogeneic stem-cell transplantation: Predictive factors for response and long-term outcome. *J. Clin. Oncol.* **2000**, *18*, 3031–3037. [CrossRef]
69. Lokhorst, H.M.; Wu, K.; Verdonck, L.F.; Laterveer, L.L.; van de Donk, N.W.; van Oers, M.H.; Cornelissen, J.J.; Schattenberg, A.V. The occurrence of graft-versus-host disease is the major predictive factor for response to donor lymphocyte infusions in multiple myeloma. *Blood* **2004**, *103*, 4362–4364. [CrossRef]
70. Van de Donk, N.W.; Kroger, N.; Hegenbart, U.; Corradini, P.; San Miguel, J.F.; Goldschmidt, H.; Perez-Simon, J.A.; Zijlmans, M.; Raymakers, R.A.; Montefusco, V.; et al. Prognostic factors for donor lymphocyte infusions following non-myeloablative allogeneic stem cell transplantation in multiple myeloma. *Bone Marrow Transplant.* **2006**, *37*, 1135–1141. [CrossRef]
71. Lokhorst, H.; Einsele, H.; Vesole, D.; Bruno, B.; San, M.J.; Perez-Simon, J.A.; Kroger, N.; Moreau, P.; Gahrton, G.; Gasparetto, C.; et al. International Myeloma Working Group consensus statement regarding the current status of allogeneic stem-cell transplantation for multiple myeloma. *J. Clin. Oncol.* **2010**, *28*, 4521–4530. [CrossRef]
72. Lin, Y.; Raje, N.; Berdeja, J.; Siegel, D.; Jagannath, S.; Madduri, D.; Liedtke, M.; Rosenblatt, J.; Maus, M.V. Idecabtagene vicleucel (ide-cel, bb2121), a BCMA-directed CAR T cell therapy, in patients with relapsed and refractory multipe myeloma: Updated results from phase 1 CRB-401 study. *Blood* **2020**, *136*, 131. [CrossRef]
73. Munshi, N.; Anderson, L.D., Jr.; Shah, N.; Jagannath, S.; Berdeja, J.; Lonial, S.; Raje, N.; Siegel, D.; Lin, Y. Idecabtagene vicleucel (ide-cel, bb2121), a BCMA-targeted CAR T-cell therapy, in patients with relapsed and refractory multiple myeloma (RRMM): Initial KarMMa results. *J. Clin. Oncol.* **2020**, *38*, 8503. [CrossRef]
74. Raje, N.; Berdeja, J.; Lin, Y.; Siegel, D.; Jagannath, S.; Madduri, D.; Liedtke, M.; Rosenblatt, J.; Maus, M.V.; Turka, A.; et al. Anti-BCMA CAR T-Cell Therapy bb2121 in Relapsed or Refractory Multiple Myeloma. *N. Engl. J. Med.* **2019**, *380*, 1726–1737. [CrossRef] [PubMed]
75. Madduri, D.; Berdeja, J.; Usmani, S.; Jakubowiak, A.; Agha, M.; Cohen, A.; Stewart, A.K.; Hari, P. CARTITUDE-1: Phase 1b/2 study of ciltacabtagene autoleucel, a B-cell maturation antigen-directed chimeric antigen receptor T-cell therapy, in relapsed/refractory multiple myeloma. *Blood* **2020**, *136*, 177. [CrossRef]
76. Zhao, W.H.; Liu, J.; Wang, B.Y.; Chen, Y.X.; Cao, X.M.; Yang, Y.; Zhang, Y.L.; Wang, F.X.; Zhang, P.Y.; Lei, B.; et al. A phase 1, open-label study of LCAR-B38M, a chimeric antigen receptor T cell therapy directed against B cell maturation antigen, in patients with relapsed or refractory multiple myeloma. *J. Hematol. Oncol.* **2018**, *11*, 141. [CrossRef]
77. Verkleij, C.P.M.; Korst, C.; van de Donk, N. Immunotherapy in multiple myeloma: When, where, and for who? *Curr. Opin. Oncol.* **2020**. [CrossRef]
78. Verkleij, C.P.M.; Frerichs, K.A.; Broekmans, M.; Absalah, S.; Maas-Bosman, P.W.C.; Kruyswijk, S.; Nijhof, I.S.; Mutis, T.; Zweegman, S.; van de Donk, N. T-cell redirecting bispecific antibodies targeting BCMA for the treatment of multiple myeloma. *Oncotarget* **2020**, *11*, 4076–4081. [CrossRef] [PubMed]
79. Topp, M.S.; Duell, J.; Zugmaier, G.; Attal, M.; Moreau, P.; Langer, C.; Kronke, J.; Facon, T.; Salnikov, A.V.; Lesley, R.; et al. Anti-B-Cell Maturation Antigen BiTE Molecule AMG 420 Induces Responses in Multiple Myeloma. *J. Clin. Oncol.* **2020**, *38*, 775–783. [CrossRef]
80. Harrison, B.; Minnema, M.; Lee, H.C.; Spencer, A.; Kapoor, P.; Madduri, D.; Larsen, J.T.; Ailawadhi, S.; Kaufman, J.L. A Phase 1 First in Human (FIH) Study of AMG 701, an Anti-B-Cell Maturation Antigen (BCMA) Half-Life Extended (HLE) BiTE® (bispecific T-cell engager) Molecule, in Relapsed/Refractory (RR) Multiple Myeloma (MM). *Blood* **2020**, *136*, 28. [CrossRef]
81. Frerichs, K.A.; Broekmans, M.E.C.; Marin Soto, J.A.; van Kessel, B.; Heymans, M.W.; Holthof, L.C.; Verkleij, C.P.M.; Boominathan, R.; Vaidya, B.; Sendecki, J.; et al. Preclinical Activity of JNJ-7957, a Novel BCMA×CD3 Bispecific Antibody for the Treatment of Multiple Myeloma, Is Potentiated by Daratumumab. *Clin. Cancer Res.* **2020**, *26*, 2203–2215. [CrossRef] [PubMed]

82. Garfall, A.L.; Usmani, S.; Mateos, M.V.; Nahi, H.; Van de Donk, N.; San-Miguel, J.; Oriol, A.; Chari, A. Updated phase 1 results of teclistamab, a B-cell maturation antigen (BCMA) x CD3 bispecific antibody, in relapsed and/or refractory multiple myeloma (RRMM). *Blood* **2020**, *136*, 27. [CrossRef]
83. Costa, L.; Wong, S.; Bermudez, A.; de la Rubia, J.; Mateos, M.V.; Ocio, E.; Rodriguez Otero, P. Interim results from the first phase 1 clinical study of the B-cell maturation antigen (BCMA) 2 + 1 T-cell engager (TCE) CC-93269 in patients (pts) with relapsed/refractory multiple myeloma (RRMM). *EHA* **2020**, 143. [CrossRef]
84. Lesokhin, A.M.; Levy, M.Y.; Dalovisio, A.P.; Bahlis, N.J.; Solh, M.; Sebag, M.; Jakubowiak, A.; Jethava, Y.S.; Costello, C.L.; Chu, M.P.; et al. Preliminary Safety, Efficacy, Pharmacokinetics, and Pharmacodynamics of Subcutaneously (SC) Administered PF-06863135, a B-Cell Maturation Antigen (BCMA)-CD3 Bispecific Antibody, in Patients with Relapsed/Refractory Multiple Myeloma (RRMM). *Blood* **2020**, *136*, 8–9. [CrossRef]
85. Madduri, D.; Rosko, A.; Brayer, J.; Zonder, J.; Bensinger, W.I.; Li, J.; Xu, L.; Adriaens, L.; Chokshi, D.; Zhang, W.; et al. REGN5458, a BCMA x CD3 Bispecific Monoclonal Antibody, Induces Deep and Durable Responses in Patients with Relapsed/Refractory Multiple Myeloma (RRMM). *Blood* **2020**, *136*, 41–42. [CrossRef]
86. Rodriguez, C.; D'Souza, A.; Shah, N.; Voorhees, P.M.; Buelow, B.; Vij, R.; Kumar, S.K. Initial Results of a Phase I Study of TNB-383B, a BCMA x CD3 Bispecific T-Cell Redirecting Antibody, in Relapsed/Refractory Multiple Myeloma. *Blood* **2020**, *136*, 43–44. [CrossRef]
87. Chari, A.; Berdeja, J.; Oriol, A.; Van de Donk, N.; Rodriguez Otero, P.; Askari, E.; Mateos, M.V.; Minnema, M.; Verona, R. A Phase 1, First-in-Human Study of Talquetamab, a G Protein-Coupled Receptor Family C Group 5 Member D (GPRC5D) x CD3 Bispecific Antibody, in Patients with Relapsed and/or Refractory Multiple Myeloma (RRMM). *Blood* **2020**, *136*, 290. [CrossRef]
88. Cohen, A.; Harrison, S.; Krishnan, A.; Fonseca, R.; Forsberg, P.; Spencer, A.; Berdeja, J.; Laubach, J. Initial Clinical Activity and Safety of BFCR4350A, a FcRH5/CD3 T-Cell-Engaging Bispecific Antibody, in Relapsed/Refractory Multiple Myeloma. *Blood* **2020**, *136*, 292. [CrossRef]

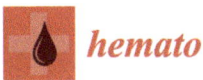 *hemato*

Review

Decades of Progress in Allogeneic Stem Cell Transplantation for Multiple Myeloma

Benedetto Bruno [1,*], Giuseppe Lia [2], Francesca Bonifazi [3] and Luisa Giaccone [2,4]

[1] Division of Hematology and Medical Oncology, NYU Grossman School of Medicine, Perlmutter Cancer Center, NYU Langone Health, New York, NY 10012, USA
[2] Department of Molecular Biotechnology and Health Sciences, University of Torino, 40138 Torino, Italy; lia.giuseppe@gmail.com (G.L.); luisa.giaccone@unito.it (L.G.)
[3] IRCCS Azienda Ospedaliero Universitaria di Bologna, 40138 Bologna, Italy; francesca.bonifazi@unibo.it
[4] Stem Cell Transplant Center, AOU Citta' della Salute e della Scienza, 40138 Turin, Italy
* Correspondence: benedetto.bruno@nyulangone.org

Abstract: Allogeneic hematopoietic cell transplantation in multiple myeloma has evolved over the decades. Myeloablative regimens have been replaced by the reduced intensity and non-myeloablative conditionings to reduce treatment-related toxicity and mortality while sparing graft-vs.-myeloma effects. Newer agents with potent anti-myeloma activity are not mutually exclusive and the combination with an allograft may improve long-term outcomes in this incurable disease especially in high-risk patients. Allografting may also be a platform for other promising new cell therapies such as CAR T-cells, NK-, and CAR NK-cells. These studies are warranted in the context of clinical trials. This review highlights the progress that has been made over the decades and possible future roles of allografting in the treatment landscape of multiple myeloma

Keywords: allogeneic transplantation; myeloablative; non-myeloablative; multiple myeloma; new drugs; CAR T

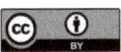

1. Introduction

In 1955, Main and Prehn by giving mice lethal irradiation and marrow from an H2 incompatible strain were able to avoid the rejection of a subsequent skin graft from the same donor strain [1]. It would be later proved that the survival of the graft was due to the persistence of donor cells leading to "tolerance". These experiments contributed to lay the foundation stone of the currently most established form of cell immunotherapy: allogeneic bone marrow transplantation. In the late 1950s, the first attempts to treat hematologic patients with irradiation and intravenous infusion of marrow from healthy donors were reported and, in 1970, approximately 200 patients had been treated. Unfortunately, all attempts had failed [2]. However, the perseverance of E.D. Thomas and his group led to the first successful reports in patients with leukemia and aplastic anemia in the mid-1970s [3,4]. Since then a history of tremendous breakthroughs unfolded in the field of allogeneic bone marrow transplantation and cell immunotherapy.

The role of allografting in multiple myeloma (MM) has always been hotly debated though it remains the only potentially curative treatment. Initially, high rates of transplant toxicity and long-term risk of relapse have prevented its widespread use. However, over time, many factors, such as greatly improved supportive care and reduced toxicity conditioning regimens, combined to significantly reduce the risk of lethal complications. So, nowadays, as for all other therapies for MM, disease recurrence is the major cause of treatment failure. In this review, we highlight the progress that has been made over the past decades, and the potential current role of allografting in combination with potent anti-MM agents and other cell therapies such as CAR T and CAR NK therapies (Figure 1).

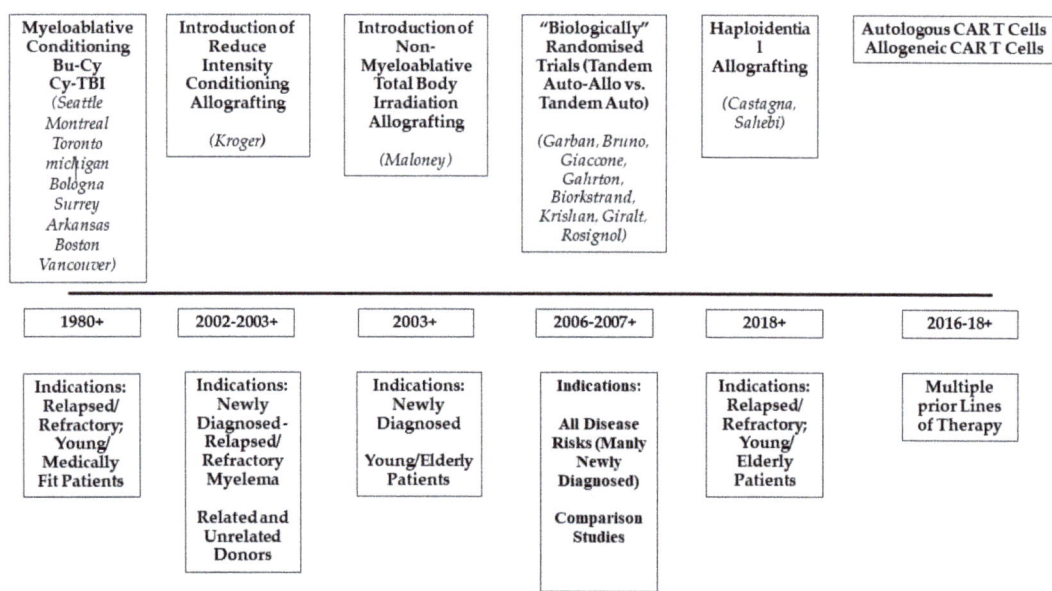

Figure 1. Timeline of allografting and cell therapies over the decades in multiple myeloma.

2. The First Reports: Myeloablative Conditionings and Their Toxicity

The very first experiences were reported by D Thomas from Seattle in 1957, as part of a transplant series of six patients with hematologic malignancies [4]. All patients died, and only one showed signs of engraftment. In the mid-'80s a few other centers presented case reports with encouraging results. Impressive was the report by Garthon et al. from the Karolinska Institute, in 1983, where a woman with refractory MM was treated with an allograft [5]. The patient achieved complete remission (CR) that lasted for longer than 3 years. Though the patient was not cured, the interest in allografting for MM was growing. The reports from the late 1980s/early 1990s included only myeloablative conditioning regimens. Cyclophosphamide was used in association with total body irradiation (TBI) or busulfan, or melphalan with TBI [6–17]. At that time, these conditions were limited to young medically fit patients. However, in MM patients, transplant-related mortality (TRM) up to 60% was clearly higher if compared to other diseases. Reasons for these unacceptable toxicity rates were somehow difficult to find. The profound immunodeficiency typical of all plasma cell dyscrasias may have been responsible for the TRM observed in MM. Most representative reports are illustrated in Table 1. Among them, the US intergroup trial (S9321) was of particular interest given its prospective design comparing autografting with myeloablative allografting [10]. This study enrolled newly diagnosed MM patients and compared early vs. late autografting, but also included a third arm that allowed patients, under the age of 55, with HLA-identical siblings to undergo myeloablative allografts. This arm was prematurely closed given an excessively high early TRM of 53% in the first 36 patients enrolled. However, after a follow-up of 7 years, overall survival (OS) was overlapping in both autologous and allogeneic recipients with progression-free survival (PFS) of 15% and 22%, respectively. However, while the risk of relapse progressively continued in the autograft patients, OS for the allograft cohort reached a plateau with follow up extending to 10 years. Despite the higher risk of toxicity, the conclusion drawn by the Authors was that allografting was the only curative treatment for MM.

Table 1. Myeloablative conditioning regimens for allografting in multiple myeloma.

Reference	Conditioning	Transplant-Related Mortality %	Complete Remission %	Overall Survival %
11	Mel (100 mg/m^2), TBI (12 Gy)	53 (at 1 year)	—	39 (at 7 years)
12	Bu, Cy, ±TBI	48 (at day 100) 63 (at 1 year)	34	22 (at 5 years)
13	Cy, TBI Bu, Cy Mel (100 mg/m^2), TBI	19 (at day 100)	62	47 (at 3 years)
14	Cy, TBI (14Gy) Bu, Cy	10	—	55 (at 2 years)
15	Mel (110 mg/m^2), TBI (10.5Gy) Cy, TBI Cy, Mel Bu, Cy	54	37	36 (at 3 years)
16	Cy, TBI (12Gy) Mel (140 mg/m^2), TBI (10.5Gy) Bu, Cy Others	22	57	32 (at 40 months)
17	Mel (160 mg/m^2), TBI (12Gy) Cy, TBI (12Gy) Bu, Cy	59	50	32 (at 3 years)
18	Cy, TBI Mel, TBI Bu, Cy, TBI Others	25	—	40 (at 3 years)

Abbreviations: Bu: Busulfan; Cy: cyclophosphamide; TBI: total body irradiation; Mel: melphalan.

Over the years, toxicity appeared to be gradually reducing. A retrospective registry analysis from the European Bone Marrow Transplant (EBMT) group reported a significant improvement in OS in the late 1990s owing to a reduction in transplant-related mortality [18]. Six-hundred-ninety patients, median age 44 years, who underwent myeloablative allografts were divided into two groups depending on the year of transplant: 1983 through 1993 versus 1994 through 1998. TRM rates at 6 months and 2 years were lower in the period 1994–1998 than between 1983–1993, 21% versus 38% and 30% versus 46%, respectively. Reduced toxicity correlated with better OS and PFR at 3 years from 35% to 55% and from 7 to 19 months for the period 1994–1998. Undoubtedly, the reduction in TRM was at least partly due to improved supportive care and better patient and donor selections.

Overall, the retrospective nature of most of these studies prevented determining the real role of myeloablative allografting in MM. Of note, most patients were heavily pretreated, had the chemo-resistant disease at transplant, and received a variety of conditionings and GvHD prophylaxes. Despite selection bias, however, it was clear that better clinical outcomes were associated with patients with chemo-sensitive MM. In most studies, only 10–25% of patients eventually became long-term disease-free survivors, but those were potentially cured.

3. The Concept of Tandem Autologous-Allogeneic Transplantation and Reduced-Intensity Conditioning Regimens

The use of myeloablation prior to transplant was commonly limited to young medically fit patients. This prevented many elderly patients from receiving potentially curative treatment for their hematological malignancy. In the late 1990s, investigators were prompted to explore highly immunosuppressive, but less myelosuppressive, conditionings that could establish stable donor engraftment, reduce transplant-related organ toxicities, and spare graft-vs.-tumor effects (Table 2). A series of pioneering preclinical studies, soon translated into clinical practice, was carried out by the Seattle group where it was shown that stable donor engraftment could be obtained with a combination of low dose non-myeloablative TBI (200 cGy) and fludarabine, followed by unmanipulated G-CSF mobilized donor peripheral blood stem cells and potent immunosuppression with cyclosporine and mycophenolate mofetil [19]. However, the risk of engraftment failure and rejection was higher in those patients, including MM patients, who had not received prior intensive chemotherapy for the treatment of their underlying malignancies. The hypothesis that the risk of graft-failure and the TRM of myeloablative conditionings could be circumvented by introducing a tandem approach of an autologous transplant followed, 2–4 months later, by a non-myeloablative TBI based allograft was clinically investigated. The rationale for this tandem autologous-allogeneic approach was to separate in time the high-dose cytoreduction with melphalan (200 mg/m^2) and the curative graft-vs.-myeloma with the potential of drastically reducing TRM and mortality. Of note, the burden of tumor eradication was almost totally shifted to donor-derived T cells. Initially, the Seattle group reported 52 newly diagnosed MM patients, treated with this tandem modality, with a complete remission rate of 48% while PFS and OS were 48% and 69% respectively [20]. The same tandem concept was also developed by Kroger et al. in Germany with the conditioning of melphalan, fludarabine, and anti-thymocyte globulin using both related and unrelated donors [21,22]. In the early 2000s, the tandem autologous-allogeneic approach was the only innovative procedure in the armamentarium of MM treatments that could be clinically investigated. Thus, before the era of so-called new drugs with potent anti-myeloma effects, prospective randomized clinical trials comparing allografting after non-myeloablative/reduced-intensity conditioning and double autologous transplantation were designed. The concept of Mendelian or genetic randomization was applied. This concept relies on the biological process through which offspring inherit genetic traits half from each parent. One in four siblings is then expected to have a potential HLA-identical sibling donor. Comparing by the intention-to-treat analysis patients with HLA-identical siblings, who could be assigned to allografting, and those without such siblings, who could only receive an autograft, was a surrogate for an unbiased randomization.

Table 2. Allografting in multiple myeloma after the introduction of non-myeloablative/reduced intensity conditionings.

Reference	Type of Conditioning/ Study Design	Transplant-Related Mortality	Event Free Survival or Progression-Free Survival	Overall Survival
[21]	Non-myeloablative/Prospective Phase II Auto-Allo in Newly Diagnosed MM	0% at 100 days	NR	78% at 552 days
[22]	Reduced-Intensity/Prospective Phase II Auto-Allo in Newly Diagnosed MM	11% at 100 days	70% at 13 months	76% at 13 months
[23]	Reduced Intensity/Prospective Phase II Auto-Allo from Unrelated Donors	10% at 100 days	53% at 2 years	74% at 2 years
[24,25]	Reduced Intensity/Prospective Comparison Auto-Allo vs. Tandem Auto in High Risk Newly Diagnosed MM	11% vs. NR	19 vs. 22 months	34 vs. 49 months
[26,27]	Non-myeloablative/Prospective Randomised Auto-Allo vs. Tandem Auto in Newly Diagnosed MM	16% vs. 2% at 6.5 years	35 vs. 29 months	80 vs. 54 months
[28]	Reduced Intensity/Prospective Comparison Auto-Allo vs. Tandem Auto in High Risk Newly Diagnosed MM	16% vs. 5%	Not reached vs. 31 months	Not reached vs. 58 months

Table 2. Cont.

Reference	Type of Conditioning/ Study Design	Transplant-Related Mortality	Event Free Survival or Progression-Free Survival	Overall Survival
[29,30]	Non-myeloablative/Prospective Randomised Auto-Allo vs. Tandem Auto in Newly Diagnosed MM	16% vs. 3% at 8 years	25% vs. 18% at 8 years 27% vs. 15% at 8 years	42% vs. 33% at 10 years 42% vs. 29% at 10 years
[31,32]	Non-myeloablative/Prospective Randomised Auto-Allo vs. Tandem Auto in Newly Diagnosed MM	20% vs. 9% at 6 years 20% vs. 11% at 10 years	22% vs. 25% at 6 years 18% vs. 19% at 10 years	59% vs. 60% at 6 years 44% vs. 43% at 10 years
[33,34]	Non-myeloablative/Prospective Randomised Auto-Allo vs. Tandem Auto in Newly Diagnosed MM	NR	43% vs. 39% at 3 years 22% vs. 12% at 8 years	75% vs. 68% at 3 years 49% vs. 36% at 8 years 48% vs. 27% at 10 years
[35]	Multiple regimens/Retrospective Haploidentical Allografting in MM Relapsed/Refractory Patients	10% at 18 months	33% at 18 months	63% at 18 months
[36]	Multiple regimens/Retrospective Haploidentical Allografting in MM Relapsed/Refractory Patients	21% at 1 year	17% at 2 year	48% at 2 year
[37]	Multiple regimens/Prospective Randomised Auto-Allo vs. Tandem Auto in MM Patients in First Relapse	27% at 5 years	NR	31% vs. 9% at 7 years

Abbreviations: MM multiple myeloma, NR: not reported.

A first such study comparing two trials on high-risk MM, in the light of elevated serum β2-microglobulin and del(13), was initially reported by the French group [23,24]. All patients received an autograft (melphalan 220 mg/m^2). Sixty-five with HLA-identical sibling donors were then treated with an allograft after a regimen combining busulfan, fludarabine, and high-dose anti-thymocyte globulin. Outcomes were compared with 219 high-risk patients who received a second autograft (melphalan 220 mg/m^2). TRM and response rates did not significantly differ. After a median follow-up of 2 years, OS and event-free survival (EFS) were 35% and 25%, and 41% and 30% for the double autologous and the autologous-allogeneic groups, respectively. This study was criticized for the use of high dose anti-thymocyte globulin that, though probably reduced the incidence of chronic graft vs. host disease to 7%, prevented potentially curative GvM. The first study which showed superior results with the auto-allo tandem approach was reported by the Italian group [25,26]. Two-hundred-forty-five consecutive newly diagnosed myeloma patients, up to 65 years, diagnosed between 1998–2004 were included. Patients received VAD-based regimens followed by standard autograft (melphalan 200 mg/m^2). Eighty patients with HLA-identical siblings were offered non-myeloablative TBI conditioning followed by an allograft. Eighty-two patients without HLA-identical siblings were assigned to receive a second autograft after high-dose or intermediate doses of melphalan (140–200 mg/m^2, and 100 mg/m^2, respectively). In the first report, at a median follow-up of 45 months, OS and EFS were significantly longer in patients with donors: 80 vs. 54 months and 35 vs. 29 months. Having an HLA-identical sibling was the only independent variable significantly associated with longer OS and EFS. Overall, in patients who completed the assigned treatments as per protocol arms, TRM was 10% and 2%, respectively. Median OS was not reached in the tandem auto-allo group and was 58 months in the tandem autologous group. EFS was 43 and 33 months, respectively. In the latest update, more than 7 years from diagnosis, the median OS was not reached in the auto/allo group vs. 4.2 years in the tandem auto group ($p = 0.001$) [26]. The long-term follow-up is a major strength of the study through the number of patients enrolled in the two cohorts is low. The Spanish study PETHEMA [27] enrolled only 25 patients in the auto-allo arm who were compared to 85 patients who received auto-auto. In this study design, only patients who did not reach CR or near CR after the autograft were eligible to either the allograft or a second autograft in the light of the availability of an HLA-identical sibling donor. Conditioning regimens used for the allograft were melphalan and fludarabine, while for the second autograft was cyclophosphamide, BCNU, etoposide (CBV), or high-dose melphalan. The difference was not statistically significant between the two arms, though the median time for PFS and OS were superior in the auto-allo cohort. The HOVON-50 study [28,29] enrolled 260 patients. One hundred-twenty-two had an HLA-identical sibling donor. Ninety-nine out of the 122 patients with a donor were treated with an auto/allo approach, whereas patients without a donor received a tandem auto/auto or maintenance with thalidomide after the first autograft. By intention to treat analysis, no significant differences in PFS or OS between the two groups at 8 or 10 years. However, when only the 99 patients who completed the protocol receiving the allograft ($n = 99$) were compared to the 122 who continued maintenance or received a second auto, there was a significant advantage in PFS for the allo patients at 8 years, this did not translate into a significantly better OS. The largest multicenter prospective study is the BMT-CTN 0102 trial [30]. It accrued 710 patients under the age of 70 years of age; 625 had the standard-risk disease. One hundred-fifty-six (83%) of 189 patients with the standard-risk disease were treated with the auto-allo (200 cGy TBI) in the light of absence/presence of an HLA-identical sibling donor; and 366 (84%) of 436 without donors tandem auto/auto (high-dose melphalan, 200 mg/m^2). Primary endpoints in standard-risk myeloma (β2 microglobulin < 3.0 mg/L and absence of deletion 13 by classic karyotyping) were OS and PFS. In the initial report, there was no statistically significant difference in 3-year PFS or OS between the two cohorts. In a recent update [31], there was still no significant difference between PFS and OS at 6 and 10 years, respectively, in standard-risk patients whereas allo patients with high-risk disease had better long-term clinical outcomes. The second-largest multicenter study, the EBMT study [32,33], included 357 patients from 23 European centers. Patients younger than 70 years of age with an HLA-identical sibling were allocated to auto-allo ($n = 108$) and those without to tandem auto ($n = 249$). Trial results were first published in 2011 [32] and updated in 2013 [33] with a median follow-up of 96 months. PFS and OS were significantly superior in the auto-allo cohort as compared to the single auto or tandem auto at that time (22% vs. 12% ($p = 0.027$, and 49% vs. 36% ($p = 0.030$), at 96 months). The reason for the superior PFS and OS in the auto-allo cohort was a lower relapse rate despite higher TRM. Of note, at a follow-up of 36 months, there was no significant difference in PFS or OS indicating that long-term follow-up is necessary to see the benefits of the allograft. By protocol analysis, comparing the patients who had received the auto-allo transplant ($n = 92$) with those who received tandem auto ($n = 104$), the same differences were confirmed.

Importantly, two meta-analyses which included some of these studies were carried out [34,38]. In the first one, published in 2013, Armeson et al. used a comprehensive search strategy of published and unpublished reports including six clinical trials. Their findings showed that in the upfront management of MM, auto-allo was associated with higher TRM and CR rates without improvement in clinical outcomes (OS and PFS) [34,38]. However, the most recent meta-analysis employed an individual patient data analysis that included the Italian study, the Spanish PETHEMA, the EBMT—NMAM2000, and BMT-CTN studies for a total of 1338 patients, 439 in the auto-allo group and 899 in the auto-auto group respectively [38]. At a median follow-up of 118.5 months, 5-year OS, and 10-year OS were 62% vs. 59%, and 44% vs. 36% at 10 years ($p = 0.01$) for auto-allo and tandem auto respectively, whereas 5-year PFS and 10-year PFS were 30.1% vs. 23.4% ($p = 0.01$) and 18.7% vs. 14.4% ($p = 0.06$) for auto-allo and tandem auto. Overall, this individual patient data analysis showed a significantly longer PFS and OS with the auto-allo approach. However, the study also stresses the importance of a long follow-up to evaluate the difference between the two transplant modalities. Moreover, the advantage of the allo-auto approach may partly be due to a long-term effect of GvM, but, most likely, to the synergy of the residual donor T cells at relapse and the rescue with novel anti-myeloma agents with immune-modulatory activities.

4. Haplo-Identical Transplantation

The use of post-transplant cyclophosphamide (PT-Cy) to selectively deplete allo-reactive T cells has allowed to considerably increase the number of haploidentical-HCT. The encouraging clinical findings reported in other malignancies prompted investigators to evaluate the role of haploidentical-HCT also in relapsed/refractory myeloma [35,36,39]. Castagna et al. reported on a series of 30 heavily pretreated MM patients who received haplo-HCT with PT-Cy as GVHD pro-phylaxis. Cumulative incidences of relapse/progression and non-relapse mortality at 18 months were 42% and 10%, respectively. Cumulative incidences of grade II-IV acute GVHD and chronic GVHD were 29% and 7%. After a median follow-up of 25 months, 18-month progression-free survival (PFS) and overall survival (OS) were 33% and 63%, respectively [39]. A larger series was reported in a retrospective EBMT/CIBMTR study that included 96 patients, transplanted between 2008 and 2016, who had relapsed and all had received a prior autologous transplant. PT-Cy was administered to 73 patients and the remaining patients received non-PT-Cy-based GVHD prophylaxis regimens. After a median follow-up of 2 years, 2-year progression-free survival (PFS) was 17%, and overall survival (OS) was 48%. At 2 years, the cumulative risk of relapse/progression was 56%, and 1-year non-relapse mortality (NRM) was 21%. Incidence of grade II-IV acute GVHD and chronic GVHD were 39% and 46%, respectively [35]. Though patient series were rather heterogeneous, chemo-refractory disease at transplantation was invariably associated with lower clinical outcomes. However, both studies showed an association between the use of PT-Cy and substantially improved OS, encouraging further studies of haploidentical-HCT in patients with MM. These encouraging results also led to further investigation. In a recent study, the hypothesis that natural killer (NK) cell alloreactivity may reduce MM relapse in the setting of a haploidentical-HCT was evaluated. A prospective phase 2 study using a killer cell immunoglobulin-like receptor (KIR)-ligand mismatched haploidentical donor included 12 patients with poor-risk MM. The graft source was bone marrow. The primary endpoint was 1.5-year PFS. All patients relapsed within a median time of 90 days leading to a premature study termination in the light of predefined stopping rules. In this small patient series with chemo-refractory MM, NK cell KIR mismatch was not superior to conventional allo-SCT [36].

5. Allografting in Refractory/Relapsed Myeloma and High-Risk Disease

The emergence of new agents with potent anti-myeloma activity and the conflicting results of allografting in newly diagnosed myeloma patients with the tandem auto-allo approach did not allow to identify a definite role for allografting in the upfront setting, and an allograft became more commonly used in the setting of relapsed/refractory disease [37,40–42]. Moreover, in the early 2000s disease stratification by cytogenetics analysis was not routinely carried out, and, at that time, the only del13q- was thought to be primarily associated with poor prognosis. Among others [37,40–42], a significant study was reported by Patriarca et al. where the Authors compared 79 patients who received an allograft at first relapse with 90 patients, without an available HLA-identical donor, who were then treated with combinations of bortezomib and immunomodulatory drugs. Patients who received an allograft showed a significantly better 7-year OS and PFS of 31% and 9% compared to 18% and 0%, respectively [43,44]. Of note, this study was an updated analysis of a previous report where clinical outcomes were not different between the 2 cohorts of patients stressing once more that long-term follow-up is needed to evaluate the potential effects of an allograft [43,44]. Several other studies have been reported [37,40–42]. However, the often relatively small numbers of the patient series, the retrospective nature, and a not standardized maintenance approach make it difficult to define the real role of allografting in the setting of refractory/relapsed patients. However, in the attempt to reach a consensus on clinical recommendations, members from four scientific societies (including the International Myeloma Working Group, the American Society of Blood and Marrow Transplantation and Cell Therapies (ASBMT), the European Society of Blood and Marrow Transplantation (EBMT), and the Blood and Marrow Transplant Clinical Trials Network) agreed that allografting should be considered in patients with early relapse (less than 24 months from diagnosis) after first-line treatment with an autograft or in those patients with high-risk features such as poor cytogenetics and plasma cell leukemia [45]. Preferably, patients should be enrolled in well-designed prospective trials.

Currently, cytogenetic abnormalities are routinely evaluated to establish prognosis in MM patients at diagnosis and at different follow-up timepoints. Aberrations such as del17p, t (4; 14), t (14; 16), gain (1q), and del8p have clearly been associated with poor clinical outcomes. Unfortunately, these aberrations were not known when most biological randomized studies, before the era of new drugs, were designed in newly diagnosed patients. Del13q was initially the first chromosomal abnormality that was associated with poor outcome but is now primarily considered a surrogate marker of other aberrations. Whether GvM, especially if combined with anti-myeloma agents, may overcome the poor prognosis determined by certain cytogenetic aberrations remain a matter of debate. In an update of the EBMT–NMAM2000 study, del13q-pos patients in the autograft cohort did worse than del13q-neg patients. However, there was no difference in clinical outcomes between del13q-neg patients and del13q-pos patients in the auto-allo cohort shoeing that GvM might overcome the negative effects of this aberration [33]. More recently, a phase 3 trial by Knop et al. compared tandem auto-auto vs. auto-allo (with reduced-intensity conditioning) in patients with newly diagnosed MM and del13q. The availability or absence of an HLA-identical matched donor determined the nature of the second transplant. The primary endpoint was PFS by intention-to-treat analysis. At a median follow-up of 91 months, median PFS was 34 vs. 21 months in the auto-allo cohort vs. tandem auto ($p = 0.003$), whereas OS was 70.2 versus 71.8 months ($p = 0.856$), respectively. However, in patients carrying both del13q and del17p, median PFS and OS were 37.5 and 61.5 months in the auto-allo (n = 19) vs. 6.1 and 23.4 months in the tandem auto cohort ($p = 0.0002$ and 0.032). These findings suggest a survival benefit for the first-line allografting in high-risk MM [46]. In another interesting report by Kröger et al. [47], 16 out of 73 patients carrying del17p13 and/or t (4; 14) who had received tandem auto-allo (reduced-intensity conditioning) experienced similar 5-year PFS as those without such aberrations (24% vs. 30%, respectively, $p = 0.70$) suggesting that GvM might overcome the poor prognostic impact associated with chromosomal abnormalities.

6. Allogeneic Transplantation and Novel Agents: An Immunological Synergy

Most of the randomized trials comparing auto-allo vs. auto-auto in the upfront setting were designed before the era of new drugs. However, multiple treatment choices became available at the time of relapse as newer agents, over the years, were approved for MM patients. Giaccone et al. reported for the first time the observation that OS after relapse was significantly longer in the auto-allo cohorts as compared to tandem auto [26]. These preliminary findings were also confirmed by Gahrton et al. in an update of the EBMT- NMAM 2000 experience [33]. A larger retrospective analysis was carried out at the Center for International Blood and Marrow Transplant Research (CIBMTR) [48]. Htut et al. compared post-relapse OS after auto-allo vs. tandem auto in patients prospectively reported to the CIBMTR between 2000 and 2010. Overall, after a median follow-up of 8.5 years, 404 patients (72%) had relapsed in the auto-auto cohort and 178 (67%) in the auto-allo cohort group. Interestingly, at six months after the second transplant, in the auto-allo group, 46% of the total relapses had already occurred as compared to 26% in the auto-auto group. However, 6-year post-relapse OS was 44% in the auto-allo group and 35% in the auto-auto group ($p = 0.05$). Of note, by multivariate analysis, both groups had a similar risk of death during the first year after relapse, nonetheless, for time points beyond 1 year, the auto-allo group had significantly superior OS ($p = 0.005$). The recurrent observation that there appears to be a synergy between donor-derived T cells and the immunologic effects of several anti-myeloma agents may partly be explained by recent functional studies. Wolschke et al. showed that lenalidomide enhances both NK and T cell-mediated anti-myeloma activity after allografting; while Kneppers et al. showed that lenalidomide increases HLA-DR + T cell subsets indicating T cell activation [49,50].

7. Minimal Residual Disease (MRD) and Graft-vs.-Myeloma

GvM, potentially curative for MM, consists of an immunological response of donor T cells against myeloma cells through the recognition of possibly disease-specific antigens. This evidence was initially documented by the achievement of CR following discontinuation of immunosuppression or after the infusion of donor T cells in patients with post-transplant relapse [13,51,52]. Some Investigators, however, reported that the strongest predictors for response to donor lymphocyte infusions were acute and chronic GvHD [53–56] indicating that GvHD and GvM may share the same antigenic targets (Figure 2). Bruno et al., however, reported that the development of chronic GVHD was not correlated with CR rates and response duration [26] suggesting that subclinical long-term graft-vs.-host reactions may occur in the absence of GVHD. Flow cytometry and PCR methods are more sensitive than standard immunofixation to evaluate the death of response and may help to identify treatment algorithms capable of eradicating the disease [57,58]. Thus, the application of studies on MRD is currently expanding [58]. The possible achievement of molecular remission (MR) by PCR methods is further evidence for GvM. High rates of prolonged MR, a reliable indicator of maximal reduction and potential disease eradication, were initially reported after myeloablative conditioning [59,60]. The predictive value of molecular monitoring after a myeloablative allograft was assessed by a European Group for Blood and Marrow Transplantation (EBMT) longitudinal study on patients who reached clinical CR [60]. Of 48 evaluable patients, 16 (33%) attained durable post-transplant PCR-negativity after transplantation, whereas 13 (27%) remained persistently PCR-positive and 19 (40%) showed a mixed pattern. The cumulative risk of relapse at 5 years was 0% for PCR-negative patients, 33% for PCR-mixed patients, and 100% for PCR-positive patients [60]. More recently, durable MR has also been reported with non-myeloablative conditioning where the burden of tumor eradication is completely shifted toward donor T cells and their ability to generate graft-vs.-myeloma effects. After a remarkable median follow-up of 12 years in a cohort of 26 patients treated with the tandem auto-non myeloablative allo approach, Ladetto et al. reported that the achievement of MR by nested-PCR was significantly associated with better long-term OS and EFS [61]. Not only median durations of both OS and EFS had not been reached at follow-up, but some patients had been disease-free and off-therapy up to 20 years (Figure 3). It is interesting to notice that in the EBMT study the occurrence of MR was observed in the early post-transplant follow-up whereas after the non-myeloablative conditioning patients usually achieved MR later, up to one-year post-transplant. This phenomenon may be explained by the immediate cytoreductive effect of high dose conditionings, which mainly included 12 Gy TBI or high-dose busulphan, as compared with the low dose TBI (2 Gy) non-myeloablative conditioning. Overall, these studies report MR rates second to no other treatment approaches in MM.

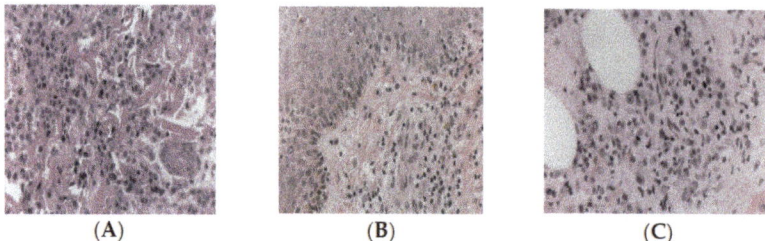

Figure 2. Graft-vs.-myeloma effect by histology (H&E staining). (**A**) biopsy proven myeloma cutis at day +19 post-allograft; (**B**) biopsy proven skin graft-vs.-host disease at day +45; (**C**) biopsy of myeloma cutis at day +60 showing lymphocyte infiltration and dying plasma cells. (Courtesy of Dr. D. Novero).

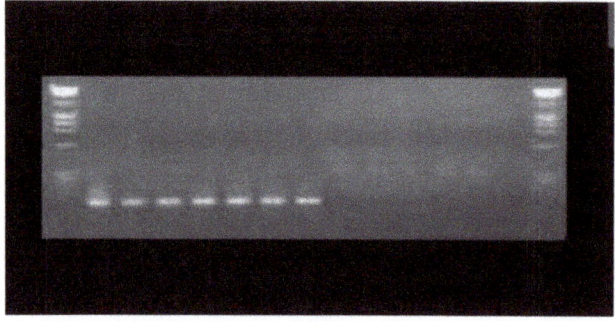

Dgn M.W. D +29 +29 +100 +100 +230 +230 +390 +390

Figure 3. Graft-vs.-myeloma (GvM) and minimal residual disease (MDR) by nested PCR analysis. The patient reached molecular remission (sensitivity $1/10^6$) in peripheral blood at one-year post-allograft and later in the bone marrow indicative of ongoing GvM. The patient has remained in continuous MDR negative remission for 20 years (Courtesy of Drs. M. Ladetto and D. Drandi) [61].

8. Graft-vs.-Myeloma Effects: The New Frontiers

In recent years, chimeric antigen receptor (CAR) T-cell therapy has changed the immunotherapy paradigm of relapsed/refractory MM with unprecedented overall response rates [62–64]. However, patients appear to ultimately relapse despite obtaining initial high CR rates and none of these current autologous therapies have been approved. Importantly, main issues such as long-term clinical outcomes, toxicities, and management of complications limit their widespread use. Moreover, autologous CAR T therapies have major limitations such as lengthy vein-to-vein turnaround time and manufacturing constraints. Thus, allogeneic CAR T therapies may then offer an alternative to these limitations. Genetically engineered "off-the-shelf" allogeneic CAR T cells may dramatically change the current CAR T-cell scenario in the future. Allogeneic CAR T cell therapies use healthy donor T cells, may decrease cost, and enable broader availability [65]. Notwithstanding, allogeneic CAR-T bears the intrinsic risk for GVHD. Thus, sophisticated technology such as TALEN- and CRISPR-based gene editing has been introduced to manufacture allogeneic CAR-T with off-the-shelf availability [66,67]. Overall, the current role of CAR-T in the treatment paradigm of MM remains to be investigated. Simpler structures and multi-target approaches may dramatically improve efficacy and safety. Long-term outcome analyses and specific detection and evaluation of CAR-T dynamics in vivo are essential to allow deeper knowledge of their potentials. Cytogenetic high-risk features, patient selection, timing of infusion during the disease phase are other factors to be strictly considered to define their role. Currently, these strategies are being investigated in preclinical and early clinical trial settings and may reshape the indications of allografting, which so far remains the most established form of cell immunotherapy with well-documented graft-vs.-leukemia/tumor effects.

9. Conclusions

Over the last two decades, dramatic improvements have been made in the treatment of MM. It is widely assumed that recent results of large randomized trials undoubtedly affirm the role of ASCT with novel potent anti-myeloma agents combined both in the pre-transplant induction and in the post-transplant maintenance/consolidation phases. Nonetheless, the disease remains fatal and in ultra-high/high-risk patients clinical outcomes are very poor with survival rates of few years. Given the remarkable concomitant reduction in toxicity of allografting in recent years, there are still areas to thoroughly investigate where the potential GVM could be of benefit for MM patients. The inclusion in control trials would be recommended. Unfortunately, large prospective control studies evaluating the combination of new drugs with allo-HSCT have never been appropriately designed. The real effects of well-designed strategies combining allografting and newer agents will regretfully remain unknown. In patient subsets where long-term disease control cannot be expected even with the current wide armamentarium of treatment options, allografting may play an important role to increase the chance of better long-term survival. Clinical trials should be considered in young newly diagnosed ultra-high-risk/high-risk patients and in those who relapse early (18 months), regardless of baseline prognostic features, from first-line treatment. In the future, an "allo" platform may be exploited in the context of other cell therapies such as donor-derived CAR T-cells and NK cell infusions or immunotherapies such as bispecific T cell engagers and bispecific killer cell engagers to evoke stronger anti-tumor effects in appropriate high risk/relapsed patient populations.

Funding: This research received no external funding.

Institutional Review Board Statement: Not applicable.

Informed Consent Statement: Not applicable.

Data Availability Statement: Not applicable.

Conflicts of Interest: The authors declare no conflict of interest.

References

1. Main, J.M.; Prehn, R.T. Success skin homografts after the administration of high dosage X radiation and homologous bone marrow. *J. Natl. Cancer Inst.* **1955**, *15*, 1023–1029.
2. Buckner, C.D.; Clift, R.A.; Fefer, A.; Neiman, P.; Storb, R.; Thomas, E.D. Human marrow transplantation–current status. *Prog. Hematol.* **1973**, *8*, 299–324.
3. Thomas, E.; Storb, R.; Clift, R.A.; Fefer, A.; Johnson, F.L.; Neiman, P.E.; Lerner, K.G.; Glucksberg, H.; Buckner, C.D. Bone-marrow transplantation (first of two parts). *N. Engl. J. Med.* **1975**, *292*, 832–843. [CrossRef]
4. Thomas, E.D. The Nobel Prize in Physiology or Medicine 1990. In *Les Prix Nobel, the Nobel Prizes 1990*; Frängsmyr, T., Ed.; Nordstedts Tryckeri AB: Stockholm, Sweden, 1991; pp. 219–221.
5. Gahrton, G.; Ringden, O.; Lönnqvist, B.; Lindquist, R.; Ljungman, P. Bone marrow transplantation in three patients with multiple myeloma. *Acta Med. Scand.* **1986**, *219*, 523–527. [CrossRef]
6. Tura, S. Bone marrow transplantation in multiple myeloma: Current status and future perspectives. *Bone Marrow Transpl.* **1986**, *1*, 17–20.
7. Gahrton, G.; Tura, S.; Ljungman, P.; Belanger, C.; Brandt, L.; Cavo, M.; Facon, T.; Granena, A.; Gore, M.; Gratwohl, A.; et al. Allogeneic bone marrow transplantation in multiple myeloma. *N. Engl. J. Med.* **1991**, *325*, 1267–1273. [CrossRef] [PubMed]
8. Bensinger, W.I.; Buckner, C.D.; Anasetti, C.; Clift, R.; Storb, R.; Barnett, T.; Chauncey, T.; Shulman, H.; Appelbaum, F.R. Allogeneic marrow transplantation for multiple myeloma: An analysis of risk factors on outcome. *Blood* **1996**, *88*, 2787–2793. [CrossRef]
9. Gahrton, G.; Tura, S.; Ljungman, P.; Biadé, J.; Brandt, L.; Cavo, M.; Façon, T.; Gratwohl, A.; Hagenbeek, A.; Jacobs, P.; et al. Prognostic factors in allogeneic bone marrow transplantation for multiple myeloma. *J. Clin. Oncol.* **1995**, *13*, 1312–1322. [CrossRef] [PubMed]

10. Barlogie, B.; Kyle, R.A.; Anderson, K.C.; Greipp, P.R.; Lazarus, H.M.; Hurd, D.D.; McCoy, J.; Moore Jr, D.F.; Dakhil, S.R.; Lanier, K.S.; et al. Standard chemotherapy compared with high-dose chemoradiotherapy for multiple myeloma: Final results of phase III US Intergroup Trial S9321. *J. Clin. Oncol.* **2006**, *24*, 929–936. [CrossRef]
11. Bensinger, W.I.; Maloney, D.; Storb, R. Allogeneic hematopoietic cell transplantation for multiple myeloma. *Semin. Hemalol.* **2001**, *38*, 243–249.
12. Reece, D.E.; Shepherd, J.D.; Klingemann, H.G.; Sutherland, H.J.; Nantel, S.H.; Barnett, M.J.; Spinelli, J.J.; Phillips, G.L. Treatment of myeloma using intensive therapy and allogeneic bone marrow transplantation. *Bone Marrow Transpl.* **1995**, *15*, 117–123.
13. Alyea, E.; Weller, E.; Schlossman, R.; Canning, C.; Webb, I.; Doss, D.; Mauch, P.; Marcus, K.; Fisher, D.; Freeman, A.; et al. T-cell-depleted allogeneic bone marrow transplantation followed by donor lymphocyte infusion in patients with multiple myeloma: Induction of graft-versus-myeloma effect. *Blood* **2001**, *98*, 934–939. [CrossRef] [PubMed]
14. Kulkarni, S.; Powles, R.L.; Treleaven, J.G.; Singhal, S.; Saso, R.; Horton, C.; Killick, S.; Tait, D.; Ramiah, V.; Mehta, J. Impact of previous high-dose therapy on outcome after allografting for multiple myeloma. *Bone Marrow Transpl.* **1999**, *23*, 675–680. [CrossRef]
15. Le Blanc, R.; Montminy-Métivier, S.; Bélanger, R.; Busque, L.; Fish, D.; Roy, D.-C.; Kassis, J.; Boileau, J.; Lavallée, R.; Bélanfer, F.; et al. Allogeneic transplantation for multiple myeloma: Further evidence for a GVHD-associated graft-versus-myeloma effect. *Bone Marrow Transpl.* **2001**, *28*, 841–848. [CrossRef]
16. Couban, S.; Stewart, A.K.; Loach, D.; Panzarella, T.; Meharchand, J. Autologous and allogeneic transplantation for multiple myeloma at a single centre. *Bone Marrow Transpl.* **1997**, *19*, 783–789. [CrossRef]
17. Varterasian, M.; Janakiraman, N.; Karanes, C.; Aberlla, E.; Uberti, J.; Dragovic, J.; Raman, S.B.K.; Al-Katib, A.; Du, W.; Silver, S.M.; et al. Transplantation in patients with multiple myeloma: A multicenter comparative analysis of peripheral blood stem cell and allogeneic transplant. *Am. J. Clin. Oncol.* **1997**, *20*, 462–466. [CrossRef]
18. Gahrton, G.; Svensson, H.; Cavo, M.; Apperley, J.; Bacigalupo, A.; Björkstrand, B.; Blade, J.; Cornelissen, J.; De Laurenzi, A.; Façon, T.; et al. Progress in allogeneic bone marrow and peripheral blood stem cell transplantation for multiple myeloma: A comparison between transplants performed 1983–93 and 1994–98 at European Group for Blood and Marrow Transplantation centres. *Br. J. Haematol.* **2001**, *113*, 209–216. [CrossRef] [PubMed]
19. McSweeney, P.A.; Niederwieser, D.; Shizuru, J.A.; Sandmaier, B.M.; Molina, A.J.; Maloney, D.G.; Chauncey, T.R.; Gooley, T.A.; Hegenbart, U.; Nash, R.A.; et al. Hematopoietic cell transplantation in older patients with hematologic malignancies: Replacing high-dose cytotoxic therapy with graft-versus-tumor effects. *Blood* **2001**, *97*, 3390–3400. [CrossRef]
20. Maloney, D.G.; Molina, A.J.; Sahebi, F.; Stockerl-Goldstein, K.E.; Sandmaier, B.M.; Bensinger, W.; Storer, B.; Hegenbart, U.; Somlo, G.; Chauncey, T.; et al. Allografting with nonmyeloablative conditioning following cytoreductive autografts for the treatment of patients with multiple myeloma. *Blood* **2003**, *102*, 3447–3454. [CrossRef]
21. Kröger, N.; Schwerdtfeger, R.; Kiehl, M.; Sayer, H.G.; Renges, H.; Zabelina, T.; Fehse, B.; Tögel, F.; Wittkowsky, G.; Kuse, R.; et al. Autologous stem cell transplantation followed by a dose-reduced allograft induces high complete remission rate in multiple myeloma. *Blood* **2002**, *100*, 755–760. [CrossRef]
22. Kröger, N.; Sayer, H.G.; Schwerdtfeger, R.; Kiehl, M.; Nagler, A.; Renges, H.; Zabelina, T.; Fehse, B.; Ayuk, F.; Wittkowsky, G.; et al. Unrelated stem cell transplantation in multiple myeloma after a reduced- intensity conditioning with pretransplantation antithymocyte globulin is highly effective with low transplantation-related mortality. *Blood* **2002**, *100*, 3919–3924. [CrossRef]
23. Garban, F.; Attal, M.; Michallet, M.; Hulin, C.; Bourhis, J.H.; Yakoub-Agha, I.; Lamy, T.; Marit, G.; Maloisel, F.; Berthou, C.; et al. Prospective comparison of autologous stem cell transplantation followed by dose-reduced allograft (IFM99-03 trial) with tandem autologous stem cell transplantation (IFM99-04 trial) in high-risk de novo multiple myeloma. *Blood* **2006**, *107*, 3474–3480. [CrossRef]
24. Moreau, P.; Garban, F.; Attal, M.; Michallet, M.; Marit, G.; Hulin, C.; Benboubker, L.; Doyen, C.; Mohty, M.; Yakoub-Agha, I.; et al. Long-term follow-up results of IFM99-03 and IFM99-04 trials comparing nonmyeloablative allotransplantation with autologous transplantation in high-risk de novo multiple myeloma. *Blood* **2008**, *112*, 3914–3915. [CrossRef]
25. Bruno, B.; Rotta, M.; Patriarca, F.; Mordini, N.; Allione, B.; Carnevale-Schianca, F.; Giaccone, L.; Sorasio, R.; Omedé, P.; Baldi, I.; et al. A Comparison of allografting with autografting for newly diagnosed myeloma. *N. Engl. J. Med.* **2007**, *356*, 1110–1120. [CrossRef] [PubMed]
26. Giaccone, L.; Storer, B.; Patriarca, F.; Rotta, M.; Sorasio, R.; Allione, B.; Carnevale-Schianca, F.; Festuccia, M.; Brunello, L.; Omedè, P.; et al. Long-term follow-up of a comparison of nonmyeloablative allografting with autografting for newly diagnosed myeloma. *Blood* **2011**, *117*, 6721–6727. [CrossRef]
27. Rosiñol, L.; Perez-Simón, J.A.; Sureda, A.; Rubia, J.D.L.; De Arriba, F.; Lahuerta, J.J.; González, J.D.; Diaz-Mediavilla, J.; Hernández, B.; García-Frade, J.; et al. A prospective PETHEMA study of tandem autologous transplantation versus autograft followed by reduced-intensity conditioning allogeneic transplantation in newly diagnosed multiple myeloma. *Blood* **2008**, *112*, 3591–3593. [CrossRef]
28. Lokhorst, H.M.; Van Der Holt, B.; Cornelissen, J.J.; Kersten, M.J.; Van Oers, M.; Raymakers, R.; Minnema, M.C.; Zweegman, S.; Janssen, J.J.; Zijlmans, M.; et al. Donor versus no-donor comparison of newly diagnosed myeloma patients included in the HOVON-50 multiple myeloma study. *Blood* **2012**, *119*, 6219–6225. [CrossRef] [PubMed]

29. Lokhorst, H.M.; Van Der Holt, B.; Cornelissen, J.J.; Kersten, M.J.; Van Oers, M.; Raymakers, R.; Minnema, M.C.; Zweegman, S.; Bos, G.; Schaap, N.; et al. Reduced relapse rate in upfront tandem autologous/reduced-intensity allogeneic transplantation in multiple myeloma only results in borderline non-significant prolongation of progression-free but not overall survival. *Haematologica* **2015**, *100*, e508–e510. [CrossRef] [PubMed]
30. Krishnan, A.; Pasquini, M.C.; Logan, B.; Stadtmauer, E.A.; Vesole, D.H.; Alyea, E.; Antin, J.H.; Comenzo, R.; Goodman, S.; Hari, P.; et al. Autologous haemopoietic stem-cell transplantation followed by allogeneic or autologous haemopoietic stem-cell transplantation in patients with multiple myeloma (BMT CTN 0102): A phase 3 biological assignment trial. *Lancet Oncol.* **2011**, *12*, 1195–1203. [CrossRef]
31. Giralt, S.A.; Costa, L.J.; Maloney, D.; Krishnan, A.; Fei, M.; Antin, J.H.; Brunstein, C.; Geller, N.; Goodman, S.; Hari, P.; et al. Tandem autologous-autologous versus autologous-allogeneic hematopoietic stem cell transplant for patients with multiple myeloma: Long-term follow-up results from the Blood and Marrow Transplant Clinical Trials Network 0102 Trial. *Biol. Blood Marrow Transpl.* **2020**, *26*, 798–804. [CrossRef]
32. Björkstrand, B.; Iacobelli, S.; Hegenbart, U.; Gruber, A.; Greinix, H.; Volin, L.; Narni, F.; Musto, P.; Beksac, M.; Bosi, A.; et al. Tandem autologous/reduced-intensity conditioning allogeneic stem-cell transplantation versus autologous transplantation in myeloma: Long-term follow-up. *J. Clin. Oncol.* **2011**, *29*, 3016–3022. [CrossRef]
33. Gahrton, G.; Iacobelli, S.; Björkstrand, B.; Hegenbart, U.; Gruber, A.; Greinix, H.; Volin, L.; Narni, F.; Carella, A.M.; Beksac, M.; et al. Autologous/reduced-intensity allogeneic stem cell transplantation vs autologous transplantation in multiple myeloma: Long-term results of the EBMT-NMAM2000 study. *Blood* **2013**, *121*, 5055–5063. [CrossRef]
34. Armenson, K.E.; Hill, E.G.; Costa, L.J. Tandem autologous vs autologous plus reduced intensity allogeneic transplantation in the upfront management of multiple myeloma: Meta-analysis of trials with biological assignment. *Bone Marrow Transpl.* **2013**, *48*, 562–567. [CrossRef]
35. Sahebi, F.; Garderet, L.; Kanate, A.S.; Eikema, D.J.; Knelange, N.S.; Alvelo, O.F.D.; Koc, Y.; Blaise, D.; Bashir, Q.; Moraleda, J.M.; et al. Outcomes of Haploidentical Transplantation in Patients with elapsed Multiple Myeloma: An EBMT/CIBMTR Report. *Biol. Blood Marrow Transpl.* **2019**, *25*, 335–342. [CrossRef]
36. Jaiswal, S.R.; Chakrabarti, S. Natural killer cell-based immunotherapy with CTLA4Ig-primed donor lymphocytes following haploidentical transplantation. *Immunotherapy* **2019**, *11*, 1221–1230. [CrossRef] [PubMed]
37. Sobh, M.; Michallet, M.; Gahrton, G.; Iacobelli, S.; Van Biezen, A.; Schönland, S.O.; Petersen, E.; Schaap, N.; Bonifazi, F.; Volin, L.; et al. Allogeneic hematopoietic cell transplantation for multiple myeloma in Europe: Trends and outcomes over 25 years. A study by the EBMT Chronic Malignancies Working Party. *Leukemia* **2016**, *30*, 2047–2054. [CrossRef] [PubMed]
38. Costa, L.J.M.; Iacobelli, S.; Pasquini, M.C.; Modi, R.; Giaccone, L.; Blade, J.; Schonland, S.; Evangelista, A.; Perez-Simon, J.A.; Hari, P.; et al. Long-term survival of 1338 MM patients treated with tandem autologous vs. autologous-allogeneic transplantation. *Bone Marrow Transpl.* **2020**, *55*, 1–7. [CrossRef] [PubMed]
39. Castagna, L.; Mussetti, A.; DeVillier, R.; Dominietto, A.; Marcatti, M.; Milone, G.; Maura, F.; De Philippis, C.; Bruno, B.; Furst, S.; et al. Haploidentical allogeneic hematopoietic cell transplantation for multiple myeloma using post-transplantation cyclophosphamide graft-versus-host disease prophylaxis. *Biol. Blood Marrow Transpl.* **2017**, *23*, 1549–1554. [CrossRef] [PubMed]
40. Efebera, Y.A.; Qureshi, S.R.; Cole, S.M.; Saliba, R.; Pelosini, M.; Patel, R.M.; Koca, E.; Mendoza, F.L.; Wang, M.; Shah, J.; et al. Reduced-intensity allogeneic hematopoietic stem cell transplantation for relapsed multiple myeloma. *Biol. Blood Marrow Transpl.* **2010**, *16*, 1122–1129. [CrossRef] [PubMed]
41. Karlin, L.; Arnulf, B.; Chevret, S.; Ades, L.; Robin, M.; De Latour, R.P.; Malphettes, M.; Kabbara, N.; Asli, B.; Rocha, V.; et al. Tandem autologous non-myeloablative allogeneic transplantation in patients with multiple myeloma relapsing after a first high dose therapy. *Bone Marrow Transpl.* **2010**, *46*, 250–256. [CrossRef]
42. Shimoni, A.; Hardan, I.; Ayuk, F.; Schilling, G.; Atanackovic, D.; Zeller, W.; Yerushalmi, R.; Zander, A.R.; Kröger, N.; Nagler, A. Allogenic hematopoietic stem-cell transplantation with reduced-intensity conditioning in patients with refractory and recurrent multiple myeloma. *Cancer* **2010**, *116*, 3621–3630. [CrossRef]
43. Patriarca, F.; Einsele, H.; Spina, F.; Bruno, B.; Isola, M.; Nozzoli, C.; Nozza, A.; Sperotto, A.; Morabito, F.; Stuhler, G.; et al. Allogeneic stem cell transplantation in multiple myeloma relapsed after autograft: A multicenter retrospective study based on donor availability. *Biol Blood Marrow Transpl.* **2012**, *18*, 617–626. [CrossRef]
44. Patriarca, F.; Bruno, B.; Einsele, H.; Spina, F.; Giaccone, L.; Montefusco, V.; Isola, M.; Nozzoli, C.; Nozza, A.; Morabito, F.; et al. Long-term follow-up of a Donor versus No-Donor Comparison in patients with multiple myeloma in first relapse after failing autologous transplantation. *Biol. Blood Marrow Transpl.* **2018**, *24*, 406–409. [CrossRef]
45. Giralt, S.A.; Garderet, L.; Durie, B.; Cook, G.; Gahrton, G.; Bruno, B.; Hari, P.; Lokhorst, H.; McCarthy, P.; Krishnan, A.; et al. American Society of Blood and Marrow Transplantation, European Society of Blood and Marrow Transplantation, Blood and Marrow Transplant Clinical Trials Network, and International Myeloma Working Group Consensus Conference on salvage hematopoietic cell transplantation in patients with relapsed multiple myeloma. *Biol. Blood Marrow Transpl.* **2015**, *21*, 2039–2051.
46. Knop, S.; Engelhardt, M.; Liebisch, P.; Meisner, C.; Holler, E.; Metzner, B.; Peest, D.; Kaufmann, M.; Bunjes, D.; Straka, C.; et al. Allogeneic transplantation in multiple myeloma: Long-term follow-up and cytogenetic subgroup analysis. *SSRN Electron. J.* **2019**, *33*, 2710–2719.

47. Kröger, N.; Badbaran, A.; Zabelina, T.; Ayuk, F.; Wolschke, C.; Alchalby, H.; Klyuchnikov, E.; Atanackovic, D.; Schilling, G.; Hansen, T.; et al. Impact of high-risk cytogenetics and achievement of molecular remission on long-term freedom from disease after autologous-allogeneic tandem transplantation in patients with multiple myeloma. *Biol. Blood Marrow Transpl.* **2013**, *19*, 398–404. [CrossRef] [PubMed]
48. Htut, M.; D'Souza, A.; Krishnan, A.; Bruno, B.; Zhang, M.-J.; Fei, M.; González-Díaz, M.; Copelan, E.; Ganguly, S.; Hamadani, M.; et al. Autologous/Allogeneic hematopoietic cell transplantation versus tandem autologous transplantation for multiple myeloma: Comparison of long-term postrelapse survival. *Biol. Blood Marrow Transpl.* **2018**, *24*, 478–485. [CrossRef]
49. Kneppers, E.; Van Der Holt, B.; Kersten, M.J.; Zweegman, S.; Meijer, E.; Huls, G.; Cornelissen, J.J.; Janssen, J.J.; Huisman, C.; Cornelisse, P.B.; et al. Lenalidomide maintenance after nonmyeloablative allogeneic stem cell transplantation in multiple myeloma is not feasible: Results of the HOVON 76 Trial. *Blood* **2011**, *118*, 2413–2419. [CrossRef] [PubMed]
50. Wolschke, C.; Stübig, T.; Hegenbart, U.; Schönland, S.O.; Heinzelmann, M.; Hildebrandt, Y.; Ayuk, F.; Atanackovic, D.; Dreger, P.; Zander, A.; et al. Postallograft lenalidomide induces strong NK cell–mediated antimyeloma activity and risk for T cell-mediated GvHD: Results from a phase I/II dose-finding study. *Exp. Hematol.* **2013**, *41*, 134–142.e3. [CrossRef]
51. Libura, J.; Hoffmann, T.; Passweg, J.R.; Gregor, M.; Favre, G.; Tichelli, A.; Gratwohl, A. Graft-versusmyeloma after withdrawal of immunosuppression following allogeneic peripheral stem cell transplantation. *Bone Marrow Transpl.* **1999**, *24*, 925–927. [CrossRef]
52. Verdonck, L.F.; Lokhorst, H.M.; Dekker, A.W.; Nieuwenhuis, H.K.; Petersen, E.J. Graft-versus-myeloma effect in two cases. *Lancet* **1996**, *347*, 800–801. [CrossRef]
53. Lokhorst, H.M.; Schattenberg, A.; Cornelissen, J.J.; Thomas, L.L.M.; Verdonck, L.F. Donor leukocyte infusions are effective in relapsed multiple myeloma after allogeneic bone marrow transplantation. *Blood* **1997**, *90*, 4206–4211. [CrossRef]
54. Lokhorst, H.M.; Schattenberg, A.; Cornelissen, J.J.; van Oers, M.H.J.; Fibbe, W.; Van De Donk, N.W.C.J.; Verdonck, L.F. Donor lymphocyte infusions for relapsed multiple myeloma after allogeneic stem-cell transplantation: Predictive factors for response and long-term outcome. *J. Clin. Oncol.* **2000**, *18*, 3031–3037. [CrossRef]
55. Lokhorst, H.; Wu, K.; Verdonck, L.F.; Laterveer, L.L.; Van De Donk, N.W.C.J.; Van Oers, M.H.J.; Cornelissen, J.J.; Schattenberg, A.V. The occurrence of graft-versus-host disease is the major predictive factor for response to donor lymphocyte infusions in multiple myeloma. *Blood* **2004**, *103*, 4362–4364. [CrossRef]
56. Van de Donk, N.W.; Kröger, N.; Hegenbart, U.; Corradini, P.; Miguel, J.F.S.; Goldschmidt, H.; Perez-Simon, J.A.; Zijlmans, M.; Raymakers, R.A.; Montefusco, V.; et al. Prognostic factors for donor lymphocyte infusions following nonmyeloablative allogeneic stem cell transplantation in multiple myeloma. *Bone Marrow Transpl.* **2006**, *37*, 1135–1141. [CrossRef]
57. Rawstron, A.C.; Davies, F.E.; DasGupta, R.; Ashcroft, A.J.; Patmore, R.; Drayson, M.T.; Owen, R.G.; Jack, A.S.; Child, J.A.; Morgan, G.J. Flow cytometric disease monitoring in multiple myeloma: The elationship between normal and neoplastic plasma cells predicts outcome after transplantation. *Blood* **2002**, *100*, 3095–3100. [CrossRef]
58. Costa, L.J.; Derman, B.A.; Bal, S.; Sidana, S.; Chhabra, S.; Silbermann, R.; Ye, J.C.; Cook, G.; Cornell, R.F.; Holstein, S.A.; et al. International harmonization in performing and reporting minimal residual disease assessment in multiple myeloma trials. *Leukemia* **2021**, *35*, 18–30. [CrossRef]
59. Corradini, P.; Voena, C.; Tarella, C.; Astolfi, M.; Ladetto, M.; Palumbo, A.; Van Lint, M.T.; Bacigalupo, A.; Santoro, A.; Musso, M.; et al. Molecular and clinical remissions in multiple myeloma: Role of autologous and allogeneic transplantation of hematopoietic cells. *J. Clin. Oncol.* **1999**, *17*, 208–215. [CrossRef]
60. Corradini, P.; Cavo, M.; Lokhorst, H.; Martinelli, G.; Terragna, C.; Majolino, I.; Valagussa, P.; Boccadoro, M.; Samson, D.; Bacigalupo, A.; et al. Molecular remission after myeloablative allogeneic stem cell transplantation predicts a better relapse-free survival in patients with multiple myeloma. *Blood* **2003**, *102*, 1927–1929. [CrossRef]
61. Ladetto, M.; Ferrero, S.; Drandi, D.; Festuccia, M.; Patriarca, F.; Mordini, N.; Cena, S.; Benedetto, R.; Guarona, G.; Ferrando, F.; et al. Prospective molecular monitoring of minimal residual disease after non-myeloablative allografting in newly diagnosed multiple myeloma. *Leukemia* **2016**, *30*, 1211–1214. [CrossRef]
62. Garfall, A.L.; Maus, M.V.; Hwang, W.T.; Lacey, S.F.; Mahnke, Y.D.; Melenhorst, J.J.; Zheng, Z.; Vogl, D.T.; Cohen, A.D.; Weiss, B.M.; et al. Chimeric Antigen Receptor T Cells against CD19 for Multiple Myeloma. *N. Engl. J. Med.* **2015**, *373*, 1040–1047. [CrossRef]
63. Cohen, A.D.; Garfall, A.L.; Stadtmauer, E.A.; Melenhorst, J.J.; Lacey, S.F.; Lancaster, E.; Vogl, D.T.; Weiss, B.M.; Dengel, K.; Nelson, A.; et al. B cell maturation antigen-specific CAR T cells are clinically active in multiple myeloma. *J. Clin. Investig.* **2019**, *129*, 2210–2221. [CrossRef]
64. Raje, N.; Berdeja, J.; Lin, Y.; Chhabra, S.; Silbermann, R.; Ye, J.C.; Cook, G.; Cornell, R.F.; Holstein, S.A.; Shi, Q.; et al. Anti-BCMA CAR T-Cell Therapy bb2121 in Relapsed or Refractory Multiple Myeloma. *N. Engl. J. Med.* **2019**, *380*, 1726–1737. [CrossRef]
65. Depil, S.; Duchateau, P.; Grupp, S.A.; Mufti, G.; Poirot, L. "Off-the-shelf" allogeneic CAR T cells: Development and challenges. *Nat. Rev. Drug Discov.* **2020**, *19*, 185–199. [CrossRef]
66. Gagelmann, N.; Riecken, K.; Wolschke, C.; Berger, C.; Ayuk, F.A.; Fehse, B.; Kröger, N. Development of CAR-T cell therapies for multiple myeloma. *Leukemia* **2020**, *34*, 2317–2332. [CrossRef]
67. Wagner, V.; Gil, J. T cells engineered to target senescence. *Nature* **2020**, *583*, 37–38. [CrossRef]

MDPI
St. Alban-Anlage 66
4052 Basel
Switzerland
Tel. +41 61 683 77 34
Fax +41 61 302 89 18
www.mdpi.com

Hemato Editorial Office
E-mail: hemato@mdpi.com
www.mdpi.com/journal/hemato